BASIC AND
CLINICAL ASPECTS OF
GROWTH HORMONE

SERONO SYMPOSIA, USA

Series Editor: James Posillico

A Continuation Order Plan is available for this series. A continuation order will bring delivery of each new volume immediately upon publication. Volumes are billed only upon actual shipment. For further information please contact the publisher.

BASIC AND CLINICAL ASPECTS OF GROWTH HORMONE

Edited by
Barry B. Bercu

University of South Florida
Tampa, Florida

PLENUM PRESS • NEW YORK AND LONDON

Library of Congress Cataloging in Publication Data

International Symposium on Growth Hormone (1987: Tampa, Fla.)
  Basic and clinical aspects of growth hormone.

  "Proceedings of the International Symposium on Growth Hormone, sponsored by Serono Symposia, USA, held June 14–18, 1987, in Tampa, Florida"—T.p. verso.
  Includes bibliographies and indexes.
  1. Somatotropin—Physiological effect—Congresses. 2. Somatotropin—Therapeutic use—Congresses. I. Bercu, Barry B. II. Serono symposia, USA. III. Title. [DNLM: 1. Somatotropin—congresses. WK 515 I6094b 1987]
QP572.S6I54   1987   615'.363   88-12527
ISBN 978-1-4684-5507-6   ISBN 978-1-4684-5505-2 (eBook)
DOI 10.1007/978-1-4684-5505-2

Proceedings of the International Symposium on Growth Hormone, sponsored by Serono Symposia, USA, held June 14–18, 1987, in Tampa, Florida

© 1988 Plenum Press, New York
Softcover reprint of the hardcover 1st edition 1988
A Division of Plenum Publishing Corporation
233 Spring Street, New York, N.Y. 10013

SCIENTIFIC COMMITTEE

Barry B. Bercu, Chairman
Tampa, FL

Gerhard Baumann
Chicago, IL

Jurgen R. Bierich
Tubingen, West Germany

Selna Kaplan
San Francisco, CA

Urban Lewis
San Diego, CA

Andrea Prader
Zurich, Switzerland

Raphael Rappaport
Paris, France

Alan D. Rogol
Charlottesville, VA

Allen W. Root
Tampa, FL

Louis E. Underwood
Chapel Hill, NC

Wylie Vale
La Jolla, CA

ORGANIZING SECRETARY

Dr. James T. Posillico
Serono Symposia, USA
Randolph, Massachusetts

PREFACE

In this era of proliferation of synthetic growth hormone in the marketplace, there is a parallel and accentuated interest in growth hormone in the scientific arena. Because many more people can be treated with available growth hormone, clinicians must be prepared to answer hard questions regarding appropriate therapeutic usage and their decisions should be based on substantiated research in growth hormone.

In June 1987, an international group of basic and clinical investigators gathered in Tampa, Florida, to address these issues and to further explore the very nature of growth hormone. The presentations contained within this book bring together their most current and vital research related to growth hormone. Section I deals with an examination of the molecular and biochemical events which define the growth hormone process. In Section II the neuroregulation of growth hormone secretion is highlighted from contrasting perspectives. The third section emphasizes and defines methods of diagnosis of growth hormone deficiency states. Section IV reviews the physiology, biochemistry and molecular actions of growth hormone and somatomedin. Section V represents an assessment of growth hormone treatment for various disorders, and the sixth section expands current uses of growth hormone therapy as it evolves into the next decade.

The symposium upon which this book is based proved to be a dynamic blending of scholarly interaction between basic and clinical scientists. I am indebted to the participants whose worthy contributions are reflected in these pages.

Barry B. Bercu

ABSTRACT

CONTENTS

III. ASSESSMENT OF GROWTH HORMONE SECRETION IN CHILDREN

IV. GROWTH HORMONE ACTION

V. THERAPEUTIC EFFECTS OF GROWTH HORMONE

VI. NEW APPLICATIONS OF GROWTH HORMONE TREATMENT

I. PROCESSING OF GROWTH HORMONE

GROWTH HORMONE GENE EXPRESSION:

HORMONAL REGULATION AND TISSUE-SPECIFIC EXPRESSION

*Norman L. Eberhardt, [2]Peter A. Cattini, *Linda N. Peritz,
*[3]John D. Baxter, *Randy Isaacs, [4]Daniel F. Catanzaro,
*Brian L. West, and *Timothy L. Reudelhuber

*Metabolic Research Unit and [3]Department of Biochemistry
and Biophysics, University of California, San Francisco, CA
94143. [2]Department of Physiology, University of Manitoba,
Winnepeg, Manitoba, Canada R3E 0W3. [4]Department of
Biological Sciences, University of Sydney, New South Wales
2006, Australia

INTRODUCTION

Growth hormone (GH) belongs to a family of polypeptide hormones that includes chorionic somatomammotropin (CS, placental lactogen), prolactin (Prl) and proliferin. This hormone family is related by structural homology (1-5), immunoreactivity and partially overlapping biological functions (6). GH and Prl are essential for the normal growth and development of mammals (7,8). GH is required for statural growth and maintenance of nitrogen, mineral, lipid and carbohydrate metabolism (7). Prl is required for the initiation and maintenance of lactation (8). Proliferin may be involved in cellular growth as it occurs in increased concentrations prior to cell division (5,9). The function of CS has been postulated to provide GH-like activities for the developing fetus (10,11); however, it does not appear to have essential functions in man. It appears that a common function of the various members of the growth hormone family may be at the level of control of cellular differentiation and proliferation.

All of the members of the GH gene family appear to have evolved from a single primordial gene (12). The human (h) GH and CS genes reside on chromosome 17 (13,14). This locus contains 5 genes: the hGH-1 gene encoding pituitary growth hormone (15,16), the hGH-2 gene, an hGH variant containing 13 amino acid differences (16) which is expressed in the placenta (17), the hCS-5 gene which appears to be a pseudogene (18) and the hCS-1 and hCS-2 genes which are both expressed in the placenta and encode identical polypeptides (16,19). The hGH/hCS locus spans about 50 kb of DNA and the genes are arranged: 5'-(hGH-1/hCS-5/hCS-1/hGH-2/hCS-2)-3' (18,20). Interestingly, the rat (r) GH and CS genes are not members of a linked gene family. In addition, the two rCS cDNAs which have been cloned to date (21,22) are more related to rPrl than rGH. Although the functions of rCS and hCS are not known and it is not clear that the two hormones have similar activities, it appears that these placental-specific gene products have independently evolved from separate precursors, both of which are members of the GH gene family. The individual members of the GH gene family are expressed in a tissue-specific manner; GH and Prl are expressed in pituitary somatotrophs and lactotrophs, respectively, and CS is expressed in the placenta. At least some of the members of the growth hormone gene family are regulated by a variety of hormones. In the case of GH, abundant evidence indicates that thyroid and glucocorticoid hormones regulate rGH mRNA levels at the level of transcription (23,24). Knowledge of these various regulatory mechanisms is essential for the understanding of growth and developmental processes affected by these hormones.

Our laboratories have been interested in studying the regulation of the various members of the GH gene family. Currently, we will review three experimental areas that are being investigated to provide a more detailed understanding of GH gene expression. First, we are utilizing transient gene transfer techniques to study the regulation of the rGH gene in transfected rat anterior pituitary cells (GC) to define cis-acting elements involved in the tissue-specific and hormonal control of this gene. These functional studies are subsequently correlated with DNase I footprinting assays of the 5'-flanking DNA after interaction with nuclear proteins from various eukaryotic cells. These studies will be able to identify specific trans-acting factors that interact with the various cis-acting elements and mediate the specific responses. Second, we are performing similar studies with the hGH and hCS genes; in addition to defining the tissue-specific and hormonal control elements, these studies may provide some information about the physiological control of the hGH and hCS genes. Finally, hormonal control of the hGH gene in primary cultures of human hGH-secreting pituitary adenomas is being investigated to provide more direct information about physiological control of the hGH genes and to provide a background of information from which the utility of transfection experiments involving the hGH gene in rat pituitary cells can be assessed.

RAT GH GENE EXPRESSION IN TRANSFECTED GC CELLS

Most of our knowledge of GH gene expression has been derived from studies in the rat. These studies have been facilitated by the availability of cultured rat pituitary tumor cell lines (GC, GH1, GH3 and GH4) that synthesize rGH and rPrl. In these cells, rGH is secreted and its synthesis is positively regulated by thyroid and glucocorticoid hormones at the level of gene transcription (23,24).

Hormonal Regulation

The studies discussed above have suggested that the cultured cell lines may be an excellent model system to study the tissue-specific and hormonal control of transfected genes. In order to distinguish the transfected and endogenous rGH mRNA by S1 analysis, a Bam HI decanucleotide linker was inserted in the 5'-untranslated region of the rGH gene (25). This modified rGH gene (rGH$_m$) contains the entire rGH structural gene sequences and 1.7 and 2.0 kb of 5'- and 3'-flanking sequences, respectively. The rGH$_m$ gene was introduced into a vector containing the gene for neomycin resistance (neo^r) driven by the SV40 promoter but lacking the SV40 enhancer. The rGH$_m$ gene was then introduced into GC cells by protoplast fusion, and cell lines containing the stably integrated rGH$_m$ gene were obtained by selection of neo^{r+} cells using the neomycin analog, G-418. S1 analysis of total cytoplasmic RNA from six of the selected cell lines using a ^{32}P-labeled Pst I fragment from the rGH$_m$ gene (nucleotides (nts) -530/+79) revealed that the rGH$_m$ mRNA can be clearly distinguished from the endogenous rGH mRNA and that it is regulated analogous to the endogenous rGH mRNA, exhibiting an induced response in the presence of dexamethasone (DEX, 10^{-6} M), triiodothyronine (T$_3$, 10^{-8} M) and DEX plus T$_3$

4

(10^{-6} and 10^{-8} M, respectively). The data indicate that the transfected rGH$_m$ gene contains the necessary control elements required for positive thyroid and glucocorticoid regulation and that GC cells provide an excellent model system to study the hormonal regulation of the transfected rGH gene.

Studies from a number of laboratories have now established that the sequences required for thyroid regulation reside on the 5'-flanking DNA of the rGH gene (26-30). The general approach for these experiments has been to fuse the 5'-flanking sequences of the rGH gene to a reporter gene, e.g., chloramphenicol acetyl transferase (cat) and neo^r, and introduce the resultant chimaeric genes into GC cells either stably or transiently and analyze the influences of T_3 on the reporter gene. Using deletion analysis of the rGH gene's 5'-flanking sequences, a sequence(s) located between nts -235/-183 has been shown to contain a thyroid hormone response element (TRE). In all cases, this TRE appears to mediate the positive regulation of the gene by thyroid hormones. Flug et al. (30) have also presented evidence that sequences containing the TRE appear to function more efficiently with the homologous rGH promoter, since sequences between nts -236/-146 of the rGH gene ligated upstream from the SV40 promoter did not confer T_3 regulation onto the viral promoter. This suggests that additional sequences located in the proximal promoter may be required for T_3 regulation. Wright et al. (29) have presented evidence that a thyroid hormone-responsive transcription inhibitory element (TIE) is located in the proximal rGH promoter region (nts -46/-21); however, the relationship of this downstream element to the overall function of thyroid hormone regulation is not currently understood.

Tissue-Specific Regulation

Rat GH gene expression is regulated in a tissue-specific manner; it is expressed at 10^8- to 10^9-fold higher levels in anterior pituitary somatotrophs than in rat hepatoma cells (31). Transfer of the intact rGH gene into mouse fibroblast cells (L cells) results in an aberrant pattern of rGH transcription in which the normal promoter appears to be inactive (32). By contrast, transfer of the rGH$_m$ gene into GC cells results in appropriate expression (25), suggesting that the rGH gene contains sequences required for its tissue-specific expression. In addition, sequences located within 235 bp 5' to the transcription initiation site appear to direct correct initiation of transcripts from chimaeric genes containing 5'-flanking sequences of the rGH gene fused to xanthine-guanine phosphoribosyl transferase (26), the neo^r gene (27), or the cat gene (33) after stable introduction into GC cells. Consequently, studies were initiated to localize the important response elements and to identify the trans-acting factors which are involved in mediating the tissue-specific regulation of the rGH gene. Analysis of deletion mutants of the 5'-flanking DNA of the rGH gene fused to the cat gene in transfected GC cells indicated that deletion of rGH 5'-flanking sequences from nt -195 to nt -141 gradually decreased, but did not abolish, expression of CAT activity in GC cells (Table 1) (33). None of the deletion mutants of the rGH gene could be expressed in Rat2 cells. These data suggest that the element(s) conferring tissue-specific expression of the rGH gene in GC cells lies within 141 bp from the transcription initiation site. To determine if the transient expression data discussed above could be correlated with the interaction of specific trans-acting factors with the rGH 5'-flanking DNA, DNase I footprinting assays using nuclear extracts from GC and Rat2 cells were performed (33,34). Two regions of rGH 5'-flanking DNA, designated GC1 and GC2, respectively, were protected from DNase I treatment after interaction of DNA with GC cell nuclear proteins. The GC1 domain is located between nts -97/-62 and the GC2 domain is located between nts -144/-106. In both cases, nuclear proteins that were present in GC cells but not in Rat2 cells or rat liver were capable of producing these footprints. Subsequent oligonucleotide-directed mutagenesis of the GC1 and GC2 binding domains resulted in a complete loss of promoter activity in the case of the GC2 binding site and a 30% reduction in promoter activity in the case of the GC1 binding site (33,34). It has also been shown that oligonucleotides containing the GC1 and GC2 binding domains compete for one another using the DNase I footprinting assay (Reudelhuber T, unpublished results), suggesting that an identical factor(s) binds to these sequences. A similar conclusion has been reached by Lefevre et al. (35) from an analysis of the hGH gene which exhibits very similar DNase I footprints in the corresponding regions using nuclear extracts of GC cells. These data provide strong support for the concept that both of these sites may be involved in mediating the tissue-specific expression of the GH genes in GC cells. In the case of the rGH gene, the GC2 binding domain appears to be the most important element.

HUMAN GH GENE EXPRESSION IN TRANSFECTED GC CELLS

Studies of hGH gene expression have been hampered by a lack of cultured cell model systems. Although some studies have been performed in primary cultures of human acromegalic hGH-secreting pituitary tumors (discussed below), these cells do not divide and, therefore, are not suitable for a variety of experimental approaches. Current knowledge of hGH regulation is derived largely from measurements of plasma hGH levels in humans who have been treated with hormones, who suffer from fundamental endocrine disorders or both. In such studies, it is impossible to distinguish primary versus secondary hormonal influences or whether the effects are exerted at the level of synthesis and/or secretion. In contrast to the case with rGH (36), glucocorticoids suppress plasma hGH levels (37). Available data on thyroid hormone regulation of plasma hGH levels are less clear. Whereas plasma hGH levels are nearly normal in hypo- and hyperthyroid individuals, there is evidence that in both of these states there is decreased release of hGH in response to provocative stimuli such as insulin-induced hypoglycemia and arginine infusion (38,39). In addition, T_3 has been reported to inhibit hGH release from primary cultures of human pituitary adenomas (40). Thus, thyroid hormone might exert negative control over hGH production; however, as discussed later, the influence of T_3 on hGH secretion may be mediated by other cellular effectors that could also modulate the effects of T_3. Consequently, the overall influence of T_3 on hGH production is unknown.

To provide a readily manipulated model system to study the hormonal regulation of hGH synthesis and its tissue-specific expression, we have been introducing the intact hGH gene and chimaeric genes containing hGH or hCS 5'-flanking DNA fused to the cat gene into GC cells (25,41,42). Based on the information gained in this system, it appears that this model system will enable us to define cis-acting elements associated with the thyroid and glucocorticoid hormonal regulation (25,42) and tissue-specific expression of the hGH gene (35,41). Nevertheless, the relevance of these studies to the regulation of the hGH gene in human somatotropic cells must be regarded with reservation, since definitive studies which would allow an assessment of this heterologous model system are not yet available.

The intact hGH gene containing complete structural sequences (exons and introns) and 496 and 628 bp of 5'- and 3'-flanking DNA, respectively, was inserted in a vector containing the neo^r gene under the direction of the SV40 promoter and lacking the SV40 enhancer (25). This plasmid was introduced into GC cells and stable transfectants were obtained with the use of the neomycin analog, G-418. RNA blotting (Northern) analysis of total RNA derived from four individual cell lines indicated that the size

Table 1. Expression of rGH.cat genes in
transfected GC and Rat2 cells.

Plasmid	GC Cell Expression (% Control)	Rat2 Cell Expression (% Control)
rGH237CAT	100	<1
rGH195CAT	40.6	<1
rGH141CAT	27.6	<1
rGH106CAT	5.7	<1
p Cat	7.2	<1

of the hGH mRNA in the transfected GC cells was the same as RNA derived
from a human acromegalic pituitary tumor, suggesting that initiation of
transcription and poly A processing are similar in the two cell types. S1
nuclease analysis of RNA derived from several of the cell lines indicated
that hGH gene transcription was correctly initiated in GC cells,
indicating that the rat cells contained transcription factors that recognized the essential elements in the hGH gene required for faithful
transcription (25). Treatment of the transfected cells with DEX resulted
in enhanced levels of hGH and rGH mRNAs in the same cells; however,
treatment with T_3 resulted in diminished levels of hGH mRNA and increased
levels of rGH mRNA. In addition, T_3 treatment abolished the positive
induction of hGH mRNA levels by glucocorticoids when both hormones were
present simultaneously. These data demonstrate that glucocorticoid
response elements (GREs) and TREs are present in the hGH gene. Robins et
al. (43) have presented evidence that a GRE is present in the 5'-flanking
DNA of the hGH gene, and Slater et al. (44) have shown that a functional
GRE is present in Intron A of the hGH gene. Since it was shown that a
transfected rGH_m gene (25) was regulated by T_3 exactly like the endogenous
rGH gene, the transfection event alone cannot account for the observed
negative T_3 regulation of the transfected hGH gene. These data, therefore, suggest that structural differences in the rGH and hGH genes account
for their differential regulation by thyroid hormones in transfected GC
cells.

To understand the nature of the potential differences in the rGH and
hGH genes, a study of the 5'-flanking DNA of the hGH gene was undertaken
to determine if different regulatory elements could be identified.
Initially, the 5'-flanking regions of the hGH and the highly related hCS
genes were fused upstream of the cat gene and these hybrid genes were
introduced into GC cells under transient transfection conditions and the
influence of T_3 and DEX treatment was examined (Table 2) (42). DEX was
found to have a modest stimulatory response (1.3- to 1.4-fold) on CAT
activity for both the hGHp.cat and hCSp.cat genes. These data support the
concept that a GRE is contained within the 5'-flanking DNA of these genes
as originally proposed by Robins et al. (43). T_3 treatment of the transfected GC cells led to a marked increase (4- to 5-fold) in CAT expression
from the hCSp.cat gene; however, CAT activity was decreased (0.7- to
0.9-fold) from the hGHp.cat gene. The rGHp.cat gene was positively
regulated (2- to 3-fold) with T_3 treatment. These data clearly show that
the 5'-flanking DNA of the hCS and rGH genes contained TREs; however, it
was surprising that the hGH gene appeared to lack a TRE in the 5'-flanking
DNA, since it has 96% homology with the hCS gene. These data could be
explained most simply by the possibilities that the hGH gene either: (1)
lacks TREs; (2) lacks a control element distinct from the TRE which is
required for T_3 response; or, (3) contains a modulatory element that

Table 2. CAT activity directed by 5'-flanking DNA of
hGH and hCS genes in transiently transfected
GC cells treated with T_3 and DEX.

Hybrid Gene	DEX		T_3	
	+BUT[a]	-BUT	+BUT	-BUT
-470hGHp.cat	1.3[b]	--	0.7	0.9
-496hCSp.cat	1.4	--	4.1	5.4
-109TKp.cat	0.9	--	1.0	--

[a] Experiments performed in the presence of 0.5 mM
sodium butyrate (BUT).
[b] All values represent fold increase above the control
which was arbitrarily set at 1.0.

exerts negative control over the TRE; in this latter case, the function of
the modulatory element might be mediated by T_3 itself.

To test these latter possibilities, hGH/hCS hybrid promoters were
fused upstream of the cat gene and tested in the transient transfection
assay in GC cells. Interestingly, the hybrid promoter containing nts
-450/-85 of the hGH 5'-flanking DNA fused to the proximal hCS promoter
(nts -85/+2) was positively regulated by T_3 to the same extent as the
hCSp.cat gene. However, the corresponding hCS/hGH hybrid promoter and the
-85hCSp.cat and -85hGHp.cat genes were not regulated by T_3 treatment
(Cattini PA, Silversides D, Eberhardt NL, unpublished results). These
data indicate that the 5'-flanking DNA of the hGH gene contains a TRE, but
it either lacks an element required for T_3 regulation or contains an ele
ment that exerts a negative modulatory effect on the TRE. These results
support the concept that differences in the structure of the rGH and hGH
genes account for their differential T_3 regulation in transfected GC
cells. The data also indicate that the structural difference is located
in the proximal promoter region of the hGH gene between nts -85/+2.

Tissue-Specific Expression

To determine if the GC cell model system could also provide information about the tissue-specific expression of the hGH gene, the hGHp.cat
gene was transiently transfected into a number of different cell lines and
the relative expression of the gene was determined (41). Efficient
expression was observed in GC cells but not Rat2, HeLa or KB cells,
suggesting that the factors present in GC cells which account for cell-
specific expression of the rGH gene can recognize elements present on the
hGH gene. Analysis of deletion mutants indicated that sequences between
nts -230 and -180 contain an element(s) that is required for efficient
expression in GC cells. In addition, Nelson et al. (45) have presented
evidence that a cell-specific control element is located about 200 bp
upstream from the transcription initiation site of the rGH gene. This
region is highly conserved between the rGH and hGH genes. As discussed
previously, this region (nts -230/-180) of the rGH gene also contains a
TRE and we have localized the TREs present in the hGH and hCS genes to the
same region (Cattini PA, Silversides D, Eberhardt NL, unpublished
results). As a consequence, deletion of the TRE could result in loss of
promoter activity that might not necessarily reflect loss of a tissue-
specific element (30). Thus, it is impossible at the present time to
ascertain whether this region contains elements in addition to the TRE
which may be involved in tissue-specific regulation. Utilizing DNase I

footprinting analyses, two regions of the hGH 5'-flanking DNA have been identified that interact specifically with GC cell nuclear proteins. The GC cell-specific nuclear proteins interact at sites between nts -144/-108 and -96/-62 (35, Catanzaro D, Reudelhuber TL, Eberhardt NL, unpublished results). These sites correspond to identical regions in the rGH gene (discussed previously), designated GC2 and GC1, respectively, which have been shown to be important for rGH gene cell-specific expression (33,34). Lefevre et al. (35) have also presented evidence that mutation of either of the sites in the hGH gene that correspond to GC1 and GC2 in the rGH gene results in loss of hGH promoter activity. These data indicate that these two regions appear to be dominantly involved in cell-specific expression. The relation of these proximal promoter sites to the more upstream site(s) at nts -230/-180 (41,45) that exert a dominant effect on basal promoter activity and their influence on tissue-specific expression remains to be determined.

HORMONAL REGULATION OF HUMAN GH GENE EXPRESSION IN ACROMEGALIC TUMORS

In order to determine if the negative regulation of the hGH gene by T_3 represented a physiologically relevant effect, studies of the regulation of the hGH gene in primary cultures of dispersed human acromegalic pituitary tumor cells were performed (46). Based on Northern analyses, it was shown that the mature hGH mRNA from acromegalic pituitary tumor cells and from normal pituitary tissue were the same size (ca. 1100 bp), suggesting that the transcription initiation and processing of the hGH mRNA were identical in normal and acromegalic pituitary tumor tissue. Four of five adenomas exhibited 2- to 4-fold increases in hGH mRNA levels with DEX treatment (Table 3); in one tumor, DEX decreased hGH mRNA levels slightly. T_3 treatment resulted in no significant effect on hGH mRNA levels (Table 3). These results indicate that unlike the regulation of the rGH gene in rat cells, T_3 does not affect hGH mRNA levels in human acromegalic pituitary cells.

Interestingly, T_3 treatment of the human pituitary cells did result in significant increases in the amount of hGH secreted into the medium (Table 4). These data suggest that in human somatotrophs T_3 may not play a significant role in the maintenance of hGH mRNA levels, but may act as a positive stimulus to increase hGH secretion. Nevertheless, in similar studies Adams et al. (40) reported that T_3 exerted a negative regulatory influence on hGH secretion from primary cultures of human acromegalic tumor cells. Although the exact reason for the differences in the results of Adams et al. (40) and those of Isaacs et al. (46) are not known, it is likely that differences in the culture conditions account for the differences. For example, the data in Table 4 indicate that insulin has a

Table 3. Regulation of hGH mRNA levels in
human pituitary tumor cells.

Adenoma	DEX	T_3	INS	DEX/INS
1	3.5*	1.1	1.2	2.0
2	2.5	1.0	1.0	2.5
3	2.0	ND**	2.1	0.6
4	2.8	1.1	1.3	1.4
5	0.8	ND	1.1	1.4

*All values expressed as fold change compared to
control values.
**ND = Not determined.

Table 4. Regulation of hGH secretion in human pituitary tumor cells.

Adenoma	Control	DEX	T_3	Insulin	DEX/Insulin
1	1.39*	4.70	5.25	1.00	0.74
2	0.35	0.61	2.32	0.37	0.51
3	0.91	1.55	--	0.88	0.61
4	16.1	26.5	26.0	14.5	3.1
5	6.17	2.78	--	6.11	3.07

*All values expressed as microgram protein/24 h.

negative modulatory effect on the ability of glucocorticoids to stimulate hGH secretion. Moreover, insulin also inhibited the ability of glucocorticoids to stimulate hGH mRNA levels in the same cells. Thus, insulin or some other effector might alter the cell's responsivity to T_3; however, this remains to be established. On balance, T_3 may have an overall positive effect on GH production in humans and rats; however, the mechanisms to achieve this appear to be distinct. The absence of positive T_3 regulation of the hGH gene in transfected GC cells mimic somewhat the behavior of the hGH gene in its own cellular milieu. This suggests that a structural difference between the hGH and rGH genes accounts for their differential regulation by thyroid hormones. This suggests that transfection of the hGH gene into rat pituitary cells may represent a reasonable quasi-physiological model system to examine the regulation of this gene.

ACKNOWLEDGMENTS

This work was supported by NIH grants AM 17838 (Eberhardt NL), AM 19997 (Baxter JD), DK 35283 (Reudelhuber TL) and an award from the American Cancer Society, JFRA-123 (Reudelhuber TL).

REFERENCES

1. Catt KJ, Moffat B, Niall HD. Human growth hormone and placental lactogen: structural similarity. Science 1967; 157:321.
2. Li CH, Dixon JS, Lo TB, Pankov YM, Schmidt KD. Amino acid sequence of ovine lactogenic hormone. Nature 1967; 224:695.
3. Sherwood LM. Similarities in the chemical structure of human placental lactogen and pituitary growth hormone. Proc Natl Acad Sci USA 1967; 58:2307.
4. Niall HD, Hogan ML, Sayer R, Rosenblum IY, Greenwood FC. Sequences of pituitary and placental lactogenic and growth hormones: evolution from a primordial peptide by gene duplication. Proc Natl Acad Sci USA 1971; 68:866.
5. Linzer DIH, Nathans D. Nucleotide sequence of a growth-related mRNA encoding a member of the prolactin-growth hormone family. Proc Natl Acad Sci USA 1984; 81:4255.
6. Niall HD, Hogan ML, Tregar GW, Segre GV, Hwang P, Friesen H. The chemistry of growth hormone and the lactogenic hormones. Recent Prog Horm Res 1973; 29:387.
7. Martin JB. Neural regulation of growth hormone secretion. N Engl J Med 1973; 288:1384.
8. Bern HA, Nicoll CS. The comparative endocrinology of prolactin. Recent Prog Horm Res 1968; 24:681.
9. Linzer DIH, Nathans D. Growth-related changes in specific mRNAs of cultured mouse cells. Proc Natl Acad Sci USA 1983; 80:4271.

10. Simpson ER, MacDonald PC. Endocrine physiology of the placenta. Annu Rev Physiol 1968; 43:163.

11. Grumbach MM, Kaplan SL, Vinik A. HCS physiology: hormonal effects. In: Berson SA, Yalow RS, eds. Peptide hormones. Amsterdam: North Holland Publishing Company, 1973:797.

12. Miller WL, Eberhardt NL. Structure and evolution of the growth hormone gene family. Endocr Rev 1983; 4:97.

13. Owerbach D, Rutter WJ, Martial JA, Baxter JD, Shows TB. Genes for growth hormone, chorionic somatommamotropin and a growth hormone-like gene are located on chromosome 17 in humans. Science 1980; 209:289.

14. George DL, Phillips JA III, Francke V, Seeburg PH. The genes for growth hormone and chorionic somatomammotropin are on the long arm of human chromosome 17 in region q21-qter. Hum Genet 1981; 57:138.

15. DeNoto FM, Moore DD, Goodman HM. Human growth hormone DNA sequence and mRNA structure: possible alternative splicing. Nucleic Acids Res 1981; 9:3719.

16. Seeburg PH. The human growth hormone gene family: nucleotide sequences show recent divergence and predict a new polypeptide hormone. DNA 1982; 1:239.

17. Frankenne F, Rentier-Delrue F, Scippo M-L, Martial J, Hennen G. Expression of the growth hormone variant gene in human placenta. J Clin Endocrinol Metab 1987; 64:635.

18. Hirt H, Kimelman J, Birnbaum MJ, et al. The human growth hormone gene locus: structure, evolution, and allelic variations. DNA 1987; 6:59.

19. Selby MJ, Barta A, Baxter JD, Bell GI, Eberhardt NL. Analysis of a major human chorionic somatomammotropin gene: evidence for two functional promoter elements. J Biol Chem 1984; 259:13131.

20. Barsh GS, Seeburg PH, Gelinas RE. The human growth hormone gene family: structure and evolution of the chromosomal locus. Nucleic Acids Res 1983; 11:3939.

21. Duckworth ML, Peden LM, Friesen HG. Isolation of a novel prolactin-like cDNA clone from developing rat placenta. J Biol Chem 1986; 261:10879.

22. Duckworth ML, Kirk KL, Friesen HG. Isolation and identification of a cDNA clone of rat placental lactogen II. J Biol Chem 1986; 261:10871.

23. Spindler SR, Mellon SH, Baxter JD. Growth hormone gene transcription is regulated by thyroid and glucocorticoid hormones in cultured rat pituitary tumor cells. J Biol Chem 1982; 257:11627.

24. Evans RM, Birnberg NC, Rosenfeld MG. Glucocorticoid and thyroid hormones transcriptionally regulate growth hormone gene expression. Proc Natl Acad Sci USA 1982; 79:7659.

25. Cattini PA, Anderson TR, Baxter JD, Mellon P, Eberhardt NL. The human growth hormone gene is negatively regulated by triiodothyronine when transfected into rat pituitary tumor cells. J Biol Chem 1986; 261:13367.

26. Casanova J, Copp RP, Janocko L, Samuels HH. 5'-flanking DNA of the rat growth hormone gene mediates regulated expression by thyroid hormone. J Biol Chem 1985; 260:11744.

27. Crew MD, Spindler SR. Thyroid hormone regulation of the transfected rat growth hormone promoter. J Biol Chem 1986; 261:5018.

28. Larsen RP, Harney JW, Moore DD. Sequences required for cell-type specific thyroid hormone regulation of the rat growth hormone promoter activity. J Biol Chem 1986; 261:14373.

29. Wright PA, Crew MD, Spindler SR. Discrete positive and negative thyroid hormone-responsive transcription regulatory elements of the rat growth hormone gene. J Biol Chem 1987; 262:5659.

30. Flug F, Copp RP, Casanova J, et al. cis-Acting elements of the rat growth hormone gene which mediate basal and regulated expression by thyroid hormone. J Biol Chem 1987; 262:6373.

31. Ivarie RD, Schacter BS, O'Farrell PH. The level of expression of the rat growth hormone gene in liver tumor cells is at least eight orders of magnitude less than in anterior pituitary cells. Mol Cell Biol 1983; 3:1460.

32. Karin M, Eberhardt NL, Mellon SH, et al. Expression and hormonal regulation of the rat growth hormone gene in transfected mouse L cells. DNA 1984; 3:147.

33. West BL, Catanzaro DF, Mellon SH, Cattini PA, Baxter JD, Reudelhuber TL. Interaction of a tissue-specific factor with an essential rat growth hormone gene promoter element. Mol Cell Biol 1987; 7:1193.

34. Catanzaro DL, West BL, Baxter JD, Reudelhuber TL. A pituitary-specific factor interacts with an upstream promoter element in the rat growth hormone gene. Mol Endocrinol 1987; 1:90.

35. Lefevre C, Imagawa M, Dana S, Grindlay J, Bodner M, Karin M. Tissue-specific expression of the human growth hormone gene is conferred in part by the binding of a specific trans-acting factor. EMBO J 1987; 66:971.

36. Coiro V, Braverman LE, Christiansen D, Fang S-L, Goodman HM. Effect of hypothyroidism and thyroxine replacement on growth hormone in the rat. Endocrinology 1979; 105:641.

37. Frantz AG, Rabkin MT. Human growth hormone: clinical measurement, response to hypoglycemia and suppression by glucocorticoids. N Engl J Med 1964; 271:1375.

38. Katz HP, Youlton R, Kaplan SL, Grumbach MM. Growth and growth hormone. III. Growth hormone release in children with primary hypothyroidism and thyrotoxicosis. J Clin Endocrinol Metab 1969; 29:346.

39. MacGillvray MH, Aceto T Jr, Frohman LA. Plasma growth hormone responses and growth retardation of hypothyroidism. Am J Dis Child 1968; 115:273.

40. Adams EF, Brajkovich IE, Mashiter K. Growth hormone and prolactin secretion by dispersed cell cultures of human pituitary adenomas: long term effects of hydrocortisone, estradiol, insulin, 3,5,3'-triiodothyronine and thyroxine. J Clin Endocrinol Metab 1981; 53:381.

41. Cattini PA, Peritz LN, Anderson TR, Baxter JD, Eberhardt NL. The 5'-flanking sequences of the human growth hormone gene contain a cell-specific control element. DNA 1986; 5:503.

42. Cattini PA, Eberhardt NL. Regulated expression of chimaeric genes containing the 5'-flanking region of human growth hormone-related genes in transiently transfected rat anterior pituitary cells. Nucleic Acids Res 1987; 15:1297.

43. Robins DM, Peak I, Seeburg PH, Axel R. Regulated expression of human growth hormone gene in mouse L cells. Cell 1982; 29:623.

44. Slater EP, Rabenau O, Karin M, Baxter JD, Beato M. Glucocorticoid receptor binding and activation of a heterologous promoter by dexamethasone by the first intron of the human growth hormone gene. Mol Cell Biol 1985; 5:2984.

45. Nelson C, Crenshaw EB III, Franco R. Discrete cis-active genomic sequences dictate the pituitary cell type-specific expression of rat prolactin and growth hormone genes. Nature 1986; 322:557.

46. Isaacs RE, Findell PR, Mellon P, Wilson CB, Baxter JD. Hormonal regulation of expression of the endogenous and transfected human growth hormone gene (submitted for publication).

2

HETEROGENEITY OF GROWTH HORMONE

Gerhard Baumann, M.D.

Center for Endocrinology, Metabolism and Nutrition
Department of Medicine
Northwestern University Medical School
Chicago, IL 60611

INTRODUCTION

Heterogeneity of polypeptide hormones is a ubiquitous phenomenon related to gene multiplicity, biosynthetic precursors, aggregation, protein-protein interaction, fragment formation, differential glycosylation, derivatization of functional groups, degradative processes, and lack of complete assay specificity. Some of this heterogeneity occurs as a physiological process, and some represents a laboratory artifact. Growth hormone (GH) is no exception and its heterogeneity has been recognized for a long time, although the details have only recently become clear. This review will primarily deal with human GH (hGH), which is the best studied in terms of structure among the various animal GHs.

HISTORICAL OVERVIEW

The concept of a pituitary growth-promoting principle (1) led to the isolation of bovine GH in 1944 (2) and hGH in 1956/57 (3,4). Several laboratories participated in devising useful purification procedures for both animal GHs and hGH (5-10). In these early studies, heterogeneity of the purified product was already recognized (5,7-12), but this was either attributed to impurities or to chemical alteration of GH during the extraction procedures, such as aggregation, proteolysis and nonenzymatic deamidation (13-15). Following the isolation of hGH, a great deal of work was devoted in several laboratories at elucidating its structure, defining the bioactive site or "core," and synthesizing the hormone or potentially bioactive fragments. In the process, considerable knowledge about the chemistry of hGH was accumulated. Efforts to produce purer, less immunogenic hGH for clinical use focused on the isolation of monomeric, homogeneous hGH corresponding to the structure published in 1971 (16,17). Less "pure" side fractions were largely ignored as undesirable.

Renewed interest in the possibility that not all hGH heterogeneity may be artifactual emerged in the early to mid-1970s as a result of several independent and seemingly unrelated observations. First, following the discovery of proinsulin in 1967 (18) and "big" insulin in plasma in 1968 (19), the possible existence of hormone precursors was extended to other hormones, including GH. Size heterogeneity was shown to exist for virtually all polypeptide hormones, not only in glandular extracts, but also in plasma (20). The demonstration of "big" and "pre-big" hGH in human plasma corresponding to similar components in pituitary extracts (21,22) made it more difficult to consider the latter extraction arti- facts. Second, the discovery that some of the acidic components contained in hGH preparations had biological activity that exceeded that of "pure" hGH severalfold (23,24) suggested that these minor contaminants might be physiologically important. Third, earlier reports of a dissociation between hGH and some of its effects (e.g., diabetogenic activity) received support from studies showing that (a) such activities could be generated by proteolytic digestion of hGH; and, (b) the activity could be physically separated from hGH (25-27). Finally, the discrepancy between GH-like bio- activity and immunoreactive GH in plasma (28), although viewed with skep- ticism, had never been adequately explained and suggested the existence of GH forms with high bioactivity/immunoreactivity ratios. Following this resurgence of interest in GH heterogeneity, major efforts were concentra- ted, primarily by Lewis and co-workers, on the isolation and characteriza- tion of the various hGH forms identified in pituitary extracts, and, in my laboratory, on the nature of secreted and circulating hGH. As a result, it has become clear that hGH is, indeed, physiologically composed of several molecular forms. In addition, it has been possible to identify which forms are native and which are generated during extraction.

In recent years, further interest in hGH heterogeneity has been stim- ulated by new insights into the structure of the hGH gene family and by the discovery of circulating hGH binding proteins.

MECHANISMS RESPONSIBLE FOR HGH HETEROGENEITY

Table 1 lists various theoretical sources of GH heterogeneity. Several of these have been shown to be operative, while others are still speculative.

Obviously, there are precedents for many of these mechanisms in the case of other proteins. Thus, hGH heterogeneity is not unique and should be seen in the context of the many modifications that proteins can undergo. A conceptually more difficult issue is that regarding the physiological importance of the multiple forms of hGH. I will now briefly review each of the possibilities listed in Table 1 and the corresponding molecular forms of GH.

HETEROGENEITY ARISING FROM PRE- AND COTRANSLATIONAL MECHANISMS

Gene Multiplicity

The hGH/hPL gene cluster on chromosome 17 contains two hGH genes (named hGH-N and hGH-V for "normal" and "variant") and three hPL genes which code for hGH and the GH-related placental lactogen (hPL), respec- tively (29). The hGH-N gene codes for the 191 amino acid, 22 kD form of hGH (hGH_{22K}) originally isolated and sequenced (4,5,16,17). The hGH-V gene codes for a second hGH protein that also has 191 residues and a size of 22 kD, but differs from (mature) hGH_{22K} in 13 amino acid positions (30). The corresponding protein (hGH-V) can be predicted to be more basic than hGH_{22K} (calculated pI~8.9, vs. 5.15 for hGH_{22K}). In addition, it possesses a potential glycosylation site (Asn^{140}) and a potential proteo- lytic site ($Arg^{18} Arg^{19}$). Modification at either site could substantially change the molecular charge and size predicted from the primary sequence. The hGH-V gene has been artificially expressed (31), and the resulting product has been found to be a 22 kD protein, to react poorly with anti-

Table 1.   Theoretical sources of multiple hGH forms.

1.	Genome:	Two hGH genes: hGH-N and hGH-V*
2.	mRNA differential splicing:	hGH$_{22K}$ and hGH$_{20K}$*[2]
3.	Precursors:	Pre-hGH, but no Pro-hGH*[23]
4.	Translational errors:	not known
5.	Posttranslational processing:	a) N-acylation*
		b) deamidation*[3]
		c) phosphorylation[23]
		d) glycosylation
		e) proteolysis
6.	Polymerization, aggregation:	a) noncovalent association*[3]
		b) intermolecular disulfide bonds*
7.	Protein-protein interaction:	Carrier proteins*
8.	Metabolic conversions:	a) immunoreactive fragments*
		b) bioactive fragments
		c) inactive metabolites*
9.	Laboratory artifacts:	a) aggregation
		b) dissociation of polymers
		c) proteolysis
		d) deamidation
		e) oxidation

*Denotes mechanisms shown to be physiologically operative in man.
[2]Denotes analogous mechanisms shown to occur in murine species.
[3]Denotes analogous mechanism known to occur in hoofed animals.

hGH antibodies but near normally with GH receptors, and to be prone to aggregation (31,32).

While the hGH-N gene is obviously expressed in the pituitary, it is not known with certainty whether the hGH-V gene is also expressed. Clearly, a functional hGH-N gene is needed for normal growth, and the presence of the hGH-V gene alone does not promote growth (33). On the other hand, the absence of the hGH-V gene does not adversely affect normal growth (34). Recent evidence from RNA hybridization studies has indicated that the hGH-V gene is expressed in placenta (35,36), and that the placental GH described by Hennen et al. (37) may be the corresponding protein (36). If this identity can be proven, hGH-V must be added to the number of GH-like molecules circulating in pregnancy (38). Frankenne et al. also found evidence for the presence of hGH-V transcripts at very low levels in one GH-producing pituitary adenoma (36), raising the possibility that hGH-V may be produced by pituitary tissue under certain circumstances.

Differential mRNA Splicing

The possibility that the same gene could give rise to two polypeptide chains (i.e., hGH$_{22K}$ and its 20 kD variant hGH$_{20K}$) was first considered by Wallis (39). He proposed that hGH pre-mRNA may be processed to two different mature mRNAs during excision of introns. Thus, in addition to the normal splicing site at the transition of intron B to exon III, a secondary splice site within exon III would also be recognized, and the corresponding protein would be hGH$_{20K}$. This hypothesis was experimentally verified (40) and recently confirmed (41). Interestingly, the identical nucleotide sequence in the hGH-V transcript is not recognized as an alternative splicing site (41), presumably because of different secondary structure of hGH-V pre-mRNA. Thus, the hGH-N gene, but not the hGH-V gene, is responsible for two polypeptides, hGH$_{22K}$ and hGH$_{20K}$. Analogous 20 kD GH variants, presumably originating through the same mechanism, occur in other species (42).

HGH$_{20K}$, first isolated from pituitary extracts in 1978 (43), lacks amino acid residues 32-46 (44,45) and has a propensity to dimerize (43,45). Its immunoreactivity is about 30% compared to hGH$_{22K}$ (43), it binds to GH receptors with lower affinity than hGH$_{22K}$ (46,47), but has comparable bioactivity in vivo, at least in the rat (43,48). This apparent discrepancy is probably explained by the slower metabolic clearance of hGH$_{20K}$ (49). HGH$_{20K}$ exhibits diminished—rather than absent as originally suggested (50,51)—diabetogenic and insulin-like activities (52,53).

GH Precursors

HGH, like other secretory proteins, is first synthesized as pre-hGH with a hydrophobic leader sequence (signal peptide) at its amino-terminal end. The signal peptide is 26 amino acids long and has a mol wt of 2700 (54). It is cotranslationally cleaved from the nascent protein and is, thus, a very transitory product that need not concern us in the present context. Analogous pre-GHs have been directly demonstrated for bovine and rat GH (55,56). No other GH precursors (pro-GHs) are either predicted by the genetic code, nor have they ever been identified.

Translational errors as a source of GH heterogeneity, while theoretically conceivable, have not been identified.

HETEROGENEITY ARISING FROM POSTTRANSLATIONAL MECHANISMS

Monomeric GH

Several of the hGH forms present in pituitary extracts represent modifications of the primary peptide chain after synthesis. They must be divided into physiologically occurring events and those occurring as chemical by-products in the process of extraction. This distinction has been notoriously difficult and has only recently become transparent.

An hGH$_{22K}$ variant with a blocked aminoterminus has been described by Lewis et al. (57). This variant, termed "fast" hGH for its electrophoretic mobility, is presumed to be N$_\alpha$-acetylated. It is almost certainly a native form with full bioactivity and immunoreactivity.

Deamidation has long been suspected to be one reason for hGH heterogeneity (see above). This is a notorious chemical artifact during protein purification, and desamido-hGH was initially viewed as such (15). However, desamido-hGH can be identified even in the freshest pituitary extracts in the absence of conditions favoring deamidation, and corresponding forms are present in pituitary culture media (58,59) and in plasma (60,61). This, coupled with the fact that deamidation is apparently not random (62), suggests that desamido-hGH is a native product. The residues involved are Asn^{152} and Gln^{137}, giving rise to two deamidated variants of hGH$_{22K}$ (62). They exhibit full growth-promoting activity and full immunoreactivity compared to hGH$_{22K}$ (57). The situation is similar for bovine GH, where the homologous residues (plus a third one, Asn^{13}) have been shown to be consistently deamidated (63).

A phosphorylated form of GH has been described recently in the rat and in sheep (64,65). The precise residues that are phosphorylated are not known. The effect of phosphorylation on bioactivity is unknown. To date, no human counterpart to these GH forms has been reported.

Glycosylation is another mechanism for posttranslational protein modification. Recent evidence points to the existence of two hGH forms in pituitary that specifically bind to concanavalin A, consistent with a glycosylated nature (66). The precise structure of this material has not been elucidated. As mentioned above, hGH-V is a potential candidate for a glycosylated hGH form.

Three proteolytically cleaved hGH forms have been described in pituitary extracts (23,24,67). They were designated hGH-C, D and E by Chrambach (67) and α_1, α_2 and α_3 by Lewis (24). The cleavage points have been identified as Arg^{134}, Lys^{140} and Lys^{145} (24). There is micro heterogeneity of hGH-E (α_3) in the region of residue 146-147 (24). Because these cleavages occur in the large disulfide loop of hGH, the two resulting fragments remain covalently connected by the disulfide bridge $Cys^{53}Cys^{165}$. The tryptic-type cleavages are believed to be catalyzed by plasmin or a related enzyme, which had been shown to be present in pituitary by Ellis and co-workers (68). Indeed, the same products can be produced artificially by limited digestion of hGH with plasmin (24,69,70). Considerable interest in the cleaved hGH forms was engendered by the observation that the more highly cleaved products (i.e., those with at least an undecapeptide removed [24,70]), exhibited five- to eightfold enhanced growth-promoting activity relative to intact hGH_{22K} (24,67,69,70). Similar enhancement of somatomedin-generating activity and of metabolic activities was also shown (71,72). (Unfortunately, not all plasmin preparations yielded the same products [70], which led to difficulties in reproducing the enhancement phenomenon in some laboratories and corresponding skepticism. However, the hGH digestion products generated in the laboratories failing to show enhancement corresponded to hGH-C [α_1] [73,74], which is, indeed, not enhanced.)

Cleaved hGH forms bind to hGH receptors in a manner indistinguishable from intact hGH (75), and their enhanced bioactivity in vivo is probably related to their delayed metabolic clearance (76). Based on the observation that the cleaved two-chain hGH forms had a higher biopotency than the single-chain parent molecule, the hypothesis was advanced that hGH may have to be proteolytically processed to a two-chain form to express its full potential (70). Intact hGH would, thus, represent a storage form that would be activated to two-chain hGH shortly before or during secretion. Considerable effort went into examining this hypothesis. However, the failure to demonstrate cleaved forms in very fresh pituitary extracts (24,59), in the media of pituitary cultures (58,59) or in blood (60,61) makes it difficult to sustain the activation hypothesis. (One report of cleaved hGH in plasma was based solely on a radioimmunoassay for two-chain hGH in unextracted plasma [77]. This assay is not completely specific for two-chain hGH [78]; it probably recognized another immunoreactive substance, such as an hGH fragment, in plasma.) Thus, the cleaved forms, for all their interesting properties, are probably not native forms. Rather, they are generated during extraction and storage of hGH as a result of the action of one or more contaminating proteases.

Two additional variants of hGH have been described that can be separated from hGH in urea-PAGE (57). They were named "slow" and "slow-slow" hGH for their characteristically slow electrophoretic mobility. They exhibit normal immunoreactivity and growth-promoting bioactivity (57). We could find no evidence for their presence in plasma (60). They were recently identified as oxidation products of methionine residues generated in the course of purification of hGH from pituitary (Lewis UJ, personal communication).

It should be noted that all the modifications described in this section apply to hGH_{22K} which is most easily studied because of its abundance. It is equally possible that hGH_{20K} may undergo similar (or different) posttranslational modifications, but this has not been examined in detail yet.

Large molecular weight (i.e., >22 kD) material has been recognized in pituitary hGH extracts since the beginning of purification efforts (5,9,10). Initially, this was attributed to contaminating proteins or RNA and to artifactual aggregates of denatured hGH, produced by harsh extraction conditions (79-83). As hGH preparations containing such aggregates were immunogenic and produced antibody-mediated GH resistance when used therapeutically (83), subsequent efforts were directed at producing monomeric, nondenatured hGH (84). These early observations—while undoubtedly correct—detracted from the fact that some of the size heterogeneity of hGH reflects native oligomers. Interest in this possibility was generated by the description of immunoreactive 40-50 kD GH forms ("big hGH"), not only in fresh pituitary extracts but also in plasma (20-22, 85). The material in pituitary was shown to be dimeric hGH by several laboratories (86-90), and the material in plasma was assumed to be its equivalent, although it remained largely uncharacterized. Both noncovalently associated and disulfide-linked dimers were identified. However, only one dimer (a disulfide dimer) has been characterized in any structural detail (90). Evidence for secretion of "big" GH was then obtained in vitro (91,92), indicating that hGH dimers were probably native forms. In addition to dimeric hGH, larger mol wt immunoreactive forms (termed "big-big" or "pre-big" hGH) were also identified (20,22,91,92), but this received relatively little attention. A recent study has examined the composition of "big" and "big-big" hGH forms in plasma in detail and found them to consist of an oligomeric series up to pentameric hGH (93). Approximately two-thirds of these are noncovalently associated, one-third is disulfide-linked, and 1-2% is covalently linked by an unknown type of bond (94). The latter is also present in the pituitary (90). Immunochemical evidence indicates that the big forms in plasma and pituitary are identical (95). Thus, there is little doubt that some hGH oligomers are physiological forms. This has to be differentiated from aggregated hGH created by harsh chemical treatment.

Certain GH forms have a predilection for dimerization. For example, hGH_{20K} has such a tendency (43,45), a characteristic which is also reflected in the fact that plasma "big" hGH is enriched in hGH_{20K} (93). Chapman has identified hGH_{22K} and hGH_{20K} homodimers as well as hGH_{22K}/hGH_{20K} heterodimers in pituitary (45). Bovine, ovine and porcine GHs exist preferentially as dimers, a fact which led to erroneous initial mol wt estimates (96).

There is considerable variability among laboratories with respect to the proportional distribution of hGH among its "little," "big" and "big-big" forms. These discrepancies are explained by multiple reasons, such as different history and treatments of samples, the relative lability of noncovalent oligomers, different separation procedures, and comparison of pituitary extracts with plasma. Thus, aggregation or disaggregation may occur during extraction and analysis; certain oligomers may or may not be separated from each other; and oligomers may exhibit different immunoreactivity depending on which antibody is used, etc. In the case of big forms in plasma, the situation is even more complex. For example, different metabolic clearance rates for the various oligomers (see below) may affect their relative proportions in plasma depending on the time elapsed between secretion and blood sampling, and GH complexed with plasma GH binding proteins (see below) may be misinterpreted as oligomeric GH.

Only limited data exist on the immunoreactivity of hGH oligomers. Li reported that a dimer fraction was fully immunoreactive (86), while the disulfide dimer isolated by Lewis had only 50% immunoreactivity (90). Both of these were probably native forms. On the other hand, Moore et al.

found that aggregated hGH (probably not a native product) had only 3%
immunoreactivity (97). Solid data on immunoreactivity are important
because the great majority of data on biological potency (particularly
receptor binding studies) define the concentration of GH in the experimental system in terms of immunoreactive GH rather than an independent
estimate of GH mass, such as, e.g., protein measurements.

The growth-promoting bioactivity of dimers has been estimated at
10-20% of that of hGH monomer, lactogenic and lipolytic activity at 50-65%
(86,90). Moore has concluded that the aggregated fraction of "clinical
grade" hGH (probably a denatured rather than native aggregate) was essentially devoid of bioactivity in children (98). Receptor binding of
dimeric hGH is also decreased with respect to the monomer, at least as
defined by radioreceptor/radioimmunoassay ratios. Typically, dimers are
between 25% and 65% as active as the monomer (88-91,99,100), oligomers
about 15% (100). These figures must be viewed with some caution in the
context of their altered immunoreactivity. Even greater caution is
required with fractions derived from plasma, where the presence of GH
binding proteins (see below) further confounds the interpretation of
binding data.

HETEROGENEITY ARISING FROM POSTSECRETORY MECHANISMS

Secreted hGH, which consists of the native forms described above,
undergoes further modification after secretion in vivo. These modifications contribute to the overall heterogeneity of GH in the circulation.

Circulating GH Binding Proteins

The possibility of binding of GH (and other polypeptide hormones) to
plasma proteins was considered in the 1960s by several groups (101-104),
but largely dismissed as an artifact caused by denatured or otherwise
altered GH and insufficiently discriminating technology. The phenomenon
of conversion of radiolabeled hGH to large mol wt material when exposed to
plasma periodically resurfaced in the literature thereafter (105-107), but
was essentially ignored or interpreted as an aggregation artifact of
radiolabeled hGH. Key to the latter argument was the fact that this
phenomenon was not easily demonstrable with unlabeled hGH, which prompted
us to reach the same negative conclusion regarding protein binding as an
explanation for "big" and "big-big" hGH in plasma (93). However, lingering doubts about the nature of the macromolecular conversion phenomenon
led us to do a detailed investigation, which led to the discovery that
there exists, indeed, one (or probably two) specific binding proteins for
hGH in human plasma (108). Shortly thereafter, Herington et al. independently reported the same observation (109). Interestingly, around the same
time, a third paper appeared, reporting essentially the same finding,
although without directly demonstrating a binding protein (110).

The principal hGH binding protein is specific for human GH, has high
affinity ($K_a \sim 3 \times 10^8$/M) and limited binding capacity for hGH_{22K} and, to
a lesser extent, hGH_{20K} (108). The association rate is rapid and within a
range relevant for in vivo conditions, and the dissociation rate is
relatively slow (108,109). The binding protein is a single chain protein
with a mol wt of 60-65,000 (108,111,112); it binds one mole hGH per mole
protein (108). This binding protein complexes the majority (80-85%) of
the bound fraction of hGH in plasma.

A second binding protein (peak I) was originally deemed to be an
artifact (108). However, we have recently confirmed its specificity for
and saturability with hGH: it has a lower affinity ($K_a \sim 10^5$-10^6/M), a

mol wt of approximately 100,000, and it appears to be a single-chain protein also (111 and Baumann G, unpublished data). This minor binding protein is responsible for 15-20% of the bound fraction of hGH.

As a consequence of these binding proteins, part of the hGH in plasma exists as a complex. We determined that approximately 50% of hGH is in complexed form under physiological conditions (113). At high hGH concentrations (>20 ng/ml), the bound fraction decreases due to partial saturation of the principal binding protein (113). This is probably the reason (114) for the higher proportion of "little" (i.e., free) hGH that has been reported in acromegaly (115). Complexed hGH makes up part of the "big-big" and "big" hGH that can be recognized upon gel filtration of plasma (108). It co-elutes with true oligomeric forms of hGH, and its presence in the fractions containing oligomers is one reason for the higher proportion of "big" hGH in plasma as compared to pituitary (21,22,87,91,93,95). (Another is the slower metabolic clearance of oligomers, addressed below). This same co-elution of complexed and oligomeric hGH is responsible for the fact that the existence of the GH binding proteins was not recognized for many years. Upon fractionation of plasma, the hGH binding protein complex partially dissociates (108), which leads to underestimation of the bound hGH fraction by conventional techniques (113).

HGH complexed with the main (smaller) binding protein retains full immunoreactivity, whereas hGH complexed with the larger binding protein is only partially immunoreactive (108).

Little is known to date about the origin or physiological importance of the hGH binding proteins. One demonstrated action is to delay the metabolic clearance and degradation of hGH, and to restrict its distribution in vivo by sequestering part of the hormone in the circulation (116). Another documented effect is the modulation of the interaction of hGH with tissue receptors by competing for hGH binding (109). The principal GH binding protein is completely absent in Laron-type dwarfism (117,118), suggesting that the binding protein and the receptor are somehow related. A great deal more work is required to delineate the physiological meaning of these newly discovered binding proteins.

Metabolic Conversions

As with any protein, GH is metabolized after secretion. While inert metabolites result quite obviously from this process, the question whether bioactive or immunoreactive metabolites may also be generated has been of some interest to workers in this field. The reason for this question lies in the multiple, seemingly unrelated activities of GH on the one hand, and in the disparity between GH-like bioactivity and immunoreactive GH levels in plasma (28) on the other. Bioactive GH fragments could be one explanation for both phenomena.

In the context of the plasmin-catalyzed cleavage/activation of hGH (see above), the question was raised whether hGH could be converted intravascularly to more active two-chain forms by circulating plasmin. This was answered in the negative (119), presumably because of the large excess of plasmin inhibitors in blood. Similarly, we found no evidence for recirculating two-chain conversion products that might be generated in peripheral tissues (120). On the other hand, Schepper et al. reported that a similar cleavage occurred in vitro when hGH was incubated with liver plasma membranes (121). The failure to demonstrate these cleavage products in vivo suggests that they are locally retained and/or further degraded.

Analysis of plasma under basal conditions (i.e., at a time of low or absent pituitary GH secretion) has revealed immunoreactive hGH fragments in plasma (61). Fragments with mol wt of 12 kD, 16 kD and 30 kD were identified. The 30 kD component is probably derived from an hGH dimer and may represent a dimer of the 16 kD fragment. The same fragments have been observed in plasma after stimulation of hGH secretion, although they are more difficult to recognize in the presence of a large excess of hGH (61). The precise plasma concentration of these fragments cannot be estimated at present as their inherent immunoreactivity is unknown. It is also not known whether these fragments exhibit any bioactivity of their own.

Degradation of the various hGH forms proceeds at different rates. hGH_{20K} is degraded more slowly than hGH_{22K} (49), and dimeric forms of both of these variants are degraded more slowly than their monomeric counterparts (122). Higher oligomers ("pre-big" hGH) are cleared from plasma at even slower rates (123). The different clearance rates of the various GH forms affect their relative proportions in plasma depending on the sampling time. Thus, hormone metabolism becomes one parameter that affects the degree and type of heterogeneity in vivo.

CIRCULATING HGH

The state of GH in the circulation is the integral of the various factors mentioned above; it represents what peripheral tissues are ultimately exposed. A better understanding of the nature of circulating GH is also important in view of the bioassay/immunoassay discrepancy of plasma (124). Table 2 briefly lists the factors that determine the mixture of GH forms in the circulation.

We have extensively evaluated the hGH forms secreted by the pituitary under a variety of circumstances in vitro and in vivo (59-61,93-95,125). To summarize briefly, at least three monomeric hGH forms are secreted in vivo: hGH_{22K}, hGH_{20K}, and one or more acidic hGH forms. The latter may represent deamidated or N_α-acylated hGH. (Other speculative acidic modifications, such as glycosylated or phosphorylated hGH, are also possible. The small quantity of acidic hGH has not permitted positive identification of its structure.) The same molecular forms are secreted after a variety of secretory stimuli, both exogenous and endogenous, and both pharmacological and physiological (125). Children secrete the same hGH forms as adults (126), and there is no difference between the sexes or in different age groups (126). Furthermore, the same forms are elaborated in acromegaly, and we found no evidence for abnormal hGH forms in that disease (60,93,125). We have also identified hGH_{22K}, hGH_{20K} and acidic hGH in urine (127). Markoff et al. have recently confirmed the fact that hGH_{20K} is a secreted form (128).

These same three monomeric forms serve as the building blocks for the hGH oligomers that also circulate after a secretory stimulus (93). We found hGH di-, tri-, tetra- and pentamers in plasma, of which approximately one-third was disulfide-linked (93). HGH_{20K} was more preponderant in the dimeric than in the other fractions. Both theoretical considerations (see below) and experimental evidence (95) suggest that these oligomers are secreted as such by the pituitary rather than aggregation products formed after secretion.

As already mentioned, the metabolic clearance of the various hGH forms differs, with hGH_{20K} and oligomeric forms being cleared more slowly than hGH_{22K} (49,122,123). This is presumably the reason for the relatively high proportions of hGH_{20K} and oligomers in plasma compared to pituitary (see 122 for review).

Table 2. Factors affecting
circulating GH forms.

- Pituitary secretory products
- Metabolic clearance of individual forms
- Protein binding
- Aggregation
- Intravascular degradation
- Recirculating tissue degradation products
- Artifacts (e.g., spurious immunoreactivity)

Binding of hGH to specific hGH binding proteins has been discussed
above. It is estimated that in vivo about half of hGH_{22K} and one-third of
hGH_{20K} is protein-bound. Little is known today about the binding of
oligomeric hGH to the binding proteins.

Aggregation of hGH after secretion is deemed to be negligible as its
low concentration in plasma does not favor it, and in vitro evidence does
not indicate that native hGH aggregates in plasma. However, it should
also be mentioned that this possibility has not been rigorously excluded
in vivo.

There is no evidence of intravascular degradation of hGH (119). HGH
appears to be very stable in plasma.

Tissue degradation products may in part reenter the circulation and
contribute to hGH heterogeneity (120). We have hypothesized that the
immunoreactive hGH fragments we identified in plasma are derived from
peripheral metabolism of hGH (61), but we cannot exclude that they are
directly secreted by the pituitary.

Spurious immunoreactivity comprises a variety of nonspecific effects
caused by plasma components in radioimmunoassays. These have to be
guarded against by using several antibodies, alternative procedures for
separation of free from bound ligand and, most importantly, some physicochemical recognition procedure or partial purification of GH from plasma
whenever unexpected or aberrant results are obtained. We know of at least
one instance where a suspected "bioinactive" GH turned out to be such a
nonspecific effect masquerading as hGH.

In summary, circulating hGH is a highly heterogeneous mixture of at
least 20 molecular forms which have been identified to date. They are
listed, together with their relative proportions, in Table 3. The primary
structural variants or building blocks are hGH_{22K} (~76%), hGH_{20K} (~16%),
acidic hGH (~8%) and the three hGH fragments mentioned earlier (61,125).
Approximately 40% of total plasma hGH exists as oligomeric forms, of which
2/3 are noncovalently associated and 1/3 disulfide-linked. HGH associates
with binding proteins in plasma, giving rise to additional molecular
states.

I wish to emphasize that the data given in Table 3 are expressed in
terms of immunoreactivity. Since for many of the circulating hGH forms
the precise immunopotency is not known, their actual proportions in terms
of mass may deviate from the figures in Table 3. This is particularly
true in the case of hGH fragments, whose concentration may be substantially underestimated due to poor immunoreactivity. The peak I binding
protein complex is another example of poorly immunoreactive hGH (108), but
this has been corrected for in the table based on the known partition of
hGH between peak II and peak I binding protein.

Table 3. Circulating immunoreactive hGH forms (percent of total).

Monomers	
Free hGH_{22K} monomer	24%
Bound hGH_{22K} monomer (to peak II binding protein)	18%
Bound hGH_{22K} monomer (to peak I binding protein)	4%
Free hGH_{20K} monomer	6%
Bound hGH_{20K} monomer (to peak II binding protein)	2%
Bound hGH_{20K} monomer (to peak I binding protein)	1%
Acidic hGH monomer (free and ? bound)	5%
Dimers (free and ? bound)	
Simple hGH_{22K} dimer	14%
Disulfide hGH_{22K} dimer	6%
Simple hGH_{20K} dimer	5%
Disulfide hGH_{20K} dimer	2%
Simple acidic hGH dimer	1.5%
Disulfide-linked acidic hGH dimer	0.6%
Oligomers (Tri-, tetra- and pentamers) (free and ? bound)	
Simple hGH_{22K} oligomers	7%
Disulfide hGH_{22K} oligomers	3%
hGH_{20K} oligomers (simple and disulfide)	1.5%
acidic hGH oligomers (simple and disulfide)	1%
Nondissociable oligomers	0.8%
Fragments	
16 kD, 12 kD and 30 kD fragments	variable

Percentages are estimates derived from data given in references 61,93,94,125, and unpublished results. The total is not 100% due to rounding out of the figures. Tri-, tetra-, and pentamers have not been separately measured to date.

It appears likely that the multiple molecular forms of hGH in the circulation contribute to a complex interplay between tissue GH receptors and both agonistic and antagonistic GH-like principles in plasma. In view of this complexity, it is not surprising that there is a less than perfect correlation between the "GH level" measured by radioimmunoassay and biological effects. (There are, of course, additional reasons for this poor correlation, such as the long delay between the chemical presence of GH and its biological effect, participation of somatomedins, etc.)

Does the complexity of GH forms in plasma explain the bioactivity/immunoreactivity paradox? This question can be answered both on theoretical and experimental grounds. The ratio between GH-like bioactivity and immunoreactive GH (bio/immuno ratio) in plasma is at least one hundredfold or higher (28,124). Among the pituitary hGH forms known to circulate, none exhibits such a high bio/immuno ratio. Conceivably, GH complexed with peak I binding protein could contribute to nonimmunoreactive plasma bioactivity, but it represents only a small part of circulating GH. Another possibility is that the GH fragments identified in plasma have bioactivity of their own, but this remains speculative. To address the above question experimentally, we examined the growth-promoting activity of plasma samples from which all immunoreactive GH in its various forms had been removed by extensive immuno-extraction on anti-hGH antibody columns in a double blind study (129). To our surprise, we found considerable growth-promoting activity, even exceeding the levels reported by Ellis et al. The bioactivity roughly paralleled the hGH level originally present in the plasma samples. The somatomedin (both IGF-I and IGF-II) quantities in these samples were insufficient to explain the observed GH-like (i.e., rat tibial line) bioactivity. It thus appears that none of the immunoreactive hGH forms listed above is directly responsible for the excess bioactivity as the bio/immuno dichotomy persists in the absence of any immunoreactive material. On the basis of these data, it is more likely that GH generates as yet unidentified mediators that contribute to the overall growth-promoting bioactivity in plasma.

PHYSIOLOGICAL SIGNIFICANCE

The physiological meaning of the multiple forms of GH remains to be defined. One interpretation is that individual forms have specific functions within the spectrum of GH actions. Another view is that the particular structure of a variant dictates the sites at which proteolysis can occur, thereby giving rise to diverse fragments depending on the parent compound (62,130). Such fragments may then carry out some of the functions that we ordinarily attribute to GH itself (see above). A third possibility is that the various forms modulate each others' actions in a way that ensures optimal biological outcome. The binding proteins, for example, serve such a modulating function. Finally, GH heterogeneity may be one expression of nature's way to generate diversity in order to allow for continued evolution. The recent availability of pure GH forms in greater abundance should facilitate delineation of the biological significance of GH heterogeneity.

ACKNOWLEDGMENT

This work was supported by grants DK10699 and DK38128 from the National Institutes of Health, and by a McGaw Medical Center Interinstitutional Grant.

REFERENCES

1. Evans HM, Long JA. The effect of the anterior lobe administered intraperitoneally upon growth, maturity and oestrus cycles of the rat. Anat Rec 1921; 21:62-3.
2. Li CH, Evans HM. The isolation of pituitary growth hormone. Science 1944; 99:183-4.
3. Li CH, Papkoff H. Preparation and properties of growth hormone from human and monkey pituitary glands. Science 1956; 124:1293-4.
4. Raben MS. Preparation of growth hormone from pituitaries of man and monkey. Science 1957; 125:883-4.
5. Li CH, Liu WK, Dixon JS. Human pituitary growth hormone. VI. Modified procedure of isolation and NH_2-terminal amino acid sequence. Arch Biochem Biophys 1962(suppl 1):327-32.
6. Wilhelmi AE, Fishman JB, Russell JA. A new preparation of crystalline anterior pituitary growth hormone. J Biol Chem 1948; 176:735-45.
7. Lewis UJ, Brink NC. Crystalline human growth hormone. J Amer Chem Soc 1958; 80:4429-30.
8. Wallace ALC, Ferguson KA. Preparation of human growth hormone. J Endocrinol 1961; 23:285-90.
9. Reisfeld RA, Hallows BG, Williams DE, Brink NG, Steelman SL.

Purification of human growth hormone on 'Sephadex G-200.' Nature 1963; 197:1206-7.

10. Roos P, Fevold HR, Gemzell CA. Preparation of human growth hormone by gel filtration. Biochim Biophys Acta 1963; 74:525-31.

11. Ferguson KA, Wallace ALC. Prolactin activity of human growth hormone. Nature 1961; 190:632-3.

12. Barrett RJ, Friesen H, Astwood EB. Characterization of pituitary and peptide hormones by electrophoresis in starch gel. J Biol Chem 1962; 237:432-9.

13. Kaplan SL, Grumbach MM. Electrophoretic and immunological characteristics of native and purified human growth hormone. Nature 1962; 196:336-8.

14. Lewis UJ. Enzymatic transformations of growth hormone and prolactin. J Biol Chem 1962; 237:3141-5.

15. Lewis UJ, Cheever EV, Hopkins WC. Kinetic study of the deamidation of growth hormone and prolactin. Biochim Biophys Acta 1970; 214:498-508.

16. Niall HD. Revised primary structure for human growth hormone. Nature New Biol 1971; 230:90-1.

17. Li CH, Dixon JS. Human pituitary growth hormone. XXXII. The primary structure of the hormone: revision. Arch Biochem Biophys 1971; 146:233-6.

18. Steiner DF, Oyer PE. The biosynthesis of insulin and probable precursor of insulin by a human islet cell adenoma. Proc Natl Acad Sci USA 1967; 57:473-80.

19. Roth J, Gorden P, Pastan I. "Big insulin": a new component of plasma insulin detected by immunoassay. Proc Natl Acad Sci USA 1968; 61:138-45.

20. Yalow RS. Heterogeneity of peptide hormones. Recent Prog Horm Res 1974; 30:597-633.

21. Goodman AD, Tanenbaum R, Rabinowitz D. Existence of two forms of immunoreactive growth hormone in human plasma. J Clin Endocrinol Metab 1972; 35:868-78.

22. Gorden P, Hendricks CM, Roth J. Evidence for "big" and "little" components of human plasma and pituitary growth hormone. J Clin Endocrinol Metab 1973; 36:178-84.

23. Yadley RA, Rodbard D, Chrambach A. Isohormones of human growth hormone. III. Isolation by preparative polyacrylamide gel electrophoresis and characterization. Endocrinology 1973; 93:866-73.

24. Singh RNP, Seavey BK, Rice VP, Lindsey TT, Lewis UJ. Modified forms of human growth hormone with increased biological activities. Endocrinology 1974; 94:883-91.

25. Lewis UJ, Singh RNP, Lindsey TT, Seavey BK, Lambert TH. Enzymically modified growth hormones and the diabetogenic activity of human growth hormone. In: Raiti S, ed. Advances in human growth hormone research. Washington, DC: DHEW Publication No. (NIH) 74-612, 1974:349-63.

26. Lostroh AJ, Krahl ME. A hyperglycemic peptide from pituitary growth hormone: preparation with pepsin and assay in ob/ob mice. Proc Natl Acad Sci USA 1974; 71:1244-6.

27. Louis LH, Conn JW. Diabetogenic polypeptide from human pituitaries similar to that excreted by proteinuric diabetic patients. Metabolism 1972; 21:1-9.

28. Ellis S, Grindeland RE. Dichotomy between bio and immunoassayable growth hormone. In: Raiti S, ed. Advances in human growth hormone research. Washington, DC: DHEW Publication No. (NIH) 74-612, 1974:409-24.

29. Barsh GS, Seeburg PH, Gelinas RE. The human growth hormone gene family: structure and evolution of the chromosomal locus. Nucleic Acids Res 1983; 11:3939-59

25

30. Seeburg PH. The human growth hormone gene family: nucleotide sequences show recent divergence and predict a new polypeptide hormone. DNA 1982; 1:239-49.

31. Pavlakis GN, Hizuka M, Gorden P, Seeburg P, Hamer DH. Expression of two human growth hormone genes in monkey cells infected with simian virus 40 recombinants. Proc Natl Acad Sci USA 1981; 78:7398-402.

32. Hizuka N, Hendricks CM, Pavlakis GN, Hamer DH, Gorden P. Properties of human growth hormone polypeptides purified from pituitary extracts and synthesized in monkey kidney cells and bacteria. J Clin Endocrinol Metab 1982; 55:545-50.

33. Phillips JA III, Parks JS, Hjelle BL, et al. Genetic analysis of familial isolated growth hormone deficiency type I. J Clin Invest 1982; 70:489-95.

34. Wurzel J, Parks JS, Herd JE, Nielsen PV. A gene deletion is responsible for absence of human chorionic somatomammotropin. DNA 1982; 1:251-7.

35. Seeburg PH. Growth hormone gene structure and regulation. Presented at Acromegaly Centennial Symposium, San Francisco, CA, June 29-July 1, 1986.

36. Frankenne F, Rentier-Delrue F, Scippo M-L, Martial J, Hennen G. Expression of the growth hormone variant gene in human placenta. J Clin Endocrinol Metab 1987; 64:635-7.

37. Hennen G, Frankenne F, Pirens G, et al. New chorionic GH-like antigen revealed by monoclonal antibody radioimunoassay. Lancet 1985; 1:399.

38. Hennen G, Frankenne F, Closset J, Gomez F, Pirens G, El Khayat N. A chorionic GH-like antigen: increasing levels during second half of pregnancy with pituitary GH suppression as revealed by monoclonal antibody radioimmunoassay. Int J Fertil 1985; 30:27-33.

39. Wallis M. Growth hormone: deletions in the protein and introns in the gene. Nature 1980; 284:512.

40. DeNoto FM, Moore DD, Goodman HM. Human growth hormone DNA sequence and mRNA structure: possible alternative splicing. Nucleic Acids Res 1981; 9:3719-30.

41. Cooke NE, Ray J, Watson MA, Kuo BA, Liebhaber SA. Alternative splicing of the hGH gene: an unexpected difference between the splicing patterns of the hGH and the highly homologous hGH-variant gene transcripts. Clin Res 1987; 35:394A.

42. Sinha YN, Gilligan TA. A "20K" form of growth hormone in the murine pituitary gland. Proc Soc Exp Biol Med 1984; 177:465-74.

43. Lewis UJ, Dunn JT, Bonewald LF, Seavey BK, VanderLaan WP. A naturally occurring variant of human growth hormone. J Biol Chem 1978; 253:2679-87.

44. Lewis UJ, Bonewald LF, Lewis LJ. The 20,000 dalton variant of human growth hormone: location of the amino acid deletions. Biochem Biophys Res Commun 1980; 92:511-6.

45. Chapman GE, Rogers KM, Brittain Y, et al. The 20,000 molecular weight variant of human growth hormone: preparation and some physical and chemical properties. J Biol Chem 1981; 256:2395-401.

46. Sigel MB, Thorpe NA, Kobrin MS, Lewis UJ, VanderLaan WP. Binding characteristics of a biologically active variant of human growth hormone (20K) to growth hormone and lactogen receptors. Endocrinology 1981; 108:1600-3.

47. Smal J, Closset J, Hennen G, DeMeyts P. Receptor-binding and down-regulatory properties of the $22000-M_r$ human growth hormone and its natural $20000-M_r$ variant on IM-9 human lymphocytes. Biochem J 1985; 225:283-9.

48. Spencer EM, Lewis LJ, Lewis UJ. Somatomedin generating activity of the 20,000 dalton variant of human growth hormone. Endocrinology 1981; 109:1301-2.

49. Baumann G, Stolar MW, Buchanan TA. Slow metabolic clearance of the

20,000-dalton variant of human growth hormone: implications for biological activity. Endocrinology 1985; 117:1309-13.

50. Lewis UJ, Singh RNP, Tutweiler GF. Hyperglycemic activity of the 20,000-dalton variant of human growth hormone. Endocr Res Commun 1981; 8:155-64.

51. Frigeri LG, Peterson SM, Lewis UJ. The 20,000-dalton structural variant of human growth hormone: lack of some early insulin-like effects. Biochem Biophys Res Commun 1979; 91:778-82.

52. Kostyo JL, Cameron CM, Olson KC, Jones AJS, Pai R-C. Biosynthetic 20-kilodalton methionyl-human growth hormone has diabetogenic and insulin-like activities. Proc Natl Acad Sci USA 1985; 82:4250-3.

53. Ader M, Agajanian T, Finegood DT, Bergman RN. Recombinant deoxyribonucleic acid-derived 22K- and 20K-human growth hormone generate equivalent diabetogenic effects during chronic infusion in dogs. Endocrinology 1987; 120:725-31.

54. Martial JA. Hallewell RA, Baxter JD, Goodman HM. Human growth hormone: complementary DNA cloning and expression in bacteria. Science 1979; 205:602-7.

55. Sussman PM, Tushinski RJ, Bancroft FC. Pregrowth hormone: product of the translation in vitro of messenger RNA coding for growth hormone. Proc Natl Acad Sci USA 1976; 73:29-33.

56. Lingappa VR, Devillers-Thiery A, Blobel G. Nascent prehormones are intermediates in the biosynthesis of authentic bovine pituitary growth hormone and prolactin. Proc Natl Acad Sci USA 1977; 74:2432-6.

57. Lewis UJ, Singh RNP, Bonewald LF, Lewis LJ, VanderLaan WP. Human growth hormone: additional members of the complex. Endocrinology 1979; 104:1256-65.

58. Talamantes F, Lopez J, Lewis UJ, Wilson CB. Multiple forms of growth hormone: detection in medium from cultured pituitary adenoma explants. Acta Endocrinol (Copenh) 1981; 98:8-13.

59. Baumann G, MacCart J. Growth hormone production by human pituitary glands in organ culture: evidence for predominant secretion of the single-chain 22,000 molecular weight form (isohormone B). J Clin Endocrinol Metab 1982; 55:611-8.

60. Baumann G, MacCart JG, Amburn K. The molecular nature of circulating growth hormone in normal and acromegalic man: evidence for a principal and minor monomeric forms. J Clin Endocrinol Metab 1983; 56:946-52.

61. Baumann G, Stolar MW, Amburn K. Molecular forms of circulating growth hormone during spontaneous secretory episodes and in the basal state. J Clin Endocrinol Metab 1985; 60:1216-20.

62. Lewis UJ, Singh RNP, Bonewald LF, Seavey BK. Altered proteolytic cleavage of human growth hormone as a result of deamidation. J Biol Chem 1981; 256:11645-50.

63. Secchi C, Biondi PA, Negri A, Borroni R, Ronchi S. Detection of desamido forms of purified bovine growth hormone. Int J Pept Protein Res 1986; 28:298-306.

64. Liberti JP, Joshi GS. Synthesis and secretion of phosphorylated growth hormone by rat pituitary glands in vitro. Biochem Biophys Res Commun 1986; 137:806-12.

65. Liberti JP, Antoni BA, Chlebowsk JF. Naturally-occurring pituitary growth hormone is phosphorylated. Biochem Biophys Res Commun 1985; 128:713-4.

66. Sinha YN, Lewis UJ. A lectin-binding immunoassay indicates a possible glycosylated growth hormone in the human pituitary gland. Biochem Biophys Res Commun 1986; 140:491-7.

67. Chrambach A, Yadley RA, Ben-David M, Rodbard D. Isohormones of human growth hormone. I. Characterization by electrophoresis and isoelectric focusing in polyacrylamide gel. Endocrinology 1973; 93:848-57.

68. Ellis S, Nuenke JM, Grindeland RE. Identity between the growth hormone degrading activity of the pituitary gland and plasmin. Endocrinology 1968; 93:1029-42.

69. Yadley RA, Chrambach A. Isohormones of human growth hormone. II. Plasmin-catalyzed transformation and increase in prolactin biological activity. Endocrinology 1973; 93:858-65.

70. Lewis UJ, Pence SJ, Singh RNP, VanderLaan WP. Enhancement of the growth promoting activity of human growth hormone. Biochem Biophys Res Commun 1975; 67:617-24.

71. Baumann G, Nissley SP. Somatomedin generation in response to "activated" and "non-activated" isohormones of human growth hormone. J Clin Endocrinol Metab 1979; 48:246-50.

72. Bunner DL, Lewis UJ, VanderLaan WP. Comparative potency of subtilisin-cleaved and intact human growth hormone measured in growth hormone-deficient human subjects. J Clin Endocrinol Metab 1979; 48:293-6.

73. Li CH, Graf L. Human pituitary growth hormone: isolation and properties of two biologically active fragments from plasmin digests. Proc Natl Acad Sci USA 1974; 71:1197-1201.

74. Reagan CR, Mills JB, Kostyo JL, Wilhelmi AE. Isolation and biological characterization of human growth hormone produced by digestion with plasmin. Endocrinology 1975; 96:625-36.

75. Baumann G, Skyler JS, Chrambach A. Preparation of isohormones of human growth hormone in milligram amounts by isoelectric focusing [Abstract]. Progr 57th Meet Endocr Soc, 1975.

76. Baumann G. Metabolic clearance rates of isohormones of human growth hormone in man. J Clin Endocrinol Metab 1979; 49:495-9.

77. VanderLaan WP, Sigel MB, Singh RNP, VanderLaan EF, Lewis UJ. Radioimmunoassay evidence that 2 chain hGH circulates in blood [Abstract]. Progr 60th Meet Endocr Soc, 1978.

78. Sigel MB, VanderLaan WP, VanderLaan EF, Lewis UJ. Measurement of multiple forms of human growth hormone: cross-reactivities in conventional and two-chain radioimmunoassays. Endocrinology 1980; 106:92-7.

79. Leaver FW. Evidence for the existence of human growth hormone-ribonucleic acid complex in the pituitary. Proc Soc Exp Biol Med 1966; 122:188-96.

80. Sluyser M. Possible cause of electrophoretic and chromatographic heterogeneity of pituitary hormones. Nature 1964; 204:574-5.

81. Hunter WM. Homogeneity studies on human growth hormone. Biochem J 1965; 97:199-208.

82. Saxena BB, Henneman PH. Isolation and properties of the electrophoretic components of human growth hormone by Sephadex-gel filtration and preparative polyacrylamide gel electrophoresis. Biochem J 1966; 100:711-7.

83. Hanson LA, Roos P, Rymo L. Heterogeneity of human growth hormone preparations by immuno-gel filtration and gel filtration electrophoresis. Nature 1966; 212:948-9.

84. Lewis UJ, Cheever EV, Seavey BK. Aggregate-free human growth hormone. I. Isolation by ultrafiltration. Endocrinology 1969; 84:325-31.

85. Bala RM, Ferguson KA, Beck JC. Plasma biological and immunoreactive human growth hormone-like activity. Endocrinology 1970; 87:506-16.

86. Li CH. Human growth hormone: perspectives on its chemistry and biology. In: Raiti S, ed. Advances in human growth hormone research. Washington, DC: DHEW Publication No. (NIH) 74-612, 1974:321-41.

87. Wright DR, Goodman AD, Trimble KD. Studies on "big" growth hormone from human plasma and pituitary. J Clin Invest 1974; 54:1064-73.

88. Benveniste R, Stachura ME, Szabo M, Frohman LA. Big growth hormone (GH): conversion to small GH without peptide bond cleavage. J Clin

Endocrinol Metab 1975; 41:422–5.

89. Soman V, Goodman AD. Studies of the composition and radioreceptor activity of "big" and "little" human growth hormone. J Clin Endocrinol Metab 1977; 44:569–81.

90. Lewis UJ, Peterson SM, Bonewald LF, Seavey BK, VanderLaan WP. An interchain disulfide dimer of human growth hormone. J Biol Chem 1977; 252:3697–702.

91. Guyda HJ. Heterogeneity of human growth hormone and prolactin secreted in vitro: immunoassay and radioreceptor assay correlations. J Clin Endocrinol Metab 1975; 41:953–67.

92. Skyler JS, Rogol AD, Lovenberg W, Knazek R. Characterization of growth hormone and prolactin produced by human pituitary in culture. Endocrinology 1977; 100:283–91.

93. Stolar MW, Amburn K, Baumann G. Plasma "big" and "big-big" growth hormone (GH) in man: an oligomeric series composed of structurally diverse GH monomers. J Clin Endocrinol Metab 1984; 59:212–8.

94. Stolar MW, Baumann G, Vance ML, Thorner MO. Circulating growth hormone forms after stimulation of pituitary secretion with growth hormone releasing factor in man. J Clin Endocrinol Metab 1986; 59:235–9.

95. Stolar MW, Baumann G. Big growth hormone forms in human plasma: immunochemical evidence for their pituitary origin. Metabolism 1986; 35:75–7.

96. Evans HM, Briggs JH, Dixon JS. The physiology and chemistry of growth hormone. In: Harris GW, Donovan BT, eds. The pituitary gland; vol 1. Berkeley: Univ Cal Press, 1966:439–91.

97. Moore WV, Jin D. Polymeric and monomeric human growth hormone binding to rat liver plasma membranes. J Clin Endocrinol Metab 1978; 46:374–80.

98. Moore WV. The role of aggregated hGH in the therapy of hGH-deficient children. J Clin Endocrinol Metab 1978; 46:20–7.

99. Gorden P, Lesniak MA, Hendricks CM, Roth J. "Big" growth hormone components from human plasma: decreased reactivity demonstrated by radioreceptor assay. Science 1973; 182:829–31.

100. Eastman RC, Lesniak MA, Hendricks CM, Gorden P. Radioreceptor assay (RRA) of endogenous and exogenous hGH components in pathologic states: evidence for increased RRA of little hGH in acromegaly [Abstract]. Progr 58th Meet Endocr Soc, 1976.

101. Touber JL, Maingay D. Heterogeneity of human growth hormone. Its influence on a radio-immunoassay of the hormone in serum. Lancet 1963; 1:403–5.

102. Hadden DR, Prout TE. A growth hormone binding protein in normal human serum. Nature 1964; 202:1342–3.

103. Collipp PJ, Kaplan SA, Boyle DC, Shimizu CSN. Protein-bound human growth hormone. Metabolism 1964; 13:532–8.

104. MacMillan DR, Schmid JM, Eash SA, Read CH. Studies on the heterogeneity and serum binding of human growth hormone. J Clin Endocrinol Metab 1967; 27:1090–4.

105. Antoniades H. Conversion of [^{125}I]growth hormone into high molecular weight forms in vivo. Endocrinology 1975; 96:799–802.

106. Beitins IZ, Rattazzi MC, MacGillivray MH. Conversion of radiolabeled human growth hormone into higher molecular weight moieties in human plasma in vivo and in vitro. Endocrinology 1977; 101:350–9.

107. Peeters S, Friesen HG. A growth hormone binding factor in the serum of pregnant mice. Endocrinology 1977; 101:1164–83.

108. Baumann G, Stolar MW, Amburn K, Barsano CP, DeVries BC. A specific growth hormone-binding protein in human plasma: initial characterization. J Clin Endocrinol Metab 1986; 62:134–41.

109. Herington AC, Ymer S, Stevenson J. Identification and characterization of specific binding proteins for growth hormone in normal human

sera. J Clin Invest 1986; 77:1817-23.

110. Nixon DA, Jordan RM. Conversion of CSF monomeric growth hormone to large growth hormone with exposure to serum. Acta Endocrinol (Copenh) 1986; 111:289-95.

111. Baumann G, Shaw MA. The circulating growth hormone binding proteins: partial purification and structural characterization by affinity crosslinking. Clin Res 1986; 34:949A.

112. Herington AC, Ymer SI, Stevenson JL. Affinity purification and structural characterization of a specific binding protein for human growth hormone in human serum. Biochem Biophys Res Commun 1986; 139:150-5.

113. Baumann G, Amburn K. Human growth hormone circulates in large part as a complex associated with (a) plasma protein(s). Clin Res 1986; 34:681A.

114. Baumann G. Molecular heterogeneity of circulating growth hormone in acromegaly. Acromegaly: a century of scientific and clinical progress. New York: Plenum Press, 1987; 35-43.

115. Gorden P, Lesniak MA, Eastman R, Hendricks CM, Roth J. Evidence for higher proportion of "little" growth hormone with increased radioreceptor activity in acromegalic plasma. J Clin Endocrinol Metab 1976; 43:364-73.

116. Baumann G, Amburn KD, Buchanan TA. The effect of circulating growth hormone-binding protein on metabolic clearance, distribution, and degradation of human growth hormone. J Clin Endocrinol Metab 1987; 64:657-60.

117. Baumann G, Shaw MA, Winter RJ. Absence of circulating growth hormone binding protein in Laron-type dwarfism. Clin Res 1987; 35:582A.

118. Daughaday WH, Trivedi B. Absence of serum growth hormone binding protein of Laron dwarfs links the binding protein with the cellular growth hormone receptor. Clin Res 1987; 35:646A.

119. Baumann G. Failure of endogenous plasmin to convert human growth hormone to its "activated" isohormones. J Clin Endocrinol Metab 1976; 43:222-5.

120. Baumann G, Hodgen G. Lack of in vivo transformation of human growth hormone to its "activated" isohormones in peripheral tissues of the rhesus monkey. J Clin Endocrinol Metab 1976; 43:1009-14.

121. Schepper JM, Hughes EF, Postel-Vinay M-C, Hughes JP. Cleavage of growth hormone by rabbit liver plasmalemma enhances binding. J Biol Chem 1984; 259:12945-8.

122. Baumann G, Stolar MW, Buchanan TA. The metabolic clearance, distribution, and degradation of dimeric and monomeric growth hormone (GH): implications for the pattern of circulating GH forms. J Clin Endocrinol Metab 1986; 119:1497-1501.

123. Hendricks CM, Eastman RC, Takeda S, Asakawa K, Gorden P. Plasma clearance of intravenously administered pituitary human growth hormone: gel filtration studies of heterogeneous components. J Clin Endocrinol Metab 1985; 60:864-7.

124. Ellis S, Vodian MA, Grindeland RE. Studies on the bioassayable growth hormone-like activity of plasma. Recent Prog Horm Res 1978; 34:213-38.

125. Baumann G, Stolar MW. Molecular forms of human growth hormone secreted in vivo: non-specificity of secretory stimuli. J Clin Endocrinol Metab 1986; 62:789-90.

126. Baumann G, Winter RJ, Shaw M. Circulating molecular variants of growth hormone in childhood. Pediatr Res 1987; 21 (in press).

127. Baumann G, Abramson EC. Urinary growth hormone in man: evidence for multiple molecular forms. J Clin Endocrinol Metab 1983; 56:305-11.

128. Markoff E, Lee DW, Culler FL, Jones KL, Lewis UJ. Release of the 22,000- and 20,000-dalton variants of growth hormone in vivo and in

vitro by human anterior pituitary cells. J Clin Endocrinol Metab 1986; 62:664-9.

129. Baumann G, Stolar MW, Grindeland RE. Growth-promoting bioactivity in human plasma depleted of immunoreactive growth hormone [Abstract]. Progr 67th Meet Endocr Soc, 1985.

130. Lewis UJ. Variants of growth hormone and prolactin and their posttranslational modifications. Annu Rev Physiol 1984; 46:33-42.

3

SOME ASPECTS ON THE BIOCHEMISTRY OF GROWTH HORMONE

Choh Hao Li

Laboratory of Molecular Endocrinology
University of California
San Francisco, CA 94143

HISTORICAL PERSPECTIVE

In 1921, Evans and Long (1) injected a saline extract of anterior lobes of bovine pituitaries into normal rats and the growth of these animals was accelerated. Later experiments by Smith in 1927 (2) showed that the growth of hypophysectomized rats was resumed on administration of the same anterior pituitary extract. Thus, the existence of growth-promoting activities in these extracts was indicated. In 1944, Li and Evans reported the isolation of a protein from bovine pituitary extracts with a molecular weight of 44,250 in solutions of pH 6.64-7.00 and an isoelectric point of pH 6.85 having growth-promoting activity in hypophysectomized rats and devoid of other pituitary hormone activities (3,4). The protein was identified as the growth hormone (GH) of bovine pituitary gland or bGH.

Highly purified bGH was first administered in the spring of 1947 to a girl judged clinically to be a hypopituitary dwarf. At a dose level approaching 5 mg per kg of body weight, it was without effect upon nitrogen balance (5). This led to the concept of species specificity of protein hormones that bGH is chemically different from the human hormone and does not exhibit growth-promoting activity in man. One of our co-workers at that time was pathologist Dr. Henry D. Moon who was asked to obtain human pituitary glands at autopsy. In the meantime, I asked Dr. Herbert Olivecrona (neurosurgeon) and Dr. Rolf Luft (clinical endocrinologist) in Stockholm to save the human pituitaries when they removed the glands from patients with breast cancer in the early 1950s. It took nearly 5 years to collect sufficient human pituitary glands for the isolation of human growth hormone (hGH) in highly purified form for biological and chemical characterizations (6,7). Indeed, it was shown that hGH is chemically distinct from bGH and hGH is active in man. It was also shown that bGH does not cross-react with rabbit antiserum to hGH (8,9).

The first metabolic studies on hGH and monkey GH (mGH) were performed by Dr. D. M. Bergenstal of the National Cancer Institute who administered the primate hormones to 2 patients (one with mild hypopituitarism and the other a hypophysectomized male subject). In both cases, a daily dose of 10 mg of either human or monkey GH, injected intramuscularly for 5 days, caused a marked retention of nitrogen and phosphorus indicative of the anabolic nature of the hormone (see data in reference 7).

Amino acid sequences of 9 mammalian GHs are known: 6 (human [10-12], bovine [13-15], ovine [16], equine [17], whale [18] and monkey [19]) obtained by direct chemical analysis and 3 (porcine [20], rat [21] and mouse [22]) derived by DNA sequence. They all contain 190-191 amino acids with a single tryptophan residue and two disulfide bridges.   Circular dichroism studies of various GHs (23-27) have reported α-helix contents of 45-55%.

A comparison of the primary structure of nonprimate GHs with that of hGH revealed that the sequence homology is 64-66% as shown in Figure 1. Table 1 lists the doublet substitutions of nonprimate sequence in the primate structure.   Each of the changes in 8 out of 9 doublets could result from single base mutations.   Among closely related species (human vs. monkey; bovine vs. ovine; rat vs. mouse), only 3 or 4 residues are not homologous.   Even in the case of porcine versus equine, 5 residues are different in residue positions 63, 71, 72, 91 and 113, as summarized in Table 2.   These changes again could result from single base mutations except residue position 185 in bovine and ovine sequences.

There are 4 half-cystine, 3 histidine and 1 tryptophan residues in each of the mammalian GH molecules. Locations of these residues in the amino acid sequence are summarized in Table 3.   Both tryptophan and half-cystine residues are in identical positions in all mammalian GHs.   Two out of three His residues are located very closely in both primate and non-primate hormones.   The regions near Trp-85, Met-125, His-18,21 and Cys-53,165,182,189 are highly conserved (see Table 4).   Among these regions, the one containing tryptophan is especially of interest.   Since all GH molecules contain a single Trp residue, it would be desirable to investigate the replacement of this residue by Phe or Tyr as to the growth-promoting activity using the protein engineering technique.

Table 1.   Doublet substitutions in nonprimate
and primate GH structure.

Residue Position*	Primate[+]	Nonprimate[+]
3-4	Thr-Ile	Ala-Met
18-19	His-Arg	Gln-His
38-39	Lys-Glu	Glu-Lys
107-108	Asn-Ser	Asp-Arg
112-113	Asp-Leu	Glu-Lys
151-152	His-Asn	Arg-Ser
170-171	Met-Asp	Leu-His
179-180	Ile-Val	Val-Met
184-185	Ser-Val	Arg-Phe

*See Figure 1.

[+]Underlined residue could result from single base mutations.

Fig. 1A — Amino acid sequence of growth hormone in different species.

Positions 5, 10, 15

		5		**10**	**15**
Human:	H-Phe-Pro-Thr-Ile-Pro-Leu-Ser-Arg-Leu-Phe-Asp-Asn-Ala-Met-Leu-				
Monkey:					
Bovine:		Ala-Met-Ser	Gly	Ala	Val
Ovine:		Ala-Met-Ser	Gly	Ala	Val
Porcine:		Ala-Met	Ser	Ala	Val
Equine:		Ala-Met	Ser	Ala	Val
Rat:	H-Leu	Ala-Met	Ser	Ala	Val
Mouse:		Ala-Met	Ser	Ser	Val
Whale:		Ala-Met	Ser	Ala	Val

Positions 20, 25, 30

	20		**25**	**30**
Human:	Arg-Ala-His-Arg-Leu-His-Gln-Leu-Ala-Phe-Asp-Thr-Tyr-Gln-Glu-			
Monkey:				
Bovine:	Gln-His		Ala	Phe-Lys
Ovine:	Gln-His		Ala	Phe-Lys
Porcine:	Gln-His		Ala	Lys
Equine:	Gln-His		Ala	Lys
Rat:	Gln-His		Ala	Lys
Mouse:	Gln-His		Ala	Lys
Whale:	Gln-His	Glu	Ala	Lys

Positions 35, 40, 45

	35		**40**	**45**
Human:	Phe-Glu-Glu-Ala-Tyr-Ile-Pro-Lys-Glu-Gln-Lys-Tyr-Ser-Phe-Leu-			
Monkey:				
Bovine:	Arg-Thr	Glu-Gly	Arg	( ) Ile-
Ovine:	Arg-Thr	Glu-Gly	Arg	( ) Ile-
Porcine:	Arg	Glu-Gly	Arg	( ) Ile-
Equine:	Arg	Glu-Gly	Arg	( ) Ile-
Rat:	Arg	Glu-Gly	Arg	( ) Ile-
Mouse:	Arg	Glu-Gly	Arg	( ) Ile-
Whale:	Arg	Glu-Gly	Arg	( )

Positions 50, 55, 60

	50		**55**	**60**
Human:	Gln-Asn-Pro-Gln-Thr-Ser-Leu-Cys-Phe-Ser-Glu-Ser-Ile-Pro-Thr-			
Monkey:				
Bovine:	Thr	Val-Ala-Phe	Thr	Ala-
Ovine:	Thr	Val-Ala-Phe	Thr	Ala-
Porcine:	Ala	Ala-Ala-Phe	Thr	Ala-
Equine:	Ala	Ala-Ala-Phe	Thr	Ala-
Rat:	Ala	Ala-Ala-Phe	Thr	Ala-
Mouse:	Ala	Ala-Ala-Phe	Thr	Ala-
Whale:	Ala	Ser-Thr-Gly	Val	

Positions 65, 70, 75

	65		**70**	**75**
Human:	Pro-Ser-Asn-Arg-Glu-Glu-Thr-Gln-Gln-Lys-Ser-Asn-Leu-Gln-Leu-			
Monkey:				
Bovine:	Thr-Gly-Lys-Asn	Ala		Asp Glu
Ovine:	Thr-Gly-Lys-Asn	Ala		Asp Glu
Porcine:	Thr-Gly-Lys-Asp	Ala	Arg	Val-Glu
Equine:	Thr-Gly-Lys	Ala	Arg	Asp-Met-Glu
Rat:	Thr-Gly-Lys	Ala		Arg-Thr-Asp-Met-Glu
Mouse:	Thr-Gly-Lys	Ala		Arg-Thr-Asp-Met-Glu
Whale:	Ala Lys-Asp	Ala	Arg	Asp-Val-Glu

Fig. 1A. Amino acid sequence of growth hormone in different species.

BIOCHEMICAL DIFFERENCES BETWEEN HUMAN AND BOVINE GH

It is now known that nonprimate GHs are not active in man and only primate hormones possess growth-promoting activity in human subjects. Moreover, it is also known that nonprimate GHs do not exhibit lactogenic activity in addition to their growth-promoting activity. There are several biochemical characteristics which are different between primate and nonprimate GHs. Table 5 presents some biochemical properties of hGH and bGH (28,29). It is obvious that bGH has a different molecular weight and isoelectric point in comparison with that for the human hormone.

```
                      80              85              90
Human:   Leu-Arg-Ile-Ser-Leu-Leu-Leu-Ile-Gln-Ser-Trp-Leu-Glu-Pro-Val-
Monkey:
Bovine:                                             Gly       Leu-
Ovine:                                              Gly       Leu-
Porcine:         Phe                                Gly
Equine:          Phe                                Gly
Rat:             Phe                                Gly
Mouse:           Phe                                Gly
Whale:           Phe                                Gly
                 77                                 87


                      95              100             105
Human:   Gln-Phe-Leu-Arg-Ser-Val-Phe-Ala-Asn-Ser-Leu-Val-Tyr-Gly-Ala-
Monkey:                                                           Thr-
Bovine:              Ser-Arg         Thr                   Phe     Thr-
Ovine:               Ser-Arg         Thr-Asp               Phe     Thr-
Porcine:             Ser-Arg         Thr                   Phe     Thr-
Equine:        Leu   Ser-Arg         Thr                   Phe     Thr-
Rat:                 Ser-Arg-Ile     Thr               Met-Phe     Thr-
Mouse:               Ser-Arg-Ile     Thr               Met-Phe     Thr-
Whale:               Glu-Lys-Ala-Tyr          Glu         Phe     Thr-
                     93                        99


                      110             115             120
Human:   Ser-Asn-Ser-Asp-Val-Tyr-Asp-Leu-Leu-Lys-Asp-Leu-Glu-Glu-Gly-
Monkey:  Tyr
Bovine:  Asp-Arg ( )             Glu-Lys
Ovine:   Asp-Arg ( )             Glu-Lys
Porcine: Asp-Arg ( )             Glu-Lys
Equine:  Asp-Arg ( )             Glu-Lys     Arg
Rat:     Asp-Arg ( )             Glu-Lys
Mouse:   Asp-Arg ( )             Glu-Lys
Whale:   Asp-Arg ( )             Glu-Lys
                                 110


                      125             130             135
Human:   Ile-Gln-Thr-Leu-Met-Gly-Arg-Leu-Glu-Asp-Gly-Ser-Pro-Arg-Thr-
Monkey:                                                       Ser
Bovine:  Leu-Ala             Arg-Glu                Thr        Ala-
Ovine:   Leu-Ala             Arg-Glu            Val-Thr        Ala-
Porcine: Ala                 Arg-Glu                           Ala-
Equine:  Ala                 Arg-Glu                           Ala-
Rat:     Ala                 Gln-Glu                           Ile-
Mouse:   Ala                 Gln-Glu                           Val-
Whale:   Ala                 Arg-Glu                           Ala-
         121                                                  133
```

Fig. 1B

Molecular Weight

In 1953, ultracentrifugation studies indicated a molecular weight of 46,000 for bGH and the possibility of a dissociation of bGH into smaller components in highly alkaline solutions (30). Subsequently, various investigators showed that bGH dissociates from the dimeric form in neural or slightly alkali solutions to the monomer in acidic solutions of low ionic strength (24,31). Earlier studies on the sedimentation behavior of hGH indicated a molecular weight of 22,000–29,000 (32,33). It is now generally agreed that primate GHs are monomer of 22 kDA, whereas non-primate hormones are dimer of 44 kDA in solutions of pH 6–8.

Isoelectric Point

It was reported in 1945 that the isoelectric point of bGH was found to be pH 6.85 by free electrophoresis at 1.5°C (4). The isoelectric point of the primate hormones was later shown to be more acidic than that of bGH (7). The values are: human, pH 4.9; monkey, pH 5.5; and bovine, pH 6.85.

Fig. 1C — Amino acid sequence comparison

Positions 140 / 145 / 150

Human: Gly-Gln-Ile-Phe-Lys-Gln-Thr-Tyr-Ser-Lys-Phe-Asp-Thr-Asn-Ser-
Monkey:

Bovine:	Leu	Asp		Met-
Ovine:	Leu	Asp		Met-
Porcine:	Leu	Asp		Leu-
Equine:	Leu	Asp		Leu-
Rat:	Leu	Asp	Ala	Met-
Mouse:	Leu	Asp	Ala	Met-
Whale:	Leu	Asp		Met-
	137	142		148

Positions 155 / 160 / 165

Human: His-Asn-Asp-Asp-Ala-Leu-Leu-Lys-Asn-Tyr-Gly-Leu-Leu-Tyr-Cys-
Monkey:

Bovine:	Arg-Ser	Ser
Ovine:	Arg-Ser	Ser
Porcine:	Arg-Ser	Ser
Equine:	Arg-Ser	Ser
Rat:	Arg-Ser	Ser
Mouse:	Arg-Ser	Ser
Whale:	Arg-Ser	Ser
	150	162

Positions 170 / 175 / 180

Human: Phe-Arg-Lys-Asp-Met-Asp-Lys-Val-Glu-Thr-Phe-Leu-Arg-Ile-Val-

Monkey:			Ile		
Bovine:		Leu-His	Thr	Tyr	Val-Met-
Ovine:		Leu-His	Thr	Tyr	Val-Met-
Porcine:	Lys	Leu-His	Ala	Tyr	Val-Met-
Equine:	Lys	Leu-His	Ala	Tyr	Val-Met-
Rat:	Lys	Leu-His	Ala	Tyr	Val-Met-
Mouse:	Lys	Leu-His	Ala	Tyr	Val-Met-
Whale:	Lys	Leu-His	Ala	Tyr	Val-Met-
	165	169	171		178

Positions 185 / 191

Human: Gln-Cys-Arg-Ser-Val-Glu-Gly ( ) Ser-Cys-Gly-Phe-OH
Monkey:

Bovine:	Lys	Arg-Phe-Gly-Gln-Ala	Ala
Ovine:	Lys	Arg-Phe-Gly Ala	Ala
Porcine:	Lys	Arg-Phe-Val-Glu-Ser	Ala
Equine:	Lys	Arg-Phe-Val-Glu-Ser	Ala
Rat:	Lys	Arg-Phe-Ala-Glu-Ser	Ala
Mouse:	Lys	Arg-Phe-Val-Glu-Ser	Ala
Whale:	Lys	Arg-Phe-Val-Glu-Ser	Ala
		183	190

Fig. 1C

Solubility

It was estimated from the data obtained in 1947 (29) that the solubility of bGH in distilled H_2O of pH 7.1 at 5°C is 0.21 mg protein per ml. Under the same conditions, the solubility of hGH is at least 10 mg protein per ml (unpublished observations). Subsequent studies on the solubility of hGH, hCS, bGH and sGH in ammonium sulfate solution of pH 6.60 as a function of ionic strength showed that hGH is more soluble as compared with the nonprimate hormones (34).

Disulfide Bridges

The two disulfide bridges in hGH can be reduced by β-mecaptoethanol and alkylated by iodoacetamide in the presence of 8 M urea without loss of growth-promoting and lactogenic activities (35). It was found subsequently that reduction of the two disulfide bonds may be achieved by dithiothreitol (DTT) in the absence of urea (36). In addition, the DTT-reduced hGH can be autooxidized at pH 8.4 and the reoxidized hormone

Table 2. Nonhomologous residues in closely
related species among GH structures.

Species	Residue Position*				
	105	107	133	173	
Human	Ala	Asn	Pro	Val	
Monkey	Thr	Tyr	Ser	Ile	
	98	129	185		
Bovine	Asn	Gly	Gln		
Ovine	Asp	Val	Gly		
	1	133	184		
Rat	Leu	Ile	Ala		
Mouse	Phe	Val	Val		
	63	71	72	91	113
Porcine	Asp	Asn	Val	Phe	Lys
Equine	Glu	Asp	Met	Leu	Arg

*Underlined residue could result from
single base mutations. For residue
position, see Figure 1.

retains the full biological potency of the native hormone (37). It is
impossible to perform these reduction/reoxidization experiments with the
bovine hormone; the hormone becomes completely insoluble as soon as it is
reduced by DTT or β–mecaptoethanol unless in the presence of denaturant.

Two Contiguous Thrombin Fragments of hGH Form an Active Recombinant,
But the Two Homologous Fragments from Ovine Hormone Do Not

From plasmin digests of hGH, two peptide fragments were isolated from
reduction and alkylation with iodoacetamide: [Cys(Cam)[53]]–hGH–(1–134) and
[Cys(Cam)[165,182,189]]–hGH–(141–191). The NH_2–terminal fragment possesses
approximately 14% growth-promoting and lactogenic activities when compared
with the native hormone, whereas the COOH-terminal fragment has only measurable activities (38). These two fragments interact noncovalently to
form a fully active complex conformationally indistinguishable from intact

Table 3. Location of Trp, His and 1/2 Cys
residues in mammalian GHs.

Amino Acid Residues	Total Number		Residue Positions	
	Primate	Nonprimate	Primate	Nonprimate
Trp	1	1	86	86
His	3	3	18,21,151	19,21,169
1/2 Cys	4	4	53,165	53,163
			182,189	180,188

Table 4. Conserved regions in the amino acid
sequence of mammalian GHs[a].

1) -Glu-Thr-Gln-Gln-Lys-Ser-Asn-Leu-Gln-Leu-Leu-Arg-Ile-Ser-Leu-
    (Ala)68   (Asp) (Glu)75   (Phe)   80

    Leu-Leu-Ile-Gln-Ser-Trp-Leu-
                85

2) -Leu-Phe-Asp-Asn-Ala-Met-Leu-Arg-Ala-His-Arg-Leu-His-Gln-Leu-Ala-
   10(Ala)   (Val)   17(Gln-His)   24

3) -Ser-Leu-Cys-Phe-Ser-Glu-Ser-Ile-Pro-Thr-Pro-Ser-
  (Ala-Phe)   54   (Thr)   (Ala)61

4) -Asp-Asp-Ala-Leu-Leu-Lys-Asn-Tyr-Gly-Leu-Leu-Tyr-Cys-Phe-
   154   160   (Ser) 166

    Arg-Lys-Asp-Met-Asp-Lys-
    (Lys)   (Leu-His)

5) -Glu-Thr-Phe-Leu-Arg-Ile-Val-Gln-Cys-Arg-
   175(Tyr)   (Val-Met-Lys)   183

6) -Ser-Cys-Gly-Phe-OH
  188   (Ala)191

[a]The sequence of hGH is indicated; residues in parentheses for
nonprimate hormones.

hGH (39). The structural requirements of this recombinant reaction have
been extensively studied by complementing the large NH_2-terminal fragment
(residues 1-134) with various synthetic analogs of the COOH-terminal fragment (40-45), and it has been concluded that even considerable structure
analogs of the COOH-terminal fragment, like its shortening to residues
154-187 (45) cause no significant change in the complementation reaction.

Two thrombin fragments of reduced-carbamidomethylated hGH represent-
ing the full primary structure of the native hormone (residues 1-134 and

Table 5. Some biochemical properties
of hGH and bGH.

Properties	Growth Hormone	
	Human	Bovine
Molecular weight		
osmotic pressure	22,000	44,250
ultracentrifugation	21,500	44,000
Isoelectric point, pH	4.90	6.85
Diffusion constant, $D_{20°_w} \times 10^7$	8.88	7.15
Sedimentation coefficient	2.18	3.10
α-Helix content, %	55	50

135-191) have been found to form a recombinant molecule with properties similar to those of reduced-carbamidomethylated hGH as shown by circular dichroism, two receptor-binding assays and radioimmunoassay (46). In contrast, the homologous thrombin fragments of reduced-carbamidomethylated oGH (residues 1-132 and 133-190) do not undergo recombination. Furthermore, neither the reduced-alkylated nor the reduced and nonalkylated COOH-terminal thrombin fragment of oGH is able to interact with the reduced carbamidomethylated NH$_2$-terminal thrombin fragment of hGH under conditions which favor the recombination of the two hGH fragments.

Crystallization

Since hGH was first isolated and identified in 1956, many attempts have been made to crystallize the hormone without success. Recently, bGH and pGH have been crystallized and the crystals appear suitable for use in the X-ray structure determination. Bell et al. (47) obtained single crystals of bGH by vapor diffusion techniques. The density of the bGH crystals was 1.19 g/ml from which the presence of eight 45 kDA dimers/unit cell was deduced. Abdel-Meguid et al. (48) reported crystallization of methionyl pGH by the hanging drop method of vapor diffusion and the crystals belong to the trigonal group with a = 58.7 Å and b = 58.7 Å.

SUMMARY

The presence of growth-promoting activities in an extract from anterior lobes of bovine pituitary glands was discovered in 1921. It took nearly a quarter of a century before bGH was isolated in highly purified form. Growth hormone has now been purified to nearly homogeneity from pituitary glands of many species. They all consist of approximately 190 amino acids with a single tryptophan residue and two disulfide bridges. The amino acid sequence of various GHs has been determined by chemical analysis or derived from DNA sequences. Comparison of known primary structures of mammalian GHs reveal that certain regions of the sequence are highly conserved. Biochemical characteristics of primate GHs are distinctly different from that for nonprimate hormones. The isoelectric point of the primate hormone is more acidic than that of bGH. Primate GH is a monomer in a solution of pH 7-9, whereas nonprimate GH is a dimer under the same conditions. Human GH can be reduced and alkylated in the absence of denaturant without loss of biological activities, whereas bovine GH cannot. Two contiguous thrombin fragments of human GH form a functionally active recombinant, but the two homologs from ovine GH do not. It is known that solubility of bGH in aqueous solutions is considerably less in comparison with the human hormone. Many attempts to crystallize hGH have been unsuccessful but bGH and pGH have recently been crystallized.

ACKNOWLEDGMENTS

For the last 45 years, this work was supported in part by the National Institutes of Health, American Cancer Society, Lasker Foundation, Allen-Geffen Fund and the Hormone Research Foundation.

REFERENCES

1. Evans HM, Long JA. The effect of the anterior lobe administered intraperitoneally upon growth, maturity and oestrus cycles of the rat. Anat Rec 1921; 21:62-3.
2. Smith PE. The disabilities caused by hypophysectomy and their repair. JAMA 1927; 88:158-61.

3. Li CH, Evans HM. The isolation of pituitary growth hormone. Science 1944; 99:183-4.

4. Li CH, Evans HM, Simpson ME. Isolation and properties of the anterior hypophyseal growth hormone. J Biol Chem 1945; 159:353-66.

5. Bennett LL, Weinberger H, Escamilla R, Margen S, Li CH, Evans HM. Failure of hypophyseal growth hormone to produce nitrogen storage in a girl with hypophyseal dwarfism. J Clin Endocrinol Metab 1950; 10:492-5.

6. Li CH, Papkoff H. Preparation and properties of growth hormone from human and monkey pituitary glands. Science 1956; 124:1293-4.

7. Li CH. Properties of and structural investigations on growth hormones isolated from bovine, monkey and human pituitary glands. Fed Proc 1957; 16:775-83.

8. Hayashida T, Li CH. An immunological investigation of human pituitary growth hormone. Science 1958; 128:1276-7.

9. Li CH, Moudgal RN, Papkoff H. Immunochemical investigations of human pituitary growth hormone. J Biol Chem 1960; 235:1038-42.

10. Li CH, Dixon JS, Liu W-K. Human pituitary growth hormone. XIX. The primary structure of the hormone. Arch Biochem Biophys 1969; 133:70-91.

11. Li CH, Dixon JS. Human pituitary growth hormone. XXXII. The primary structure of the hormone: revision. Arch Biochem Biophys 1971; 146:233-6.

12. Li CH. Hormones of the adenohypophysis. Proc Amer Philos Soc 1972; 116:365-82.

13. Santome JA, Dellacha JA, Paladini AC, et al. The amino acid sequence of bovine growth hormone. FEBS Lett 1971; 16:198-200.

14. Wallis M. The primary structure of bovine growth hormone. FEBS Lett 1973; 35:11-4.

15. Graf L, Li CH. On the primary structure of pituitary bovine growth hormone. Biochem Biophys Res Commun 1974; 56:168-76.

16. Li CH, Gordon D, Knorr J. The primary structure of sheep pituitary growth hormone. Arch Biochem Biophys 1973; 156:493-508.

17. Zakin MM, Poskus E, Langton AA, et al. Primary structure of equine growth hormone. Int J Pept Protein Res 1976; 8:435-44.

18. Pankov YA, Bulatov AA, Osipova TA. Primary structure of seiwhale pituitary somatotropin. Int J Pept Protein Res 1982; 30:396-9.

19. Li CH, Chung D, Lahm H-W, Stein S. The primary structure of monkey pituitary growth hormone. Arch Biochem Biophys 1986; 245:287-91.

20. Seeburg PH, Sias S, Adelman J, et al. Efficient bacterial expression of bovine and porcine growth hormone. DNA 1983; 2:37-45.

21. Seeburg PH, Shine J, Martial JA, Baxter JD, Goodman HM. Nucleotide sequence and amplification in bacteria of structural gene for rat growth hormone. 270:486-94.

22. Linzer DIH, Talamantes F. Nucleotide sequence of mouse prolactin and growth hormone mRNA and expression of these mRNAs during pregnancy. J Biol Chem 1985; 260:9574-9.

23. Aloj SM, Edelhoch H. Conformational stability of ovine prolactin and bovine growth hormone. Proc Natl Acad Sci USA 1970; 56:830-6.

24. Bewley TA, Li CH. Molecular weight and circular dichroism studies of bovine and ovine pituitary growth hormones. Biochemistry 1972; 11:927-32.

25. Holladay LA, Hammonds RG Jr, Puett D. Growth hormone conformation and conformational equilibria. Biochemistry 1974; 13:1653-61.

26. Bewley TA, Brovetto-Cruz J, Li CH. Human pituitary growth hormone. Physicochemical investigations of the native and reduced-alkylated protein. Biochemistry 1969; 8:4701-8.

27. Bewley TA, Li CH. The conformation of monkey pituitary somatotropin. Arch Biochem Biophys 1986; 248:646-51.

28. Li CH. Human growth hormone: 1974-1981. Mol Cell Biochem 1982; 46:31-41.

29. Li CH. Physicochemical characterization of pituitary growth hormone. J Phys Colloid Chem 1947; 51:218-28.

30. Li CH, Pedersen KO. Sedimentation behavior of hypophyseal growth hormone. J Biol Chem 1953; 201:595-600.

31. Dellacha JM, Santome JA, Paladini AC. Physicochemical and structure studies of bovine growth hormone. Ann NY Acad Sci 1968; 148:313-27.

32. Squire PG, Pedersen KO. The sedimentation behavior of human pituitary growth hormone. J Am Chem Soc 1961; 83:478-81.

33. Li CH, Starman B. Human pituitary growth hormone. IX. Molecular weight of the monomer. Biochim Biophys Acta 1964; 86:175-6.

34. Tarli P, Li CH. Human pituitary growth hormone: solubility in ammonium sulfate solutions. Arch Biochem Biophys 1974; 161:696-7.

35. Dixon JS, Li CH. Retention of the biological potency of human pituitary growth hormone after reduction and carbamidomethylation. Science 1966; 154:785-6.

36. Bewley TA, Dixon JS, Li CH. Human pituitary growth hormone. XVI. Reduction with dithio-threitol in the absence of urea. Biochim Biophys Acta 1968; 154:420-2.

37. Bewley TA, Li CH. Human pituitary growth hormone. XXII. The reduction and reoxidation of the hormone. Arch Biochem Biophys 1970; 138:338-46.

38. Li CH, Graf L. Human pituitary growth hormone: isolation and properties of two biologically active fragments from plasmin digests. Proc Natl Acad Sci USA 1974; 71:1197-201.

39. Li CH, Bewley TA. Human pituitary growth hormone: restoration of full biological activity by noncovalent interaction of two fragments of the hormone. Proc Natl Acad Sci USA 1976; 73:1476-9.

40. Blake J, Li CH. The synthesis and biological activity of [165,182,189-S-carbamidomethylcystein]-human growth hormone-(140-191). Int J Pept Protein Res 1975; 7:495-501.

41. Li CH, Blake J, Hayashida T. Human somatotropin: semisynthesis of the hormone by noncovalent interaction of the NH_2-terminal fragment with synthetic analogs of the COOH-terminal fragment. Biochem Biophys Res Commun 1978; 82:217-22.

42. Blake J, Li CH. Human somatotropin 55. Synthesis and growth-promoting activity of peptide analogs of the carboxyl terminal plasmin fragment. Int J Pept Protein Res 1978; 11:315-22.

43. Li CH, Blake J. Semisynthesis of human somatotropin analogs. Proc Natl Acad Sci USA 1979; 76:6124-7.

44. Li CH, Blake J, Cheng CHK, Jibson MD. Human somatotropin: synthesis of the hormone by non-covalent interaction of the natural NH_2-terminal fragment with a synthetic analog of the COOH-terminal fragment. Arch Biochem Biophys 1981; 211:338-45.

45. Li CH, Blake J, Cabrera CM. Human somatotropin: noncovalent interactions of the natural NH_2-terminal 1-134 fragment with synthetic analogs of the COOH-terminal fragment. Arch Biochem Biophys 1985; 293:12-7.

46. Graf L, Li CH, Cheng CHK, Jibson M. Two contiguous thrombin fragments of human somatotropin form a functionally active recombinant, but the two homologous fragments from sheep hormone do not. Biochemistry 1981; 20:7251-8.

47. Bell JA, Moffat K, Vonderhaas BK, Golde BW. Crystallization of preliminary X-ray characterization of bovine growth hormone. J Biol Chem 1985; 260:8520-5.

48. Abdel-Meguid SS, Smith WW, Violand BN, Bentle LA. Methionyl porcine somatotropin, a genetically engineered variant of porcine growth hormone. J Mol Biol 1986; 192:159-60.

4

MULTIPLE FORMS OF GROWTH HORMONE

U. J. Lewis, R. N. P. Singh, L. J. Lewis, and N. Abadi

The Whittier Institute for Diabetes and Endocrinology
Lutcher Brown Department of Biochemistry
9894 Genesee Avenue, La Jolla, CA 92037

INTRODUCTION

Increasingly, variant forms of growth hormone are being found, but an understanding of their significance has not kept pace with the ability to detect them. One of the problems is that the variants occur in much lower concentrations than the major form, thus making preparation of quantities for biologic testing a difficult task. In addition, availability of human pituitary glands for such studies was limited until recently, when clinical treatment with pituitary-derived growth hormone was discontinued and the glands became available for research projects concerned with identification of new substances. The low concentration of many of the forms raises a frequently asked question: can these forms have physiologic relevance when they occur in such small amounts compared to the major form? What is usually overlooked here is the fact that the major form occurs in an enormous quantity compared to the other pituitary hormones. A comparison of human pituitary hormones will illustrate this point. There are between 5000 and 7000 µg of the major form of human growth hormone (hGH_{22K}) in a pituitary gland. If the concentration of a variant of hGH is 1% of this (50 to 70 µg), its concentration would be similar to that of FSH; a 3% concentration would equal the amount of prolactin in a gland.

There are problems in expressing concentration of a variant in a biologic sample. Gel electrophoresis is the usual method of resolving mixtures of the various forms, and visualization and quantitation of a component in a gel are done on the basis of immunoreactivity or color development. These detection methods can be misleading because of different degrees of reactivity of the substances. For example, if a mixture of hGH_{20K} (80%) and hGH_{22K} (20%) is first separated by SDS gel electrophoresis and then the bands are made visible either by silver staining in the first instance or by immunoblotting with a polyclonal antiserum for hGH in the second, the silver stain will quite accurately indicate this difference in concentration. On the other hand, immunostaining will give just the opposite result, that is, 20% hGH_{20K} and 80% hGH_{22K}. Furthermore, some forms may not be immunoreactive as demonstrated by the P16 variant (1) and the 20K-dalton form of rat GH (2) which are not detected by currently available antisera. Staining with Coomassie Blue can also be misleading; reactivity of a glycosylated form can be quite different in comparison to a form without carbohydrate. Obviously, specific antisera to the variant forms are needed to accurately evaluate their concentration in pituitary extracts.

Mention should also be made of the analytical methods now available for resolving mixtures of the variants. Separation by gel electrophoresis is the most discriminating, and separation may be effected either by molecular size, by charge, or by a combination of the two techniques. Use of one approach alone can give misleading answers. Two variants could have the same size but different charges, or the opposite. Therefore, to insure optimum resolution, two-dimensional analysis (size and charge) is required. The report by Yokoya and Friesen (3) is an excellent example of resolution of variants of rat GH by two-dimensional analysis.

In the following description of the variants of growth hormone, both human and nonhuman forms will be mentioned. At this time, all the known variations of structure have not been found in a single species, but we think that occurrence in one species indicates a high probability of finding the form in others.

GROWTH HORMONE GENES

Two genes for hGH have been detected. The major form of the hormone is an expression product of the gene designated as N. The second gene, denoted as V, codes for a variant that differs from the major form at 13 positions (4). Only recently has evidence for expression of the V gene been obtained. Frankenne et al. (5) noted an increase in secretion of an hGH-like substance during pregnancy and a decrease of the hormone at term. Hybridization studies with placental mRNA and oligonucleotide probes of specific portions of the N or V genes indicated that the hGH-like substance was probably hGH-V. Although the hormone is produced in significant amounts by the placenta, only a low order of expression of the V-gene has been noted in a pituitary adenoma. Whether or not under other physiologic conditions hGH-V is produced in greater amounts must await further studies.

An interesting difference in the amino acid sequences of hGH-N and hGH-V is that the variant form has an Asn-X-Ser/Thr sequence, frequently referred to as a consensus sequence for asparagine-linked glycosylation, whereas hGH-N does not. Another result of the amino acid substitutions in hGH-V is formation of a double base (Arg-Arg) sequence at positions 18 and 19, thus providing a second location for possible proteolytic processing.

In the rat only a single gene for growth hormone has been reported (6). As a result of finding at least 16 GH-immunoreactive proteins in the pituitary gland, Yokoya and Friesen (3) raise the question of the possibility of additional genes. They point out that when looking for other genes, higher homology of the cDNA probes with the genes could result in additional hybridizations. Also, since hybridization specificity can vary with experimental conditions, changing these conditions may possibly reveal additional genes. If additional genes are not found to account for the multiple forms of rat GH, there must be multiple mRNAs for a single gene, or proteolytic processing of the major form must be considered as a source of the various substances.

Multiple forms of growth hormone can also be seen in the human pituitary gland. As shown in Figure 1, even clinical grade growth hormone prepared from pituitary extracts contains at least 12 different immunoreactive components when analyzed by 2-dimensional gel electrophoresis. High and low molecular weight substances are seen, as well as charge isomers.

44

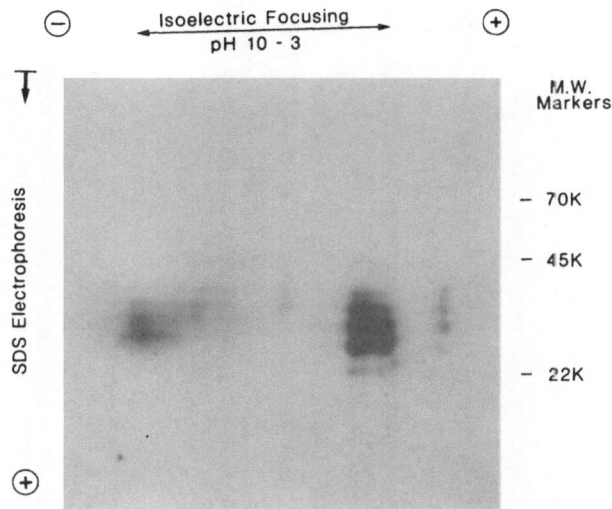

Fig. 1. Two dimensional gel electrophoresis of a sample of clinical grade hGH. The isoelectric focusing was done in a pH gradient of 4 to 6. The SDS electrophoresis was by the method of Laemmli (33). Components in the mixture were detected by immunoblotting with a polyclonal antiserum to hGH.

ALTERNATIVE mRNA SPLICING

The 20K-dalton variant of hGH is a product of alternative splicing of the precursor mRNA for hGH-N (7,8). During processing of the mRNA when the B-intron is removed, an additional 45 nucleotides are also removed. Translation of this mature mRNA results in a variant with 15 fewer amino acids (residues 32-46) (9). This smaller form is found in the circulation (10-12). It is possible that the hGH-V gene could also give rise to a similar 20K-dalton variant, thus adding to the list of multiple forms that can be produced.

Alternative splicing may involve introns other than the B sequence. Hampson and Rottman (13) found an mRNA for growth hormone in bovine pituitary glands in which the intron D had not been removed during splicing and only the first 50 nucleotides of exon 5 were retained. If translated, this mRNA would produce a growth hormone that was 42 amino acids longer than the major form, with a molecular weight near 27K. The COOH-terminal portion of this variant would be entirely different from that of the major form. The translation product of this variant mRNA for bovine GH has not yet been reported. As shown in Figure 2, we see a 27K-dalton form of hGH, but whether or not intron D is involved in its production is not yet known.

POST- AND/OR COTRANSLATIONAL MODIFICATION

Proteolytic

Several types of proteolytically cleaved hGH have been identified in the pituitary gland. Figure 3 illustrates that the region of the molecule involving residues 135-149 is susceptible to proteolytic attack. Cleavage

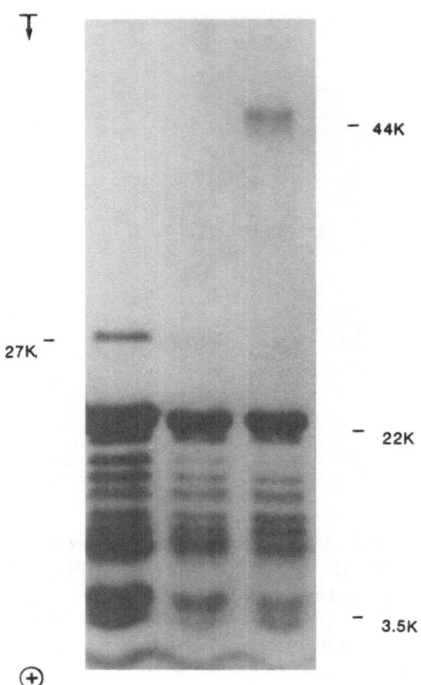

Fig. 2. SDS electrophoresis of an acidic
fraction obtained by anion exchange chromatography of a heterogeneous sample of hGH
(see Fig. 6). The gel was 12% in polyacrylamide. Note that there are both high and
low molecular weight acidic forms.

can occur at a single peptide bond, or there can be two breaks resulting
in removal of a short sequence (14). In either case, the molecule is
converted to a two-chain form because of the disulfide bridge at 55-165.
The protein retains full biologic activity (growth and lactogenic properties), and in certain cases an enhancement of activities is seen
(14,15). Although linkages involving arginine and lysine residues are the
points of attack in some of the forms, in others, such as the $_3$ modification, a phenylalanine-serine bond is cleaved. Production of a two-chain
form of rat GH results from cleavage in the region of 152 to 156 (1).
Davis et al. (1) suggest that it may be the alanine-valine at 152-153 that
is affected. For all the two-chain forms, it is not known whether after
cleavage of the peptide chain, the disulfide at 55-165 is opened to
produce two separate chains. These points are illustrated in Figure 3.

Proteolytic cleavage outside the large disulfide loop of growth
hormone can also occur (Fig. 3). The major portion of the amino terminal
sequence of hGH can be removed by cleavage at position 43 (serine). The
peptide has been isolated (16) and found to have biologic effects (17,18).
Finding hGH_{1-43} indicated that hGH_{44-191} must also be in pituitary
extracts; but only recently did we obtain evidence for that possibility.
The protein has a molecular weight near 17K. After reduction, it remains
intact and actually decreases in electrophoretic mobility, indicating
opening of a disulfide bond. Although not completely pure, peptide
mapping of a tryptic digest of the protein by HPLC indicated a decreased
amount of peptides arising from hGH_{1-43}.

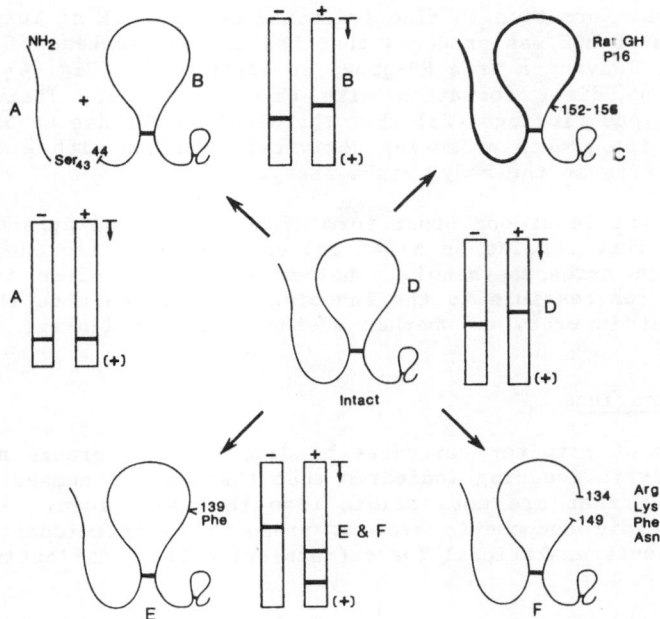

Fig. 3. Schematic representation of types of proteolytic cleavage that have been noted for hGH. A represents hGH_{1-43}; B, the remaining part of the hGH molecule after cleavage at the 43-44 linkage. No electrophoresis pattern is shown for C; a 2-dimensional gel can be found in reference 1. Forms E and F give the same electrophoresis patterns. Cleavages have been noted at Arg, Lys, Phe and Asn in these forms. The electrophoresis patterns show how the cleaved forms behave in SDS electrophoresis when analyzed with and without reduction with mercaptoethanol.

The numerous low molecular weight immunoreactive forms seen in Figure 1 indicate that there are other cleavage products in pituitary extracts. Their isolation will permit a better evaluation of their physiologic importance, especially if specific RIAs can be developed for them.

Interchain Disulfide Dimers

Two groups (19, 20) have found a "mercaptoethanol dissociable" dimer of hGH both in the pituitary gland and in serum. Even though this dimer is detected in fresh pituitary extracts, because its formation has also been detected during lyophilization of hGH, it is not known with certainty that it is formed under physiologic conditions. It is interesting that the hGH disulfide dimer has little growth promoting activity, whereas its lactogenic property as measured by the pigeon crop sac assay is retained. This could be a way for hGH to exert lactogenic actions without the activities associated with growth.

If hGH behaves as human placental lactogen, the disulfide interchange that produces the dissociable dimer occurs at the COOH-terminal disulfide (21). The bridge that forms the large disulfide loops does not appear to be involved. That the S-S linkage at 55 and 165 is not involved in disulfide dimer formation is also indicated by the work of Tokunaga et al. (22). A form of hGH was produced that had alanine instead of cysteine at position 165, leaving a free SH-group at position 55 (Fig. 4). There was no evidence of dimer formation with this substance. Their work also supports previous findings (23) that the disulfide bridge at 55 and 165 is not required for growth promoting activity. The hGH with alanine at 165 had full activity in the body weight assay.

There is at least one other form of hGH (19), and apparently of rat GH also (3), that remains as a 44K dalton immunoreactive substance after treatment with mercaptoethanol. Whether this is a dimer in which the disulfide is inaccessible to the reducing agent, even when the reduction is carried out in urea, or whether another covalent linkage is involved, is not known.

Acidic Modifications

Analysis of pituitary extracts by disc electrophoresis above pH 7.5 or by isoelectric focusing indicates that there are a number of forms of growth hormone that are more acidic than the major form. If we assume that these acidic components are not products of individual genes, but, rather, are posttranslational (or cotranslational) modifications of the

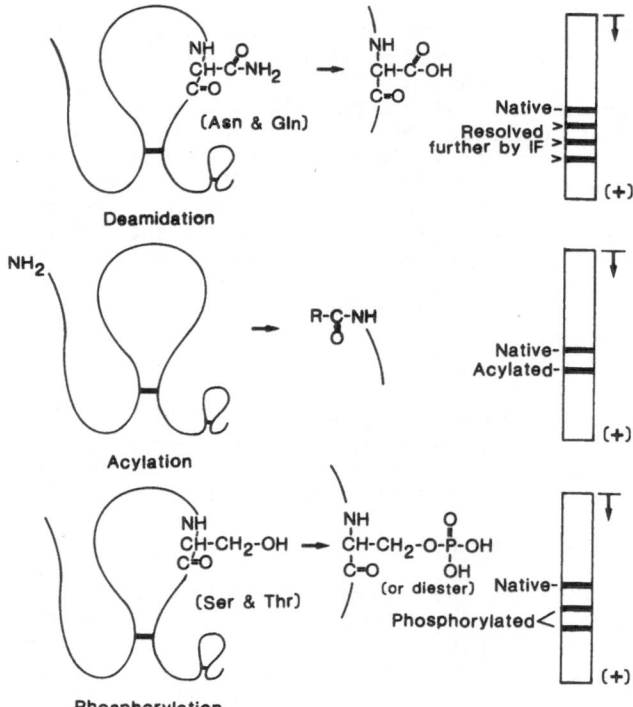

Fig. 4. Schematic representation of three acidic modifications of growth hormone that have been found. The electrophoresis patterns indicate how the substances behave during disc electrophoresis at pH 7.6. The deamidated forms can be resolved further by isoelectric focusing, depending on which Asn or Gln in the peptide chain is deamidated.

known possible forms of hGH (hGH-N, hGH-V and their 20K-dalton forms), there are at least four ways in which a more acidic protein could be produced: (1) The two-chain, proteolytic cleavage products discussed above are all more acidic than intact hGH, probably because of loss of a greater number of basic amino acids than acidic ones (14). (2) Deamidation occurs readily in the growth hormone of all species with which we have worked, but because of difficulty in identifying deamidated asparaginyl or glutaminyl residues, an unequivocal statement as to whether or not a component in an electrophoretic pattern is a desamido form is difficult to make (24). (3) Acylation of the NH_2-terminus has been suggested as a means whereby GH can assume a more acidic charge (25). Loss of the free NH_2-terminal group by acylation imparts a less basic (more acidic charge) to the protein. Here, also, identification of this form is difficult because of the relatively insensitive methods for detecting the acylating group. (4) Phosphorylation of growth hormone has been indicated (26) and may contribute to the heterogeneity of the hormone. However, if the hormone is not labeled with radioactive phosphorus, identification as a phosphorylated protein is difficult unless quite large quantities are available for analysis. Because prolactin also undergoes this modification (27), the process may be of general importance in altering biologic behavior of these pituitary hormones.

The formation of these acidic modifications of $hGH_{22}K$ and hGH_{20K} enormously complicates purification of the multiple forms. The molecular weights are almost identical, thus making separation by gel filtration poor; their similarities in charge decrease usefulness of ion exchange chromatography, and the small differences in hydrophobicity minimizes separations by reversed phase chromatography. These points are discussed in more detail below in the section dealing with purification.

Glycosylated Forms

Two recent reports reopen the question of glycosylated growth hormone. As discussed above, the expression product of the hGH-V gene would have a consensus sequence for asparagine-linked glycosylation (Asn-X-Ser/Thr), so if the placental hGH-like substance reported by Hennen et al. (5) is actually this variant, the possibility of finding a glycosylated form seems likely. In the human pituitary gland, evidence for a glycosylated growth hormone comes from a newly developed lectin-immunoassay (28) which detects substances that bind to concanavalin A and at the same time react with an antiserum to hGH. In support of a glycosylated growth hormone is the fact that prolactin, which has always been thought not to be glycosylated, has been found to have a major glycosylated form (29-31). It appears that GH and PRL must now be classified with the other glycoprotein hormones. Progress is being made on the purification of the human pituitary substance that binds to concanavalin A and that is hGH-like immunologically. Soon we should have structural data that will indicate in a more direct manner whether or not we have been successful in isolation of a glycosylated hGH.

Purification Methods

In the section above dealing with the acidic modifications of growth hormone, we alluded to the problems encountered in their purification. Here we will give specific examples of four different chromatographic procedures used in attempts at purification of the components in the preparation of heterogeneous hGH. The sample was the same as that used for the 2-dimensional electrophoresis pattern shown in Figure 1. The chromatography columns were those provided in the FPLC system of Pharmacia, Inc. Gel filtration was done with a Superose 12 column with various buffers such as 0.05 M NH_4HCO_3 with or without 8 M urea, 10% acetic acid or 0.02 M Tris-HCl, pH 8. The results of the chromatography are shown in Figure 5 where 0.05 M NH_4HCO_3 was used for the elution. The other buffers gave comparable results. There was no resolution into separate peaks. As seen in the immunoblot (hGH antiserum of the chromatogram) of a SDS electrophoresis gel, the resolution was quite poor. Separation on the basis of charge gave somewhat improved enrichment of some of the components, but there was no separation into single substances. This is shown in Figure 6 where a Mono Q column with a 0.05 M to 0.5 M linear gradient with NH_4HCO_3 was used. A 0.02 M Tris-Cl/NaCl gradient, pH 8, likewise gave similar results. To take advantage of charge differences, we also tried to purify the substances by chromatofocusing. A pH 6-4 gradient was used for elution from a Mono P column. As seen in Figure 7, there are indications that partial separations do take place but fail to give single components. Finally, we tried reversed phase chromatography on a C_{1-8} column (Pro RPC) with either a 0.1% TFA/CH_3CN or a $NaCLO_4-H_3PO_4/CH_3CN$ gradient. As seen in Figure 8, there were enrichments of components greater and smaller than 22K molecular weight, but no purification. Reluctantly, we are faced with the need to cut and elute components from the SDS-electrophoresis gels to achieve purifications of these multiple forms.

SUMMARY

We are now certain that there are multiple forms of growth hormone which are secreted from the pituitary gland but their role in biologic

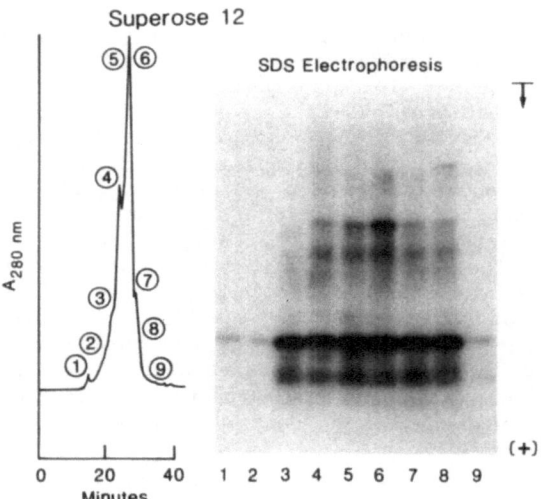

Fig. 5. Chromatography of a heterogeneous sample of hGH on a Superose 12 (HR 10) column. The sample load was 2 mg and the column was developed with 0.05 M NH_4HCO_3 at a flow rate of 20 ml/h. Various fractions along the chromatogram were analyzed by SDS electrophoresis and the components visualized by immunoblotting with a polyclonal antiserum to hGH.

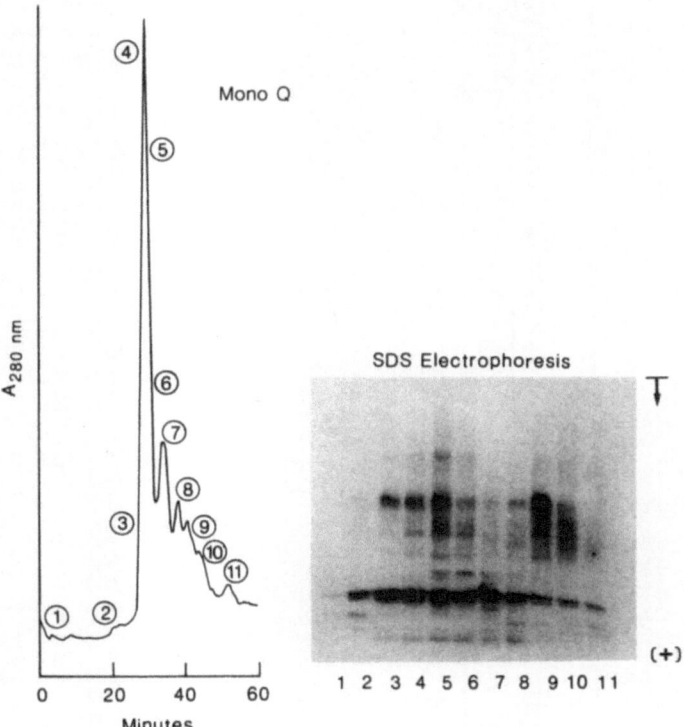

Fig. 6. Anion exchange chromatography cf a heterogeneous sample of hGH on a Mono Q (HR 5/5) column. The sample load was 5 mg and the column was developed with a linear gradient of NH_4HCO_3 (0.05 M to 0.5 M) at a flow rate of 18 ml/h. Various fractions along the chromatogram were analyzed by SDS electrophoresis and the components visualized by immunoblotting with an antiserum to hGH.

reactions is completely unknown. Although only speculating, we do have some ideas on the possible physiologic importance of the variants. First of all, we reject the suggestion that because of their low concentrations they have no physiologic relevance. In the rat de novo synthesis has been shown (3), a strong argument against the forms being artifactual. On the positive side, we suggest that the physiologic need for such an array of forms could be that, for the numerous actions of growth hormone, the variants are needed to initiate different reactions at the receptor. On the other hand, we may find that there are specific receptors for the various forms. To explain the function of the high concentration of the major form, we have postulated (32) that it serves as a prohormone for smaller forms, including physiologically active fragments. Only after purification of all the GH-related forms in the pituitary gland, will we be able to evaluate the merit of these speculations.

51

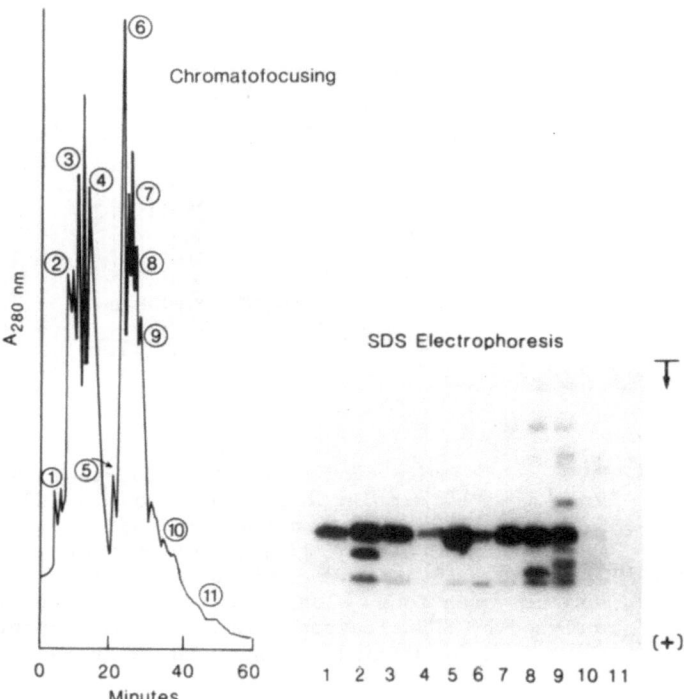

Fig. 7. Chromatofocusing of a heterogeneous sample of hGH on a Mono P (HR 5/20) column. The sample load was 2.5 mg. The column was first equilibrated with 0.025 M piperazine HCl, pH 6.3, prepared in 6 M urea. The column was developed with Polybuffer HCl, pH 4.5 made 6 M in urea, at a flow rate of 30 ml/h. Various fractions along the chromatogram were analyzed by SDS electrophoresis and the components visualized by immunoblotting with an antiserum to hGH.

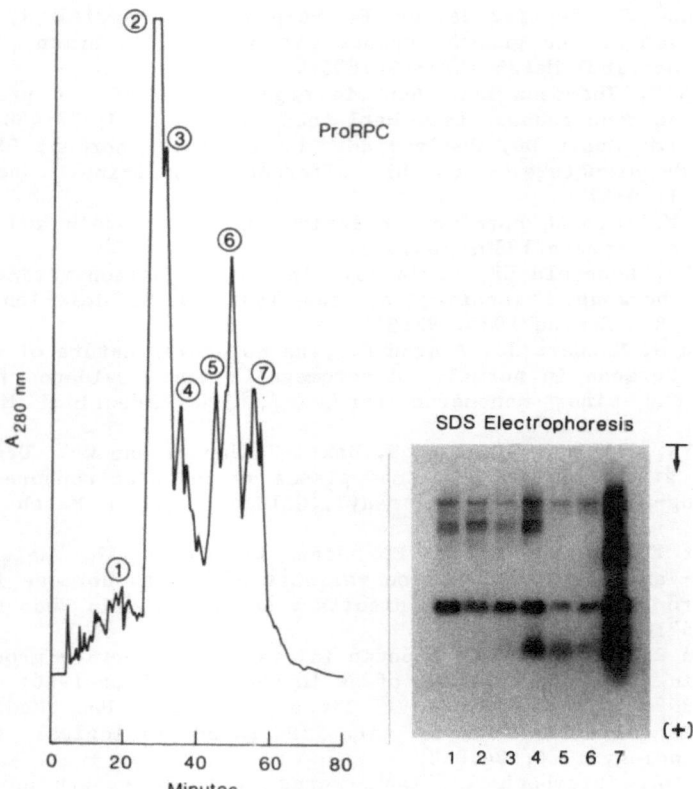

Fig. 8. Reversed phase chromatography of a heterogeneous sample of hGH on a ProRPC (HR 5/10) column. The sample load with 2 mg and the column was developed with a linear gradient of 0.01 M $NaClO_4$-0.05% H_3PO_4 and CH_3CN at a flow rate of 18 ml/h. Various fractions along the chromatogram were analyzed by SDS electrophoresis and the components visualized by immunoblotting with an antiserum to hGH.

ACKNOWLEDGMENTS

This research was supported by grants DK31416, DK31417 and BRSG RR05826 from the National Institutes of Health.

REFERENCES

1. Davis RB, Morris J, Ivarie R. The polypeptide P16 is a carboxy terminal cleavage product of rat growth hormone in anterior pituitary and GH_3 pituitary tumor cells. Mol Endocrinol 1987; 1:102.
2. Sinha YN, Gilligan TA. A "20K" form of growth hormone in the murine pituitary gland. Proc Soc Exp Biol Med 1984; 177:465.
3. Yokoya A, Friensen HG. Human growth hormone (GH)-releasing factor stimulates and somatostatin inhibits the release of rat GH variants. Endocrinology 1986; 119:2097.
4. Seeburg PH. The human growth hormone gene family: nucleotide sequences show recent divergence and predict a new polypeptide hormone. DNA 1982; 1:239.

5. Frankenne F, Rentier-Delrue F, Scippo M-L, Martial J, Hennen G. Expression of the growth hormone variant gene in human placenta. J Clin Endocrinol Metab 1987; 64:635.

6. Chien Y-H, Thompson EB. Genomic organization of rat prolactin and growth hormone genes. Proc Natl Acad Sci USA 1980; 77:4583.

7. DeNoto FM, Moore DD, Goodman HM. Human growth hormone DNA sequence and mRNA structure: possible alternative splicing. Nucleic Acids Res 1981; 9:3719.

8. Wallis M. Growth hormone: deletions in the protein and introns in the gene. Nature 1980; 284:512.

9. Lewis UJ, Bonewald LF, Lewis LJ. The 20,000-dalton variant of human growth hormone: location of the amino acid deletion. Biochem Biophys Res Commun 1980; 92:511.

10. Baumann G, MacCart JG, Ambrun K. The molecular nature of circulating growth hormone in normal and acromegalic man: evidence for a principal and minor monomeric form. J Clin Endocrinol Metab 1983; 56:946.

11. Sinha YN, Gilligan TA, Lee DW, Baxi SC, VanderLaan WP. Demonstration of 20K growth hormone in human plasma by gel electrophoretic-immuno-staining-autoradiographic assay (GEISAA). Horm Metab Res 1986; 18:402.

12. Markoff E, Lee DW, Culler FL, Jones KL, Lewis UJ. Release of the 22,000- and the 20,000-dalton variants of growth hormone in vivo and in vitro by human anterior pituitary cells. J Clin Endocrinol Metab 1986; 62:664.

13. Hampson RK, Rottman FM. A potential variant of bovine growth hormone resulting from non-splicing of an intron. Fed Proc 1986; 45:1703.

14. Singh RNP, Seavey BK, Rice VP, Lindsey TT, Lewis UJ. Modified forms of human growth hormone with increased biological activities. Endocrinology 1974; 94:883.

15. Yadley RA, Chrambach A. Isohormones of human growth hormone. II. Plasmin-catalyzed transformation and increase in prolactin biological activity. Endocrinology 1973; 93:858.

16. Singh RNP, Seavey BK, Lewis LJ, Lewis UJ. Human growth hormone peptide 1-43: isolation from pituitary glands. J Prot Chem 1983; 2:425.

17. Frigeri LG, Teguh K, Wehrenberg WB, Ling N, Lewis UJ. Enhancement of insulin action by NH_2-terminal peptides of growth hormone [Abstract]. Clin Res 1986; 34:103A.

18. Frigeri LG, Ling N, Rudman C, VanderLaan WP, Lewis UJ. Increased in vivo glucose utilization by amino terminal peptides of growth hormone [Abstract]. Burlington, Vermont: Research Symposium of Diabetes and Exercise, July, 1983.

19. Lewis UJ, Peterson SM, Bonewald LF, Seavey BK, VanderLaan WP. An interchain disulfide dimer of human growth hormone. J Biol Chem 1977; 252:3697.

20. Benveniste R, Stachura ME, Szabo M, Frohman LA. Big growth hormone (GH): conversion to small GH without peptide bond cleavage. J Clin Endocrinol Metab 1975; 41:422.

21. Schneider AB, Kowalski K, Russell J, Sherwood LM. Identification of the interchain disulfide bonds of dimeric human placental lactogen. J Biol Chem 1979; 254:3782.

22. Tokunaga T, Tanaka T, Ikehara M, Ohtsuka E. Synthesis and expression of a human growth hormone (somatotropin) gene mutated to change cysteine-165 to alanine. Eur J Biochem 1985; 153:445.

23. Dixon JS, Li CH. Retention of the biological potency of human pituitary growth hormone after reduction and carbamidomethylation. Science 1966; 154:785.

24. Lewis UJ, Singh RNP, Bonewald LF, Seavey BK. Altered proteolytic cleavage of human growth hormone as a result of deamidation. J Biol Chem 1981; 256:11645.

25. Lewis UJ, Singh RNP, Bonewald LF, Lewis LJ, VanderLaan WP. Human growth hormone: additional members of the complex. Endocrinology 1979; 104:1256.
26. Liberti JP, Antoni BA, Chlebowski JF. Naturally-occurring pituitary growth hormone is phosphorylated. Biochem Biophys Res Commun 1985; 128:713.
27. Oetting WS, Tuazon PT, Traugh JA, Walker AM. Phosphorylation of prolactin. J Biol Chem 1986; 261:1649.
28. Sinha YN, Lewis UJ. A lectin-binding immunoassay indicates a possible glycosylated growth hormone in the human pituitary gland. Biochem Biophys Res Commun 1986; 140:491.
29. Lewis UJ, Singh RNP, Lewis LJ, Seavey BK, Sinha YN. Glycosylated ovine prolactin. Proc Natl Acad Sci USA 1984; 81:385.
30. Pankov YuA, Butnev VYu. Multiple forms of pituitary prolactin. Glycosylated form of prolactin with enhanced biological activity. Int J Pept Protein Res 1986; 28:113.
31. Meuris S, Svoboda M, Christophe J, Robyn C. Evidence for a glycosylated prolactin variant in human pituitary and amniotic fluid. In: MacLeod RM, Thorner MO, Scapagnini U, eds. Prolactin, basic and clinical correlates. Padova: Livana Press, 1985:487-93.
32. Lewis UJ. Variants of growth hormone and prolactin and their post-translational modifications. Annu Rev Physiol 1984; 46:33.
33. Laemmli UK. Cleavage of structural proteins during assembly of the head of bacteriophage T_4. Nature 1970; 227:680.

5

GENETIC DEFECTS IN PROCESSING GROWTH HORMONE

John A. Phillips, III, M.D.

Professor of Pediatrics and Biochemistry
Vanderbilt University School of Medicine
Nashville, Tennessee 37232

INTRODUCTION

Progress in recombinant DNA technology has enabled characterization of the sequence and organization of the hGH gene and the hGH gene cluster. This chapter reviews these findings and their pertinence to hGH expression in normal tissues as well as their derangements in selected genetic types of hGH deficiency.

HGH BIOSYNTHESIS

HGH Gene Organization

The hGH and closely related chorionic somatomammotropin (hCS) genes reside in a 50,000 base pair (50 kb) portion of human chromosome 17 (see Figure 1). Studies of the nucleotide sequences of isolated genomic fragments containing single hGH or hCS genes or multiple, different genes indicate that only 5 loci (2 hGH, 2 hCS, and 1 hCS-like) reside within the hGH gene cluster (1-3). In the case of the hGH genes, 1 locus (GH1) encodes the known protein sequence, while the other locus (GH2) encodes a protein that differs by 13 amino acids (see Figure 2) (4,5). In the case of the hCS genes, there are 3 loci. The CSH1 and CSH2 loci encode proteins of identical sequence while the CSHP1 locus encodes a protein that differs by 13 amino acids (3). Unusual features of the hGH gene cluster are the very high degree of homology retained between its loci and their flanking regions and the large number (≥27) of Alu-type middle repetitive sequences that occur in the cluster (3).

HGH Expression and Processing

The gene organization of GH1, CSHP1, CSH1, GH2 and CSH2 are very similar with each having 5 exons interrupted at identical positions by small introns. These genes retain 92 to 98% homology in their immediate flanking, intervening and coding sequences (6). An exception to the conservation of intron/exon sequences is CSHP1 which contains 25 nucleotide substitutions in its exons and a G to A transversion in the 5' or donor splice site of its second intron (3). This substitution would prevent pre-mRNA processing at the same donor splice site utilized by the GH1, 2 and CSH1, 2 loci (7). CSHP1 specific oligonucleotides do not detect cDNA

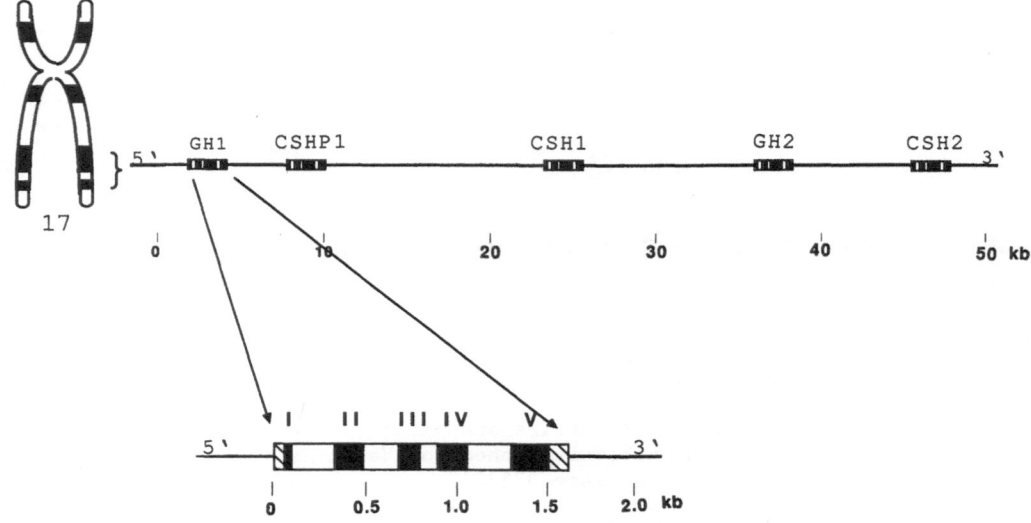

Fig. 1. Schematic representation of the hGH gene cluster and its location on chromosome 17. Exons, introns, and nontranslated sequences are depicted as solid, open, and shaded rectangles.

clones in libraries derived from human pituitary or placental mRNAs (3). These data suggest that CSHP1 is either a pseudogene (an inactive gene) or its expression only occurs in human tissues other than pituitary or placenta.

The GH1, GH2, CSH1, CSH2, and CSHP1 genes all have the CATAAA and TATAA sequences characteristic of eukaryotic promoters located 55 and 30 bp, respectively, upstream from their transcription initiation sites (see Figures 1 and 3). Each also has an AATAA sequence in the 3' regions 20 bp upstream from their transcription stop sites (3,4). The first 4 genes encode protein products of 217 amino acids which represent prehormones. The 26 additional amino acids at the N-terminus of each protein constitute signal peptide or leader sequences that are important in directing transport through the membrane of the rough endoplasmic reticulum (REF) (see Figure 3) (8). Following transport to the RER cisternae, the signal peptides are cleaved from the 24 kb pre-hGH and pre-hCS hormones to yield the 191 amino acid mature hormones which are 22k.

GENES

5'	GH1	CSHP1		CSH1	GH2	CSH2 3'

PRODUCTS

	GH1	CSHP1		CSH1	GH2	CSH2
	45K HGH	?		HCS	22K HGH	HCS
	24K HGH				variant	
	22K HGH					
	20K HGH					

TISSUE

	PITUITARY	?		PLACENTA	PLACENTA	PLACENTA

Fig. 2. The hGH gene cluster is shown above with the corresponding protein products and tissue of expression below.

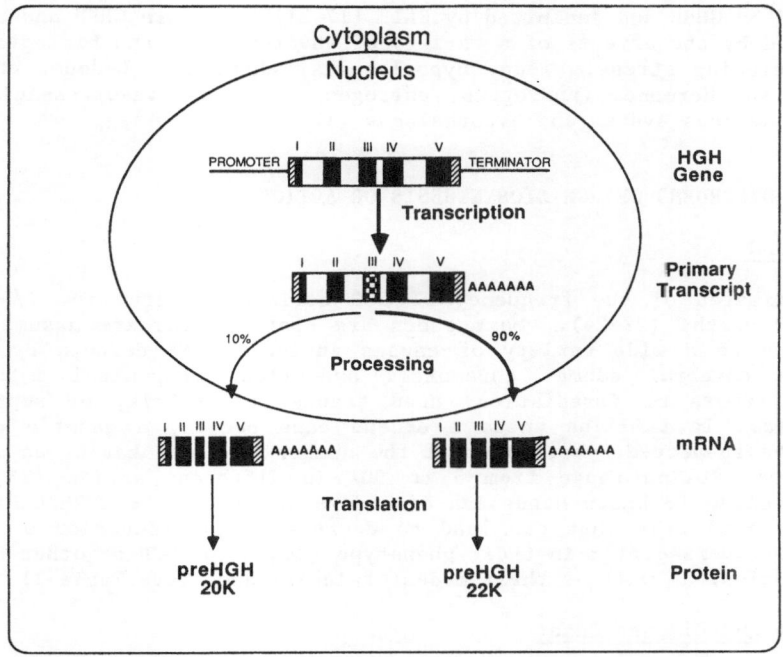

Fig. 3. Schematic representation of hGH biosynthesis in a
pituitary somatotroph.

Expression of the GH1 gene can utilize two different splicing
sequences (9,10). Alternative splicing of the primary GE1 transcripts is
the basis of the 20k hGH variant peptide (see Figures 2 and 3). The 20k
variant comprises 5 to 10% of total pituitary hGH and it differs from 22k
hGH by having an internal deletion of 15 amino acids (10,11). The codons
for these 15 amino acids begin precisely at the 5' end of Exon III (see
Figures 1-3). In addition, 45 base pairs (bp) downstream from this point
the sequences preceding the codon for amino acid 47 correspond with the
consensus sequences for splice acceptor sites (12,13). Thus, the 45
nucleotides contained in the 5' end of Exon III are deleted by alternative
splicing at the cryptic splice acceptor site which precedes codon 47
resulting in deletion of codons 32 through 46.

Additional size and charge variants of hGH include the 45 kb dimers
and two 24k variants. One 24k variant results from retention of the 26
amino acid signal peptide sequence of pre-hGH. The other results from
cleavage between residues 139 and 140 of the 22k form of hGH (9,14).

Physiologic Regulation

Human GH biosynthesis is under complex regulatory control and at the
level of transcription hGH production is increased by thyroid hormone,
glucocorticoids, and GHRH (see Figure 3) (15,16). The DNA sequences
required by thyroid and glucocorticoid hormone induction differ and the
effects of the two hormones appear to be independent and additive (15).
Secretion of hGH into the peripheral circulation is controlled by at least
2 hypothalamic factors, GHRH and somatostatin (SRIH). Secretion of hGH is

promoted by GHRH and inhibited by SRIH (17-21). In turn GHRH and SRIH are modulated by the effects of a variety of environmental and biological factors including stress, sleep, hypoglycemia, chemicals (L-dopa, chlorpromazine) and hormones (androgens, estrogens, hGH, and vasopressin) on the central nervous system and hypothalamus (17).

GENETIC DISORDERS OF HGH BIOSYNTHESIS OR ACTION

Background

Estimates of the frequency of hGH deficiency vary from 1/4,000 to 1/10,000 births (22-24). Most cases are sporadic and are assumed to be secondary to a wide variety of causes including CNS defects or insults such as cerebral edema, chromosome anomalies, congenital infections, cranial tumors or irradiation, head trauma, meningitis, or septo-optic dysplasia. In families where a second case occurs, a genetic etiology should be suspected. Estimates of the number of cases having an affected parent or sibling range from 3 to 30% in different series (23,25,26). These include 13 known Mendelian disorders involving the GHRH/hGH/Somatomedin-C (SmC) axis that can lead to decreased hGH production or action. These disorders differ in their phenotype (degree of hGH or other hormonal deficiencies) as well as their modes of inheritance (see Table 1).

Ontogeny and Disease Onset

Human GH appears in fetal serum at the end of the first trimester and increases progressively to reach a peak of 100 to 150 ng/ml at about 20 weeks gestation (27). By term, the plasma levels of hGH in the fetus are about 30 ng/ml. Plasma levels of hGH continue to decline in the first few months after birth, and in childhood the basal levels of hGH are similar to those of adults. Secretion of hGH occurs in a pulsatile pattern, primarily due to the effect of GHRH, and the frequency and amplitude of these pulses increase during puberty. Secretion of hGH continues throughout life but normally declines in old age.

Growth retardation due to hGH deficiency typically does not occur until several months after birth. Newborns who are homozygous for GH1 or CSH gene deletions have relatively normal fetal growth suggesting that other genes are responsible for stimulation of embryonic and fetal somatomedin production (28). Infants with severe hGH deficiency manifest growth retardation by 6 months of age. Children with acquired or progressive hGH deficiency may have relatively normal growth until several months or years of age. When concomitant deficiencies of other anterior pituitary hormones such as LH, FSH, TSH, and/or ACTH occur along with hGH deficiency, the severity of the retardation in growth and skeletal maturation is increased and may preclude the spontaneous onset of puberty.

Isolated HGH Deficiency (IGHD) Types 1A, 1B, II and III

Among the familial types of isolated growth hormone deficiency (IGHD), type 1A is the most severe. The disorder is characterized by occasional short body length at birth, severe dwarfism by 6 months of age, occasional hypoglycemia, strong initial anabolic response to exogenous hGH frequently followed by the development of anti-hGH antibodies in sufficient titer to cause arrest of response to hGH replacement (29,30). Studies of DNA samples have demonstrated homozygous deletions of GH1 genes in over 25 known IGHD 1A cases (see Figure 4). In the great majority of these individuals, only the 3.8 kb BamHI derived fragment is missing consistent with homozygous deletion of GH1 but retention of CSHP1-CSH1-GH2 and CSH1 (see Figures 1 and 4). Since the GH1 and CSHP1 genes both reside

Table 1. Genetic disorders of hGH production or action.

Name	Inheritance	Endogenous hGH	Response to hGH
Isolated growth hormone deficiency			
1A	AR*	Absent	Often Temporary
1B	AR	Decreased	Present
II	AD*	Decreased	Present
III	X-linked	Decreased	Present
"Bioinactive" growth hormone	? AR	? Inactive	Present
Laron dwarfism	AR	Normal or increased	Absent
Panhypopituitary dwarfism			
I	AR	Decreased	Present
II	X-linked	Decreased**	Present
Congenital absence of pituitary	? AR	Absent**	Present
EEC syndrome	AR	Deficient**	Present
Fanconi pancytopenia	AR	Deficient	Present
Holoproencephaly	AD or AR	Absent or deficient**	? Present
Rieger	AD	Deficient**	? Present

*AR = autosomal recessive; AD = autosomal dominant.

**Conditions in which deficiencies of hGH and other anterior pituitary hormones (ACTH, FSH, LH, TSH) occur.

in the same 26 kb HindIII derived fragment, the size of the GH1 deletions can be inferred by determining the amount of reduction in size of the 26 kb fragment. The majority (12/17) (71%) of deletions characterized in this way are the smaller ones of 6.7 kb depicted just below GH1 in Figure 4. A minority (5/17) (29%) of deletions are the slightly larger (7.6 kb) depicted just beneath the 6.7s (31). In these patients 14/17 (82%) have developed high titers of blocking antibodies to exogenous hGH (30,31, unpublished data). Interestingly, one of these who formed blocking antibodies to pituitary derived hGH has subsequently shown a good initial response to recombinant DNA derived methionyl hGH (32). In addition 3/17 (19%) have shown fair to good long-term growth responses despite high titers of anti-hGH antibodies. Interestingly, Laron et al. (33) have also reported cases of IGHD 1A in which no anti-hGH antibodies were detected.

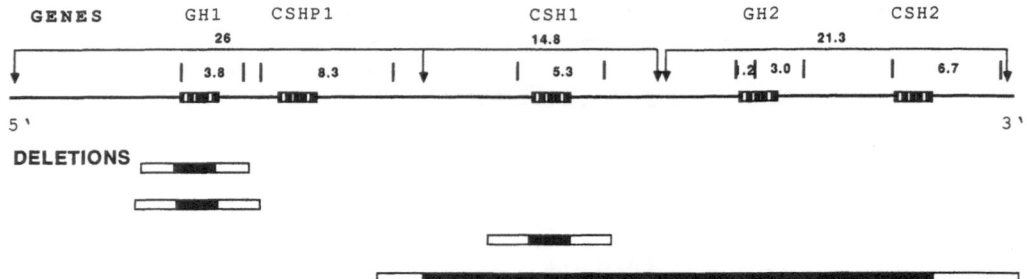

Fig. 4. Schematic representation of the hGH gene cluster
showing the location of HindIII (arrows) and selected BamHI
(lines) restriction sites above. The locations of 4 known
deletions are shown at bottom with dark and open rectangles
indicating obligatory deletions and ranges of endpoints respectively.

Further heterogeneity in the deletions beyond that demonstrated by
size differences was obtained by examining restriction fragment length
polymorphisms (RFLPs) (1). Using BglII or MspI digestions, 4 common RFLPs
near the CSHP1, CSH1, GH2, and CSH2 loci are detected (see Figure 5).
Interestingly, affected individuals from different families who appear to
have the same size deletion frequently have different patterns or haplo-
types of RFLPs (31). This finding indicates that the deletions from
different families represent recurring events and thus each may be different. Further support of this hypothesis is the finding by Goosens et
al. (34) of a double deletion in an IGHD 1A patient. This subject's GH
gene cluster contained only CSHP1 (see Figure 4) consistent with occurrence of both the top and bottom deletions in the homozygous state.
Deletions of only CSH1 or CSH1-GH2-CSH2 as depicted in the bottom of
Figure 4 have been reported (35,36).

A second type of IGHD (IGHD 1B) is characterized by production of
deficient but detectable amounts of hGH after provocative stimuli. In
contrast to IGHD 1A, those with IGHD 1B do not have detectable GH gene
deletions (1). To determine if subtle GH1 gene alterations were responsible, the RFLPs shown in Figure 5 were used in linkage analysis of
multiple IGHD 1B families. Among the 12 families studied, at least 6
demonstrated that affected siblings had inherited different GH1 alleles
from one or both parents. Since the RFLPs are very close to the GH1 locus
(see Figure 5), they should be accurate markers for following transmission
of parental GH1 alleles. The observed discordances between RFLPs in IGHD
1B sibling pairs indicates that a majority of the mutation(s) causing this
disorder segregate independently of the GH gene cluster. This suggests
that the mutations causing IGHD 1B affect a nonlinked locus (possibly one
important for GHRH production or release, or alternatively, important for
development of somatotropic cell function) rather than the GH1 structural
gene (1). In agreement IGHD 1B subjects can exhibit normal responses to
GHRH infusions (37).

A third type of IGHD (IGHD II) has an autosomal dominant mode of
inheritance. Affected individuals from different kindreds differ in the
severity of hGH deficiency, their propensity to develop hypoglycemia, and
in their response to exogenous hGH (38,39). Related individuals with IGHD
II have been tested for hGH response to GHRH infusion (37). Since all 4
related subjects failed to show significant hGH secretion, the defect in
this kindred must be distal to GHRH and include one or more steps shown in
Figure 3.

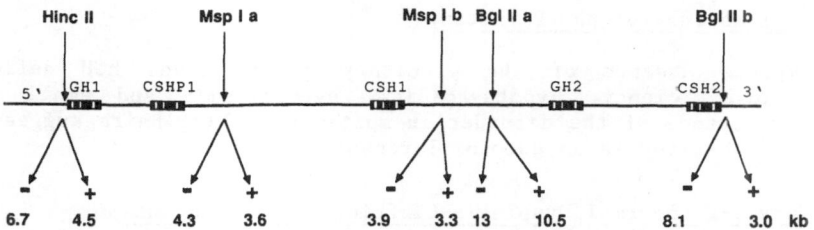

Fig. 5. Location of 5 restriction fragment length polymorphisms detected with GH1 cDNA as a probe. The location
of the polymorphic sites and the size of the alternative
alleles are shown below.

A fourth type of IGHD (IGHD III) has an X-linked mode of inheritance
(40). All 4 reported males had hypogammaglobulinemia (deficient IgG, IgA,
IgM, and IgE) as well as hGH deficiency.

Bioinactive HGH

Bioinactive hGH has been hypothesized to occur in some children who
have short stature comparable to that seen in hGH deficiency and have low
levels of SmC but normal levels of hGH by radioimmunoassay (RIA) (41). In
such cases, administration of exogenous hGH is reported to produce an
increase in SmC levels and a growth response. Since the concentration of
hGH measured by RIA exceeds that detected by radioreceptor assay, the
basis of bioinactive hGH could be production of an abnormal hGH polypeptide whose alteration causes reduced biologic activity but enables
reaction with anti-hGH antibodies. However, alterations in hGH have not
been documented in individuals with this syndrome and there is no clear
evidence of familial aggregation of "bioinactive" hGH to support clear cut
Mendelian inheritance.

Laron Dwarfism

Laron dwarfism is characterized by low SmC but normal to high levels
of hGH by RIA measurement (42). These subjects have the clinical appearance of severe IGHD with very delayed growth, abnormal facial appearance,
high-pitched voice, and small male genitalia. The disorder has an autosomal recessive mode of inheritance and affected individuals do not
respond to exogenous hGH. The hGH from Laron dwarfs reacts normally in
radioreceptor assays. This, along with their refractoriness to exogenous
hGH, suggests the primary defect may be an abnormality in the structure or
function membrane receptors for hGH (43).

Panhypopituitary Dwarfism

Panhypopituitary dwarfism is characterized by deficiency of ACTH,
FSH, LH, or TSH in addition to hGH deficiency. While most cases are
presumed to be sporadic, at least 2 Mendelian forms are recognized (Table
1). These 2 types differ in their modes of inheritance, type I having
autosomal recessive and type II having X-linked recessive modes of inheritance (31). The severity of associated trophic hormone deficiencies
exhibit inter- and intrafamilial variability in both types of panhypopituitary dwarfism. Furthermore, the hGH secretory responses to infusions of
GHRH vary from deficient to normal in different affected individuals from
the same kindreds (37). These findings suggest that the hypothalamus is
the probable site of the basic defect but a primary pituitary defect with
varying severity may also be possible.

Congenital Absence of the Pituitary

Complete absence of the pituitary gland causes hGH deficiency, adrenal insufficiency, hypothyroidism, hypoglycemia and small phallus (38). Occurrence of the disorder in multiple sibling pairs suggests that it can be inherited as an autosomal recessive trait.

Ectrodactyly-Ectodermal Dysplasia-Clefting (EEC) Syndrome

The EEC syndrome is characterized by hand and foot malformations varying from syndactyly to ectrodactyly, ectodermal dysplasia, and cleft lip and/or cleft palate. The disorder has an autosomal recessive mode of inheritance. Patients with EEC and hGH deficiency associated with absence of the septum pellucidum have been reported (44).

Fanconi Pancytopenia Syndrome

This disorder is characterized by short stature, thumb anomalies, skin hyperpigmentation, pancytopenia and occasional deficiency of hGH (38). The syndrome has an autosomal recessive mode of inheritance.

Holoprosencephaly

This disorder is characterized by the presence of median cleft lip and palate. Cases are usually sporadic but families with clear autosomal dominant or autosomal recessive modes of inheritance are reported (45). Others, due to a variety of chromosomal anomalies, usually have additional congenital malformations (38,45). Associated abnormalities or absence of the pituitary gland can cause IGHD or panhypopituitary dwarfism.

Rieger Syndrome

Rieger syndrome is characterized by iris dysplasia, hypodontia, and occasional optic atrophy and pituitary dwarfism (38,45). It has an autosomal dominant mode of inheritance and variable expression.

SUMMARY

Characterization of the sequence of the GH1 gene has given insight to some of the regulatory steps that control its expression and processing. Applications of recombinant DNA technology to familial types of hGH deficiency have clarified the basic defects causing 2 of these disorders (IGHD 1A and 1B). In IGHD 1A, the primary defect is deletion of the structural gene for hGH (GH1). In IGHD 1B, the GH1 gene is apparently intact and linkage analysis of families using RFLPs detected by GH1 cDNA have shown that the defects responsible for this disorder reside at loci far removed from the hGH gene cluster. Further studies of the various types of hGH deficiency, including "bioinactive" hGH and Laron dwarfism, should clarify genetic alterations responsible and clarify how they perturb hGH expression.

ACKNOWLEDGMENTS

The author thanks Ms. Judith Copeland for expert preparation of the manuscript. This work was supported in part by National Institutes of Health grants AM35592 and RCDA AM01434.

REFERENCES

1. Phillips JA III, Parks JS, Hjelle BL, et al. Genetic basis of familial isolated growth hormone deficiency type I. J Clin Invest 1982; 70:489.
2. Barsh GS, Seeburg PH, Gelinas RE. The human growth hormone gene family: structure and evolution of the chromosomal locus. Nucleic Acids Res 1983; 11:3939.
3. Hirt H, Kimelman J, Birnbaum MJ, et al. The human growth hormone gene locus: structure, evolution, and allelic variations. DNA 1987; 6:59.
4. Seeburg PH. The human growth hormone gene family: nucleotide sequences show recent divergence and predict a new polypeptide hormone. DNA 1982; 1:239.
5. Pavlakis GN, Hizuka N, Gorden P, Seeburg P, Hamer DH. Expression of two human growth hormone genes in monkey cells infected by simian virus 40 recombinants. Proc Natl Acad Sci USA 1981; 78:7398.
6. Miller WL, Eberhardt NL. Structure and evolution of the growth hormone gene family. Endocr Rev 1983; 4:97.
7. Wieringa B, Meyer F, Reiser J, Weissman C. Unusual splice sites revealed by mutagenic inactivation of an authentic splice site of the rabbit, β-globin gene. Nature 1983; 301:38.
8. Lingappa VR, Blobel G. Early events in the biosynthesis of secretory and membrane proteins: the signal hypothesis. Recent Prog Horm Res 1980; 36:451.
9. Lewis UJ, Singh RNP, Tutwiler GF, Sigel MB, Vanderlaan EF, Vanderlaan WP. Human growth hormone: a complex of proteins. Recent Prog Horm Res 1980; 36:477.
10. Lewis UJ, Bonewald LF, Lewis LJ. The 20,000-dalton variant of human growth hormone: location of the amino acid deletions. Biochem Biophys Res Commun 1980; 92:511.
11. Denoto F, Moore DD, Goodman HM. Human growth hormone DNA sequence and mRNA structures: possible alternative splicing. Nucleic Acids Res 1981; 9:3719.
12. Moore DD, Walker MD, Diamond DJ, Conkling MA, Goodman HM. Structure, expression, and evolution of growth hormone genes. Recent Prog Horm Res 1982; 38:197.
13. Seif I, Khoury G, Dhar R. BKV splice sequences based on analysis of preferred donor and acceptor sites. Nucleic Acids Res 1979; 6:3387.
14. Chawla RK, Parks JS, Rudman D. Structural variants of human growth hormone: biochemical, genetic, and clinical aspects. Annu Rev Med 1983; 34:519.
15. Evans RM, Birnberg NC, Rosenfeld MG. Glucocorticoid and thyroid hormones transcriptionally regulate growth hormone gene expression. Proc Natl Acad Sci USA 1982; 79:7659.
16. Barinaga M, Yamonoto G, Rivier C, Vale W, Evans E, Rosenfeld MG. Transcriptional regulation of growth hormone gene expression by growth hormone-releasing factor. Nature 1983; 306:84.
17. Martin JB. Neural regulation of growth hormone secretion. N Engl J Med 1973; 288:1384.
18. Wehrenberg WB, Ling N, Bohlen P, Esch F, Brazeau P, Guillemin R. Physiological roles of somatocrinin and somatostatin in the regulation of growth hormone secretion. Biochem Biophys Res Commun 1982; 109:562.
19. Grossman A, Savage MO, Besser GM. Growth hormone releasing hormone. Clin Endocrinol Metab 1986; 15:607.
20. Brazeau P, Epelbaum J, Tannenbaum GS, et al. Somatostatin: isolation, characterization, distribution, and blood determination. Metabolism 1978; 27:1133.
21. Kasting NW, Martin JB, Arnold MA. Pulsatile somatostatin release from the median eminence of the unanesthetized rat and its rela-

tionship to plasma growth hormone levels. Endocrinol 1981; 109:1739.

22. Vimpani GV, Vimpani AF, Lidgard GP, Cameron EHD, Farquhar JW. Prevalence of severe growth hormone deficiency. Br Med J 1977; 2:427.

23. Rona RJ, Tanner JM. Aetiology of idiopathic growth hormone deficiency in England and Wales. Arch Dis Child 1977; 52:197.

24. Lacey KA, Parkin JM. Causes of short stature—a community study of children in New Castle upon Tyne. Lancet 1974; 1:42.

25. Tanner JM. Human growth hormone. Nature 1972; 237:433.

26. Seip M, Trygstad O, Aarskog D. Comment on pituitary dwarfism in Norway, 1961-1970. Birth Defects, Original Article Series 1971; 7:33.

27. Gluckman PD, Grumbach MM, Kaplan SL. The neuroendocrine regulation and function of growth hormone and prolactin in the mammalian fetus. Endocr Rev 1981; 2:363.

28. Sara VR, Hall K, Rodeck CH, Wetterberg L. Human embryonic somatomedin. Proc Natl Acad Sci USA 1981; 78:3175.

29. Illig R, Prader A, Ferrandez A, Zachmann M. Hereditary prenatal growth hormone deficiency with increased tendency to growth hormone antibody formation ("A-type" isolated growth hormone deficiency). Acta Pediatr Scand [Suppl] 1971; 60:607.

30. Phillips JA III, Hjelle BL, Seeburg PH, Zachmann M. Molecular basis for familial isolated growth hormone deficiency. Proc Natl Acad Sci 1981; 78:6372.

31. Phillips JA III, Ferrandez A, Frisch H, Illig R, Zuppinger K. Defects of GH genes. In: Raiti S, ed. Clinical syndromes in human growth hormone. New York: Plenum Publishing Corp., 1986:211-26.

32. Hauffa BP. Personal communication.

33. Laron Z, Kelijman M, Pertzelan A, Keret R, Shoffner JM, Parks JS. Human growth hormone gene deletion without antibody formation or growth arrest during treatment—a new disease entity? Isr J Med Sci 1985; 21:999.

34. Goossens M, Brauner R, Czernichow P, Duquesnoy P, Rappaport R. Isolated growth hormone (GH) deficiency type 1A associated with a double deletion in the human GH gene cluster. J Clin Endocrinol Metab 1986; 62:712.

35. Wurzel JM, Parks JS, Herd JE, Nielsen PV. A gene deletion is responsible for absence of human chorionic somatomammotropin. DNA 1982; 1:251.

36. Parks JS, Nielsen PV, Sexton LA, Jorgensen EH. An effect of gene dosage on production of human chorionic sommatomammotropin. J Clin Endocrinol Metab 1985; 60:994.

37. Rogol AD, Blizzard RM, Foley TP Jr, et al. Growth hormone releasing hormone and growth hormone: genetic studies in familial growth hormone deficiency. Pediatr Res 1985; 19:489.

38. Rimoin DL. Genetic disorders of the pituitary gland. In: Emery AEH, Rimoin DL, eds. Principles and practice of medical genetics. Edinburgh: Churchill Livingstone, 1983:1134.

39. Van Gelderen HH, Van Der Hoog CE. Familial isolated growth hormone deficiency. Clin Genet 1981; 20:173.

40. Fleisher TA, White RM, Broder S. X-linked hypogammaglobulinemia and isolated growth hormone deficiency. N Engl J Med 1980; 302:1429.

41. Rudman D, Kutner MH, Blackston RD, Cushman RA, Bain RP, Patterson JH. Children with normal-variant short stature: treatment with human growth hormone for six months. N Engl J Med 1981; 305:123.

42. Pertzelan A, Adam A, Laron Z. Genetic aspects of pituitary dwarfism due to absence or biological inactivity of growth hormone. Isr J Med Sci 1968; 4:895.

43. Jacobs LS, Sneid SD, Garland JT, Laron Z, Daughaday WH. Receptor-active growth hormone in Laron dwarfism. J Clin Endocrinol Metab 1976; 42:403.

44. Knudtzon J, Aarskog D. Growth hormone deficiency associated with the ectrodactyly-ectodermal dysplasia-clefting syndrome and isolated absent septum pellucidum. Pediatrics 1987; 79:410.
45. McKusick VA, ed. Mendelian inheritance in man. 7th ed. Baltimore: The Johns Hopkins University Press, 1986.

6

SUMMARY OF SESSION I

PROCESSING OF GROWTH HORMONE

John A. Phillips, III, M.D.

Vanderbilt University
Nashville, Tennessee

Applications of recombinant DNA techniques have elucidated the nucleotide sequence and organization of the human growth hormone (hGH or GH1) gene. This information, while of general interest, has only provided a start in identifying sequences or elements that are important in effecting the tissue-specific expression of GH1 and its transcription, processing, and translational regulation.

To identify sequences responsible for the effects of thyroid and glucocorticoids on GH1 expression, Dr. Eberhardt has studied the expression of transvected hGH and rGH genes in murine pituitary cells. Using footprint analysis, he has found that the region between -139 and -110 bp (upstream) from the origin of transcription are responsible for tissue-specific expression. Furthermore, sequences -200 to -150 bp from the origin of transcription are important in thyroid hormone (T_3) binding and responsiveness. Finally, sequences 330 to 300 upstream contain enhancer sequences that are important in the expression of rGH genes in pituitary cells. Finally, at least two regions upstream (-140 to -100 and -90 to -60) and another downstream to the origin of transcription are responsible for responsiveness to glucocorticoids. Corresponding sequences that modulate expression of the hGH gene are somewhat more complex and the interaction of their effects are responsible for the increased hGH synthesis that occurs in pituitary cells following treatment with dexamethasone and/or T_3. Interestingly, the complex interactions responsible for the regulation of transcription are thought to be distinct from secretory mechanisms. Thus, the end result of synthetic and secretory steps involve complex interactions between the responses of promoter, enhancer, and glucocorticoid and thyroid hormone responsive elements flanking the hGH gene and other endogenous and exogenous factors.

The process of hGH gene expression becomes more complex when alternative processing, translation and secretion provide further heterogeneity in the tissue levels, the protein sequence of and the amounts of different forms of hGH. Dr. Baumann has identified nine theoretical sources of hGH diversity including: (1) genomic differences—presence of different, GH1 and GH2, loci; (2) differential splicing to give 20 and 22k species of hGH; (3) retention of the signal sequence which is normally cleaved to give 24K hGH; (4) posttranslational modifications; (5) polymerization; (6) aggregation; (7) interactions with carrier proteins; (8) metabolic conversions to active or inactive product; and, (9) laboratory artifacts.

The resulting heterogeneity is vast and analysis of the circulating immunoreactive forms of hGH indicate that less than one-quarter of the total hGH exists in the form of the 22k monomer and that 20 different forms of hGH have been identified. The physiologic significance of this heterogenous mixture is unclear. The isoforms may each have different specific functions, reflect different susceptibilities to modification, or the various forms may modulate the effect of the others so as to affect an optimal homeostasis.

Multiple forms of hGH are also found in the brain. Dr. Lewis has detected 20k, 20k variants and 22k, as well as various proteolytic products, dimers, and forms resulting from deamidation or phosphorylation. Thus, a heterogeneous array of hGH products, each potentially having a different function, has been documented in the central nervous system.

In the final analysis, the possible heterogeneity due to differences in expression, processing, and modification reaches an order of complexity that becomes difficult to comprehend. Better understanding of the biological significance of this heterogeneity of hGH products may become more clear through studies utilizing pure forms of hGH recently obtained in great abundance.

II. NEUROENDOCRINE REGULATION OF GROWTH HORMONE SECRETION

7

INTERACTIONS BETWEEN GROWTH HORMONE RELEASING HORMONE, SOMATOSTATIN AND GALANIN IN THE CONTROL OF GROWTH HORMONE SECRETION

Steven M. Gabriel, Patricia E. Marshall, and
Joseph B. Martin

Department of Neurology, Massachusetts General Hospital
and Harvard Medical School
Boston, MA 02114

Growth hormone (GH) is secreted episodically in man and animals (1,2). This rhythmic secretory pattern results from the interactions between two neuropeptides, GH-releasing hormone (GHRH) and somatostatin. Evidence supports the hypothesis that these two hypophysiotrophic factors are themselves released in an episodic manner into the portal circulation, thereby directly influencing the pituitary somatotrophs. Our understanding of the interactions between GHRH and somatostatin at both the hypothalamic and pituitary levels, although extensively investigated, is incomplete.

While GHRH and somatostatin are the primary factors that control GH release, other central and peripheral signals appear to modulate GH release by altering the activity of GHRH- or somatostatin-containing neurons, or by influencing their actions on the pituitary. These secondary elements include hormones secreted by pituitary-endocrine target organs, the biogenic amines, and several hypothalamic peptides. In this paper we discuss selected aspects of GHRH and somatostatin interactions in GH regulation, and present evidence for a direct role of galanin on GH secretion.

FUNCTIONS OF GHRH AND SOMATOSTATIN IN THE REGULATION OF GH

Anatomy of the GHRH and Somatostatin Systems in the Human Hypothalamus

We have studied the distribution of GHRH and somatostatin in the human hypothalamus and preoptic area (POA). Both somatostatin and GHRH immunoreactivity were localized in human postmortem tissue fixed by immersion in buffered 10% formalin. Somatostatin antisera were generated in rabbits (3, and Immunonuclear Corp.). An antiserum to human pancreatic GHRH(1-40) was kindly provided by Dr. Wylie Vale (4). Antibody binding was visualized with the Avidin-Biotin method (Vector Laboratories) using 3-3'-diaminobenzidine as the chromogen.

Parvicellular neurons immunoreactive (IR) for somatostatin were located principally in the periventricular zone (PVZ) of the anterior hypothalamus and POA (Fig. 1). Scattered neurons were seen in the periformical region, and rarely in the tuberal region. Somatostatin-IR fibers were densely distributed in the anterior hypothalamic PVZ and enter the infundibulum laterally, to become associated with portal vessels in the external layer of the median eminence (ME). Fewer somatostatin-IR fibers were distributed throughout the suprachiasmatic nucleus (SCN), lateral POA (LPOA), and lateral hypothalamus.

Parvicellular and bipolar GHRH-IR neurons were located more caudally in the hypothalamus than somatostatin-IR neurons (Fig. 1-3). The GHRH-IR cells were primarily in the medial basal hypothalamus (MBH), but their distribution was not restricted by conventional nuclear boundries. GHRH-IR cells occupied a broad band extending from the infundibular lip into the PVZ that included the dorso-lateral aspect of the tuberoinfundibular nucleus (TIN) and ventromedial portion of the ventromedial nucleus (VMN). Other GHRH-IR cell bodies were found in the periformical region. Immunoreactive varicose fibers were closely associated with all these neurons. Like the somatostatin-IR fibers, GHRH-IR fibers entered the infundibulum laterally to terminate in the external layer of the ME. Dense GHRH-IR fibers were seen in the PVZ, with a few extending into the dorsal hypothalamus. Additional fibers, some of which appeared to be terminal arborizations, were found in areas distant from the ME, including the SCN, medial POA (MPOA), and lateral hypothalamus.

The distribution of GHRH-IR neurons and fibers in the human hypothalamus described here is in agreement with other reports (4-6). Our observation of extensive GHRH-IR fibers and terminals outside the confines of the tuberoinfundibular region in the PVZ and dorsal hypothalamus has not been reported in human tissue. However, a recent report found GHRH-IR fibers in the PVZ and dorsal hypothalamus of the rat (7). These fibers are probably collaterals of GHRH-containing neurons that project to the ME.

Although somatostatin-IR and. GHRH-IR perikarya are differentially distributed in the hypothalamus, some somatostatin-IR fibers are found in regions containing GHRH-IR cell bodies and fibers in the medial basal hypothalamus, PVZ, and ME. It is not clear whether this overlap represents any anatomic interconnections between these two neuronal systems.

Physiological Relationships Between GHRH and Somatostatin

The interactions between GHRH and somatostatin which generate GH secretory patterns have been the subject of intense study (1,2). Evidence suggests that GH may feed back on the hypothalamus by modulating GHRH or somatostatin secretion into portal blood, thereby regulating GH release (8). During abnormally high GH secretion, such as in acromegaly, this feedback loop might be altered. Using specific radioimmunoassays (3,9),

Figures 1-3 (opposite page):
Fig. 1. The distribution of GHRH-IR and somatostatin-IR neurons (dots) and varicose fibers (dotted lines) in the POA and hypothalamus of the human. Somatostatin (SOM) immunoreactivity is shown on the left half; GHRH immunoreactivity is shown on the right. Abbreviations are: SON, supraoptic nucleus; F, fornix; OC, optic chiasm; SCN, suprachiasmitic nucleus; TIN, tuberoinfundibular nucleus; VMN, ventromedial nucleus.

Fig. 2. GHRH-IR neurons in the MBH.

Fig. 3. GHRH-IR varicose fibers and terminal arborizations lateral to the ventromedial nucleus.

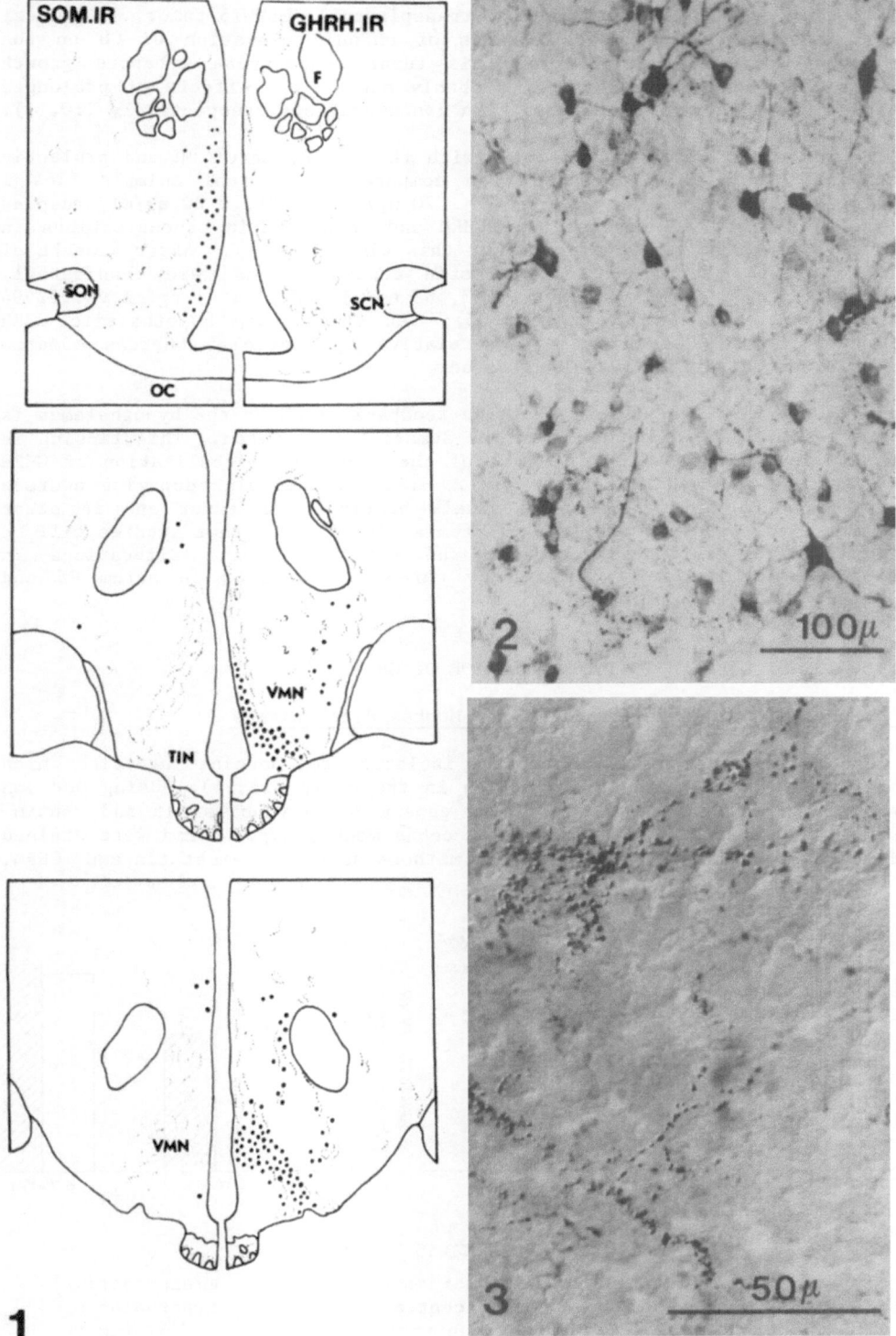

we evaluated GHRH and somatostatin concentrations in the hypothalamus of male Wistar-Furth rats bearing the transplantable MtTW15 tumor, as a model for assessing the feedback effects of chronic elevation of GH on the hypothalamus. Animals bearing this tumor demonstrate enhanced growth rates and gonadal dysfunction, probably due to the effects of prolonged elevations in serum GH and prolactin concentrations, respectively (10,11).

Two weeks after innoculation with the tumor, serum GH and prolactin concentrations were increased when compared to control animals (164 ± 97 ng/ml vs. 543 ± 106 ng/ml and 38 ± 20 ng/ml vs. 282.± 80 ng/ml, respectively, P<0.05). Immunoreactive GHRH and somatostatin concentrations in the hypothalamus were unaffected at this time (Fig. 4). After 4 weeks of tumor growth, serum GH and prolactin concentrations were considerably higher (76 ± 45 ng/ml vs. 18,972 ± 3,563 ng/ml and 11 ± 11 ng/ml vs. 1,994 ± 517 ng/ml, respectively, P<0.05). At this time, hypothalamic GHRH immunoreactivity was reduced 45% relative to controls, whereas somatostatin concentrations were unaffected.

These findings suggest that the feedback of GH on the hypothalamus is exerted on the GHRH rather than the somatostatin neuron. This finding is particularly interesting in light of the possible colocalization of GHRH in dopamine-containing neurons (12). Tuberoinfundibular dopamine neurons are known to be affected in animals bearing this tumor and in other experimental models for hyperprolactemia (10,11). Further studies will be required to distinguish between the pathophysiologic alterations in hypothalamic regulation induced by chronic elevations in serum GH and prolactin concentrations.

FUNCTION OF GALANIN IN THE REGULATION OF GH

Anatomy of Galanin in the Human and Monkey Hypothalamus

Galanin is an amidated peptide isolated from porcine intestine which appears to have a wide distribution in the brain (13,14). Using our own and commercially available antisera generated in rabbits (15 and Penninsula Labs, Torrence, CA), human and cebus monkey hypothalami were stained immunohistochemically using similar methods as for somatostatin and GHRH.

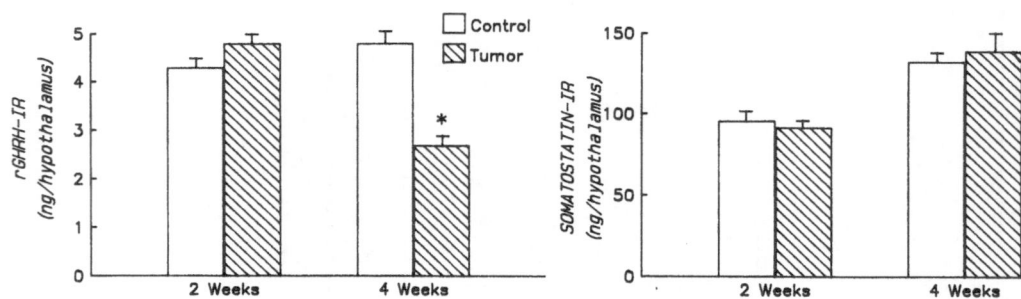

TIME AFTER MTTw15 INNOCULATION

Fig. 4. Effects of MtTW15 tumor innoculation on immunoreactive rat GHRH and somatostatin concentrations in the hypothalamus. Immunoreactive rat GHRH concentrations in control or tumor-innoculated animals are in the left panel; immunoreactive somatostatin concentrations are on the right. * denotes P<0.05 vs. control at the same time point.

All antibodies demonstrated comparable staining patterns in both human and cebus brains, although the specificity of these antisera varied, as judged by the intensity of the reaction product.

In the hypothalamus, galanin-IR cell bodies were densely distributed in the tuberoinfundibular nucleus, with some neurons extending into the pituitary stalk (Fig. 5-9). This pattern of galanin-IR cell staining was similar to that seen in the rat (16-18). Sparser cell bodies were seen medially and laterally around the VMN and dorsal to the supraoptic nucleus. A dense fiber network surrounded these neurons and extended into the PVZ. Fewer fibers appeared dorsal to the VMN, in the perifornical region, and in the anterior hypothalamus. Galanin-IR fibers extended into the stalk medially and were found in all layers of the human ME. Interestingly, in the anterior ME of the cebus monkey, galanin-IR nerve terminals were primarily localized to the internal layer. The lateral tuberal nuclei were conspicuous by a paucity of galanin-IR.

In the preoptic area, scattered galanin-IR parvicellular neurons were present in the SCN and organum vasculosum of the lamina terminalis. Dense fibers were seen in the SCN, and retrochiasmatically a few galanin-IR fibers entered the infundibulum. Larger, presumably cholinergic, neurons of the diagonal band of Broca (DBB) and basal forebrain showed less intense staining. With our fixation and incubation procedures, no neuronal processes were associated with these neurons. The immunoreactivity disappeared with preadsorption of the galanin antibody. Colocalization of galanin and acetylcholine in these neurons in the monkey brain has been described previously (19).

In addition to the hypothalamic and POA galanin-IR neurons, cells and many fibers were associated with the stria terminalis and ventral amygdalofugal systems. This was demonstrated particularly well in the cebus brain. Dense fibers and scattered cell bodies were found in the bed nucleus of the stria terminalis. Many stained fibers appeared in the stria terminalis and its projection areas—the anterior hypothalamus, MPOA, LPOA, and surrounding the VMN. Small bundles of positively stained fibers were also seen in the lateral hypothalamus and LPOA (medial and lateral to the DBB), and sparse fibers were seen throughout the medial and lateral septum.

From these data, galanin immunoreactivity appears to have a more restricted distribution in human and cebus POA and hypothalamus than in the rat using the same commercially available (17) or other independently produced antisera to porcine galanin (16,18). Whether this represents true species differences in the distribution of galanin immunoreactivity, unidentified antigens cross-reacting with the galanin antisera, or methodological differences, remains an issue to be resolved when species-specific antibodies to galanin become available. The presence of galanin-IR cell bodies and nerve terminals in the tuberoinfundibular region and ME suggests that galanin might play a role in regulating anterior pituitary function. Galanin-IR and GHRH-IR neurons in the tuberoinfundibular nucleus appear to overlap in their distribution; however, any anatomic relationships between galanin- and GHRH-containing neurons or galanin- and somatostatin-containing nerve terminals and fibers remains to be elucidated.

Comparison of GHRH, Somatostatin, and Galanin in the Median Eminence

Like GHRH and somatostatin, galanin appears to be localized in the ME. Because galanin-containing cell bodies could arise from a number of hypothalamic regions, we administered glutamate to rats during the neonatal period (monosodium salt, 4 gm/kg BW, days 1, 3, 5, 7, and 9) to pro-

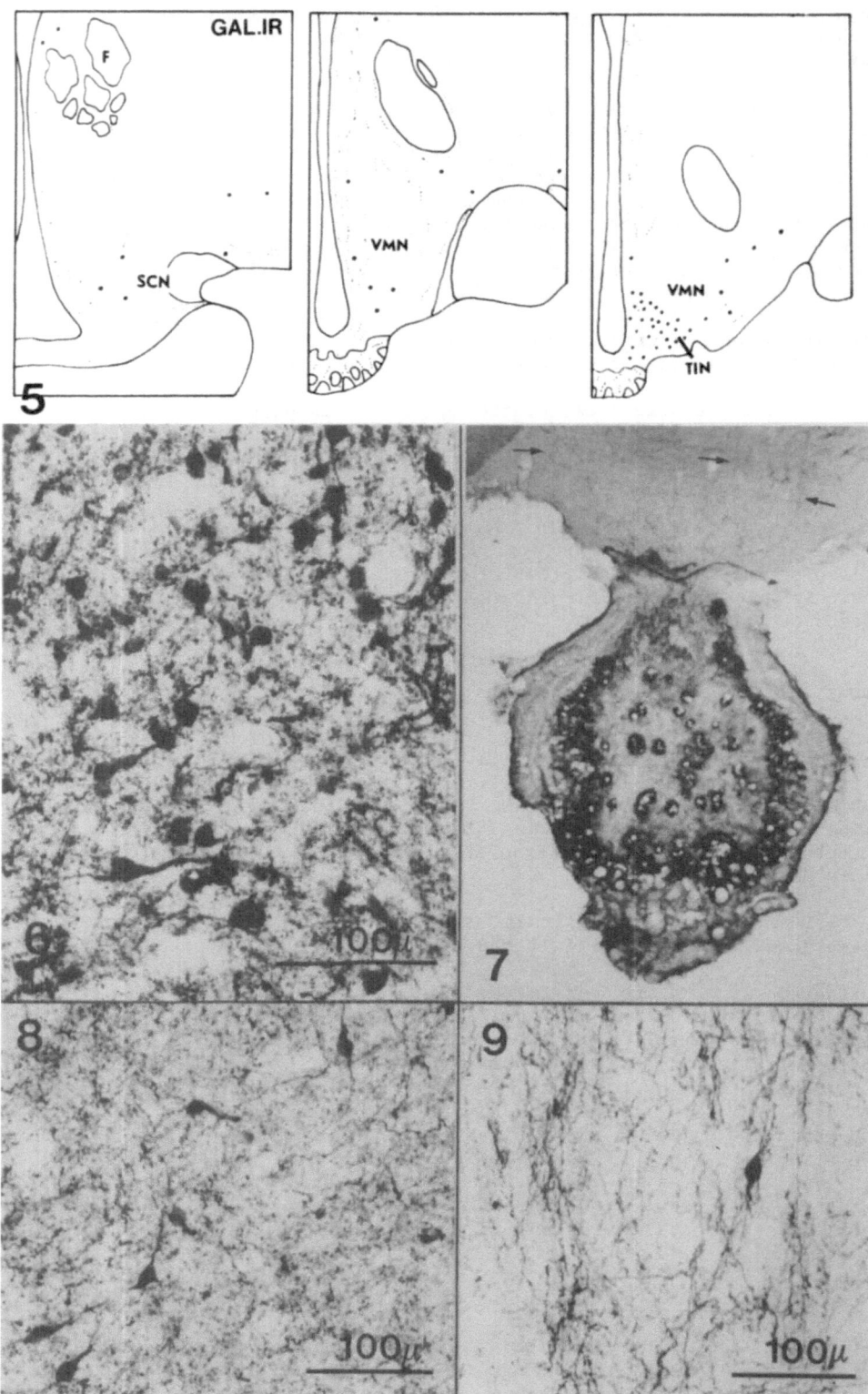

duce a cytotoxic lesion in the arcuate nucleus. This treatment causes endocrine abnormalities as a result of the loss of neurotransmitters localized within the terminal beds of arcuate nucleus neurons (20). At maturity, animals were sacrificed and MEs were removed from fresh tissues using fine iris scissors under a dissection microscope. Acid extracts were lyophilized and reconstituted in assay buffer for measurement of rat GHRH, somatostatin, and galanin by radioimmunoassay (3,9,15).

Figure 10 shows the concentrations of immunoreactive rat GHRH, somatostatin and galanin in the ME of adult male rats treated neonatally with glutamate. These peptides were differentially affected by the neonatal treatment in a manner which correlates with their differential anatomic distributions. Rat GHRH neurons are confined to the arcuate nucleus, and as a consequence GHRH concentrations in the ME were reduced more than 90% by neonatal glutamate treatment. Somatostatin neurons, which project to the ME from outside the arcuate nucleus, are unaffected by glutamate. Immunoreactive galanin concentrations in the ME were diminished more than 50%. While this could suggest that there is a glutamate-insensitive population of galanin-containing neurons in the arcuate nucleus, it is more likely that approximately one-half of the ME galanin is derived from cell bodies outside the arcuate nucleus. This source might be from other hypothalamic areas, such as the PVZ.

Effects of Galanin on GH Secretion

Recent evidence suggests that galanin may play a role in the regulation of GH secretion in man and animals (21,22). We examined the effect of synthetic porcine galanin on GH release in monolayer cultures of pituitary cells. Male Sprague-Dawley rats were sacrificed by decapitation and anterior pituitary cells were prepared as described previously (23).

Galanin caused an increase in GH concentrations in the culture medium that was maximal at 90 min incubation and was sustained for 3 h (24). The GH secretory response to galanin was greatest when the cells were grown in the presence of 25 nM dexamethasone and 30 pM thyroxine (24). Figure 11 shows the stimulatory effect of galanin on GH release. Galanin increased GH concentrations in the culture medium at all doses employed. This stimulatory effect of galanin on GH release reached significance at the 3×10^{-7} M and 1×10^{-6} M doses. Maximal effective doses of galanin and synthetic rat GHRH were additive in eliciting GH release. After 3 h incubation with either 1×10^{-6} M galanin or 1×10^{-10} M rat GHRH, GH concentrations were increased when compared to control incubations. The combination of galanin plus rat GHRH caused a greater increase in GH concentrations than either peptide elicited alone.

Figures 5-9 (opposite page):

Fig. 5. Summary of the distribution of galanin (GAL)-IR neurons (dots) and varicose fibers (dotted lines) in frontal sections of the POA and hypothalamus of the human and cebus brain.

Fig. 6. Densely packed bipolar and multipolar galanin-IR neurons in the tuberoinfundibular nucleus.

Fig. 7. Galanin-IR nerve terminals in the rostral pituitary stalk and ME of the cebus monkey. Fibers entering this zone are seen retrochiasmatically (arrows).

Fig. 8. Galanin-IR cell bodies and numerous varicose fibers in the lateral margin of the SCN.

Fig. 9. Galanin-IR fibers in the bed nucleus of the stria terminalis arising from the stria and from intrinsic neurons.

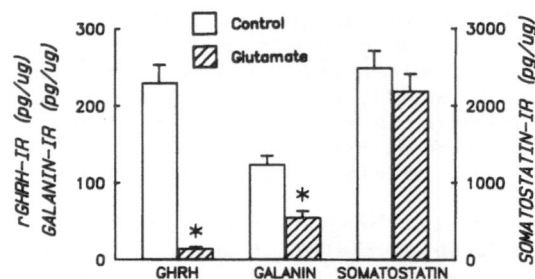

Fig. 10. Effects of neonatal glutamate treatment on immunoreactive GHRH, galanin, and somatostatin concentrations in the ME of adult male rats. * denotes P<0.05 vs. control.

These data indicate a direct effect of galanin on GH secretion in cultures of anterior pituitary cells. Radioimmunoassay characterization of porcine galanin-like immunoreactivity in several species and molecular studies with a putative rat galanin message RNA indicate that considerable molecular heterogeneity exists at the carboxy-terminus of galanin (25,26). While this would suggest that the amino-terminus of the galanin molecule is crucial for bioactivity, some studies have reported bioactivity with carboxy-terminus fragments of porcine galanin (14). These factors may contribute to the variations observed in galanin's potency between in vitro preparations (14), and its low potency in the present study. On a molar basis, galanin is less potent in eliciting GH release when compared to rat GHRH (24). It is possible that the rat form of galanin will be a more potent GH-releasing peptide than the porcine molecule.

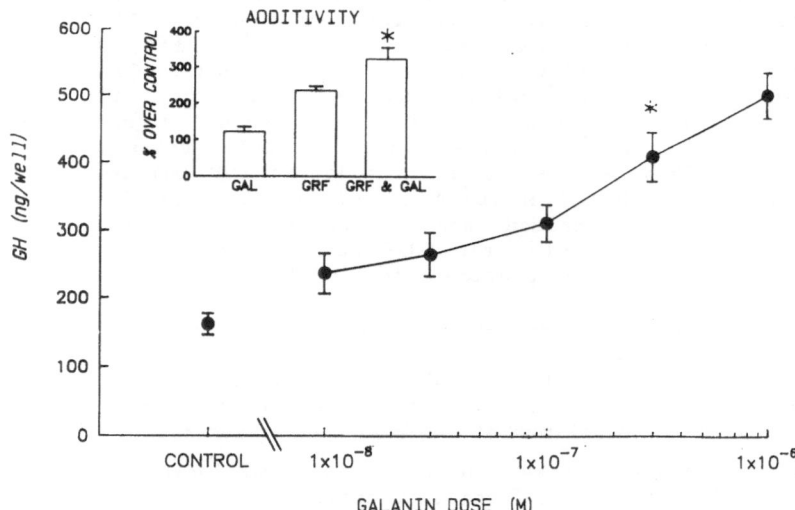

Fig. 11. Effects of galanin on GH secretion in monolayer cultures of rat anterior pituitary cells. All incubations were for 3 h. Doses in the inset were: galanin 1 x 10^{-6}M, and rat GHRH 1 x 10^{-10}M. The GH concentrations in control incubations for the inset were 473 ± 45 ng/ml. * denotes P<0.05 vs. controls. GRF = GHRH. These experiments are presented in reference 24.

The present findings agree with recent data suggesting that galanin may be important in regulating GH release (21,22). When injected intravenously, galanin stimulates GH release in man (21). While such a finding could be secondary to an effect of galanin on the brain's circumventricular organs or to its peripheral actions on the endocrine pancreas (14), our observation that galanin stimulates GH release in vitro suggests a pituitary locus for galanin's actions. Another study in rats, however, suggests that galanin acts at the hypothalamic rather than the pituitary level (22). The resolution of these differences must await the availability of rat and human forms of the galanin molecule.

It is uncertain what physiological effects galanin has on GH secretion in vitro. Perhaps galanin works in concert with GHRH or somatostatin to regulate GH release. Since galanin is present in the internal layer of the median eminence, it is possible that galanin may act both at the level of the pituitary and the hypothalamus to modulate GH release.

In summary, we have shown that GHRH-, somatostatin- and galanin-containing neurons are differentially distributed in the hypothalamus, but that all three neuropeptides share at least one common terminal bed in the median eminence. While it is the interactions between GHRH and somatostatin that produce the pulsatile pattern of GH release, the short-loop feedback of GH on the hypothalamus appears to be directed on the GHRH neuron. Finally, several central and peripheral factors may modulate the effects of GHRH and somatostatin on GH release. One of these is the newly characterized neuropeptide, galanin.

ACKNOWLEDGMENTS

The authors would like to acknowledge Dr. Neil Kowall for his generous gift of the galanin sections presented in this paper. We would also like to thank Drs. James I. Koenig, M. Flint Beal, and James A. Nathanson for their advice and help in the above studies, and Ms. Carol Millbury and Judith Audet-Arnold for technical assistance. Prolactin and GH concentrations were measured using the kits provided by the NIH pituitary hormone distribution program. This work was supported by NIH grants DK07561(SMG) and AM26252(JBM).

REFERENCES

1. Frohman LA, Jansson J-O. Growth-hormone releasing hormone. Endocr Rev 1986; 7:223-53.
2. Martin JB, Reichlin SR. Clinical neuroendocrinology. Philadelphia: Davis, 1987:233-94.
3. Arnold MA, Reppert SM, Rorstad OP, et al. Temporal pattern of somatostatin immunoreactivity in the cerebrospinal fluid of the rhesus monkey: effect of environmental lighting. J Neurosci 1982; 2:574-80.
4. Vale W, Vaughan J, Jolley D, et al. Assay of growth hormone releasing factor. Methods Enzymol 1986; 124:389-401.
5. Bloch B, Gaillard RC, Brazeau P, Lin HD, Ling N. Topographical and ontogenetic study of the neurons producing growth hormone-releasing factor in human hypothalamus. Regul Pept 1984; 8:21-31.
6. Bressen JL, Clacequin MC, Fellman D, Bugnon C. Ontogeny of the neuroglandular system revealed with hpGRF-44 antibodies in human hypothalamus. Neuroendocrinology 1984; 39:68-73.
7. Ciofi P, Croix D, Tramu G. Coexistence of hGHRH and NPY immunoreactivities in neurons of the arcuate nucleus of the rat. Neuroendocrinology 1987; 45:425-8.

8. Tannenbaum GS. Evidence for autoregulation of growth hormone secretion via the central nervous system. Endocrinology 1980; 107:2117-20.

9. Gabriel SM, Millard WJ, Badger TM, Martin JB. Measurement of growth hormone-releasing factor in male and female rats [Abstract]. Neuroscience Society 1986; 12:412.5.

10. Gudelsky GA, Simpkins JW, Pass KA, Alysworth CF, Steger RW, Meites J. Effects of a prolactin secreting tumor on hypothalamic, gonadotropic, and testicular function in male rats. Neuroendocrinology 1980; 30:7-10.

11. Simpkins JW, Gabriel SM. Chronic hyperprolactemia causes progressive changes in hypothalamic dopaminergic and noradrenergic neurons. Brain Res 1984; 309:277-82.

12. Meister B, Hokfelt T, Vale WW, Sawchenko PE, Swanson L, Goldstein M. Coexistence of tyrosine hydroxylase and growth hormone-releasing factor in a subpopulation of tuberoinfundibular neurons of the rat. Neuroendocrinology 1986; 42:237-47.

13. Tatemoto K, Rokaeus A, McDonald TJ, Mutt V. Galanin--a novel biologically active peptide from porcine intestine. FEBS Lett 1983; 164:124-8.

14. Rokaeus A. Galanin: a newly isolated biologically active peptide. TINS 1987; 10:158-64.

15. Gabriel SM, Koenig JI, McGarvey U, Swartz KJ, Martin JB, Beal MF. Effects of neonatal glutamate treatment on galanin immunoreactivity in the rat brain [Abstract]. Neuroscience Society 1987 (in press).

16. Melander T, Hokfelt T, Rokaeus A. Distribution of galaninlike immunoreactivity in the rat central nervous system. J Comp Neurol 1986; 218:175-217.

17. Skofitsch G, Jacobowitz DM. Immunohistochemical mapping of galanin-like neurons in the rat central nervous system. Peptides (Fayetteville) 1985; 6:509-46.

18. Kohler C, Ericson H, Watanabe T, Polak J, Palay SL, Chan-Palay V. Galanin immunoreactivity in hypothalamic histamine neurons: further evidence for multiple chemical messengers in the tuberomammillary nucleus. J Comp Neurol 1986; 250:58-64.

19. Melander T, Staines WA. A galanin-like peptide coexists in putative cholinergic somata of the septum-basal forebrain complex and in acetylcholinesterase containing fibers and varicosities within the hippocampus in the owl monkey (aotus trivirgatus). Neurosci Lett 1986; 68:17-22.

20. Nemeroff CB, Grant LD, Bissette G, Ervin GN, Harrell LE, Prang AJ Jr. Growth, endocrinological and behavioral deficits after monosodium L-glutamate in the neonatal rat: possible involvement of dopamine neuron damage. Psychoneuroendocrinology 1977; 2:179-93.

21. Bauer FE, Ginsberg L, Venetikou M, MacKay DJ, Burrin JM, Bloom SR. Growth hormone release induced by galanin, a new hypothalamic peptide. Lancet 1986; 2:192-5.

22. Ottlecz A, Samson WK, McCann SM. Galanin: evidence for a hypothalamic site of action to release growth hormone. Peptides 1986; 7:51-3.

23. Fukata J, Martin JB. Influence of sex steroids on rat growth hormone-releasing factor and somatostatin in dispersed pituitary cells. Endocrinology 1986; 119:2256-61.

24. Gabriel SM, Millbury CM, Nathanson JA, Martin JB. Galanin directly stimulates pituitary growth hormone secretion. Life Sci (submitted).

25. Bauer FE, Adrian TE, Christofides ND, et al. Distribution and molecular heterogeneity of galanin in human, pig, guinea pig, and rat gastrointestinal tracts. Gastroenterology 1986; 91:877-83.

26. Kaplan LM, Spindel ER, Isselbacher KJ, Chin WW. Tissue-specific expression of the rat galanin gene: isolation and characterization of cloned cDNA [Abstract]. Neuroscience Society 1987 (in press).

8

THE ROLE OF NEUROTRANSMITTERS IN GROWTH HORMONE SECRETION

Eugenio E. Muller, Vittorio Locatelli, Silvano G. Cella,
Sandro Loche, Ezio Ghigo, Daniela Cocchi, Franco Camanni,
and Carlo Pintor

Departments of Pharmacology and Biomedicine
University of Milan and Turin, Institute of Pediatrics
University of Cagliari, Italy

It is now a tenet of neuroendocrinology that the secretion of anterior pituitary (AP) hormones is regulated by the central nervous system (CNS) through a family of hypophysiotropic neuropeptides, the releasing and inhibiting hormones. In addition, the neuroregulation of a given AP hormone is influenced by a host of neurotransmitters and neuropeptides, which at hypothalamic and suprahypothalamic levels provide intermediate and obligatory links between hypophysiotropic and both exogenous and endogenous influences on hormone secretion (1,2). Figure 1 depicts schematically how neurotransmitter-neurohormonal interactions may occur at the hypothalamic level. The complexity of the system stems from the abundance of different neurotransmitter and neuropeptide neurons present in the mediobasal hypothalamus (MBH) and the various ways they may reciprocally interact. Another reason for complexity is the phenomenon of coexistence, which ultimately results from cotransmission, i.e., occurrence and then release of two transmitter substances present in the same nerve endings (3). Though cotransmission undoubtedly provides greater versatility and sophistication to the vocabulary of synaptic transmission (3), it compounds the understanding of the physiology and pathophysiology of neuroendocrine control.

In this manuscript, we consider some salient aspects of the neurotransmitter control of growth hormone (GH) secretion in both experimental animals and humans and discuss them in the light of the new knowledge relating to neurotransmitter-neuropeptide interactions. Special emphasis will be placed on catecholamine (CA) and acetylcholine (ACh) involvement, in view of the wealth of information available and the important role exerted by these neurotransmitters.

NEUROTRANSMITTERS AND NEUROPEPTIDES FOR GH SECRETION

General Premises

In the hypothalamus, two specific neuropeptides, e.g., a GH-releasing-hormone (GHRH) and a GH-release-inhibiting hormone or somatostatin (SRIH) exert a dual hypothalamic control over GH secretion and are in turn regulated by numerous neurotransmitters which may act alternatively at the level of GHRH- or SRIH-producing neurons, or both. Table 1 reviews the principal neurotransmitter influences controlling GH release, as derived from in vivo animal and human studies. Both amine (CAs, indoleamines, ACh, histamine) and amino acid (γ-hydroxybutyric acid) neurotransmitters play a role in the control of GH release by either stimulating and/or inhibiting hormone release. This is best exemplified by the action of CAs, where α_2 and $\alpha_1-\beta_2$ receptors exert stimulatory and inhibitory influences. Another example is DA, which is inhibitory to GH release in most animal species but there is a dual action in man; by the opposing effect of histamine (H), H_1 and H_2 receptors, γ-hydroxybutyric acid (GABA) can either stimulate or inhibit GH secretion in rodents (4).

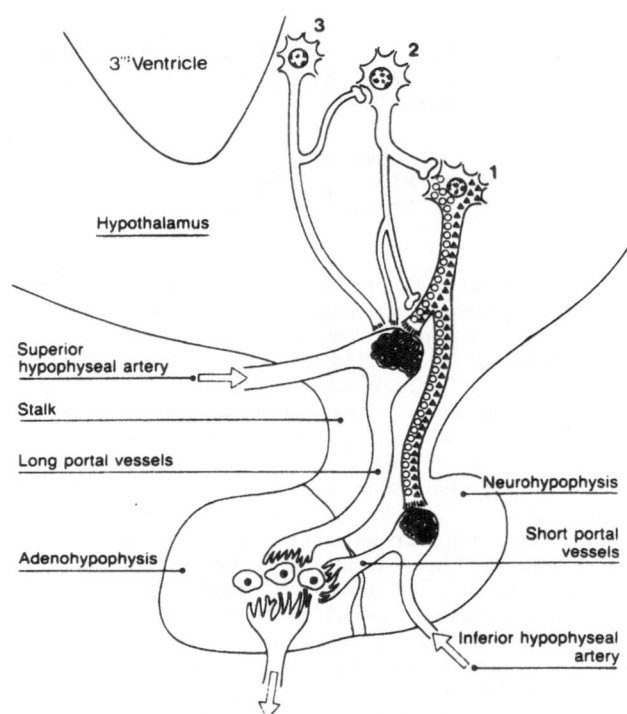

Fig. 1. Neurotransmitter-neurohormonal control of anterior pituitary secretion. The diagram demonstrates the principal neural afferents involved in pituitary hormonal regulation. Neuron 1 denotes a tuberohypophyseal peptidergic neuron which manufactures hypothalamic hormones which are then released into the hypophyseal portal vessels and are relayed to the anterior pituitary. Different symbols in the neuron (▲, o) refer to the possibility of peptide-amine, peptide-peptide co-localization. Neuron 2 denotes a neurotransmitter nerve ending in relation to a peptidergic neuron (axosomatic or axoaxonic contact). Another possibility is depicted: a neurotransmitter neuron (dopamine, epinephrine, gamma aminobutyric acid, etc.) ends directly in contact with the primary plexus of blood capillaries at the median eminence level. Neuron 3 is a nonhypophysiotropic peptidergic neuron that modulates the activity of a neurotransmitter neuron (axosomatic or axoaxonic contact). For the sake of clarity, peptidergic neurons of the supraoptic and paraventricular-hypophyseal systems with cell bodies in the hypothalamus and nerve endings in the neurohypophysis have been omitted. Reproduced with permission from reference 4.

Table 1. Effect of brain neurotransmitters on GH secretion.

Subjects	E	α₁	α₂	β₁	β₂	NE	DA	5-HT	Ach*	H₁	H₂	GABA
Experimental animal	↑	↓	↑		↓	↑	↑↓	↑↓?	↑	↑↓		↑↓
Human	↑⁺		↑	↓		↑	↑±	↑↓?	↑	↑	↓	↑

Key to symbols: ↑, stimulation; ↓, inhibition; ?, action still question-able. Where no symbol is given, action is not determined. Shorter arrows indicate effect of activation of receptor subclasses for E (epinephrine), NE (norepinephrine), and H (histamine); GH, growth hormone; DA, dopamine; 5-HT, 5-hydroxytryptamine; ACh, acetylcholine; GABA, γ-aminobutyric acid. *Muscarinic receptors. +In combination with propranolol. ±Inhibitory in acromegaly.

The main reason(s) for the dual effect of most neurotransmitters on GH secretion is that the same molecule may act either at the level of GHRH or SRIH-secretory neurons (4). Thus, endogenous neurotransmitter release and secretion may relate to accessibility and availability of receptor sites on GHRH or SRIH secretory neurons. Also, neurotransmitter effect may depend on previous receptor occupancy. Alternatively, the neuro-transmitter enters into the stalk blood to act on receptor sites located on the somatotrophs. Dopamine (and GABA?) is (are) neurotransmitter(s) which may fulfill the last prerequisite (4).

In addition to classical neurotransmitters, a host of neuropeptides which includes endogenous opioid peptides (EOPs), vasoactive intestinal polypeptide (VIP), peptide histidine isoleucine amide (PHI), neuropeptide Y (NPY), motilin, galanin, cholecystokinin (CCK), and neurotensin (NT) stimulate GH release (5). In addition, thyrotropin-releasing hormone (TRH) and luteinizing hormone releasing hormone (LHRH) are able to stim-ulate GH release; they are capable of this action in certain pathologic conditions of animals and humans (6). In general, these compounds do not act directly at the pituitary level, but via the CNS, with notable excep-tions including motilin (7), NPY (8), and secretin (9). The underlying mechanism(s) of action for these neuropeptides in vivo appear to be that they do not act directly on the hypophysiotropic neurosecretory neurons, but rather they act presynaptically through the secretion of classical neurotransmitters. This has been previously ascertained for EOPs (10) and, more recently, for galanin (see below).

Neurotransmitters and GHRH Release

Coexistence. Co-localization studies, using a sequential double staining technique, have demonstrated the presence of tyrosine hydroxylase (TH)-like immunoreactivity, a marker mainly of DA neurons, in most GHRH-immunoreactive cells in the ventral part of the arcuate (ARC) nucleus (ventral A₁₂ DA cell group) (11). Partly overlapping GHRH- and TH immuno-reactivity fibers in the median eminence (ME) occurred, indicating pos-sible coexistence of the two compounds in periportal nerve endings (11). In similar studies, it has been shown that a subset of GHRH immunoreac-tivity neurons contains NT immunoreactivity (12). Since previous studies had demonstrated coexistence of DA and NT immunoreactivity (13) or DA and glutamic acid decarboxylase (GAD) immunoreactivity (14), a marker of GABA neurons, the possibility of multiple co-localizations in GHRH neurons can be envisaged. The functional significance of co-localization of DA and NT in GHRH neurons is presently unknown; however, on theoretical grounds, the amine co-released from the GHRH neuron may act presynaptically on neighboring SRIH receptors to inhibit or stimulate SRIH release. Alternatively, the amine may enter into the hypophyseal portal vessels and be transported to the pituitary. In any event, a modulatory action of the GHRH-induced GH response may be foreseen, in agreement with results from studies on the functional role of coexistence of peptides and classical transmitters (3). More recently, the existence of a dense population of NPY immunoreactivity perikarya co-staining with about 90% of the ARC nucleus-GHRH immunoreactivity perikarya has been reported in the medial part of the ARC nucleus. Only a minority of GHRH perikarya, located ventrolaterally in the ARC nucleus, did not stain for NPY and, interestingly, those were the ones projecting to the external zone of the ME. In fact, virtually no NPY immunoreactivity was detected at the level of the ME, suggesting that the majority of the GHRH neurons in the rat ARC nucleus constitutes a tubero-extra-infundibular projecting system (15). This would not be involved in the direct control of the anterior pituitary, but may rather have neuromodulatory functions.

In vivo and in vitro studies. Only recently, data are available on the effects of neurotransmitters or agonist and antagonist drugs on the release of hypothalamic GHRH release, though most of the evidence is only inferential and derived mainly from in vivo experiments (Table 2). In urethane-anesthetized rats pretreated with a SRIH-antiserum, intracerebroventricular (icv) administration of 10 nmole of either epinephrine (E) or norepinephrine (NE) stimulated a rise in plasma GH, an effect which, unexpectedly, was not shared by the α_2-adrenoceptor agonist, clonidine (16). In this system, DA, ACh and serotonin (5-HT) were ineffective (16) which would suggest that the action of these compounds on GH release was mainly mediated through inhibition of hypothalamic SRIH release. It is also difficult to interpret the inhibitory effect of the α_1-receptor agonist, phenylephrine, on GH release (16) since we have recently shown that infant rats pretreated with SRIH-antiserum failed to suppress plasma GH levels following administration of another α_1-adrenoceptor agonist, methoxamine (17). Moreover, freely moving rats pretreated with GHRH-antiserum failed to exhibit a GH response following icv administration of GABA or 5-HT, which would imply for both transmitters an action mediated via GHRH release (but for 5-HT, see below). It must be noted, however, that in all the experiments in which we used an antiserum raised against GHRH, the effect of a given GH secretagogue was invariably suppressed, thus casting doubts on the discriminatory ability of this approach (17).

Clonidine

Despite clonidine's failure to cause GH release in the above experiments (Table 2), evidence is accumulating that the GH release induced by clonidine occurs via a GHRH-mediated mechanism. The evidence includes: (1) the ability of clonidine to elicit GH release in reserpinized rats pretreated with SRIH-antiserum (20); (2) failure of clonidine to trigger GH release in adult rats pretreated with a GHRH-antiserum (23); or (3) in rats with monosodium glutamate-induced destruction of GHRH-secretory structures (22); and, finally, (4) the ability of clonidine to cause GHRH release from rat hypothalami perfused in vitro (21) (Table 2).

We have recently studied the effects of clonidine on GH release in neonatal and infant rats, comparing them with the effects elicited by GHRH stimulation. Briefly, our data can be summarized as follows: clonidine (150 µg kg/ip) increased plasma GH in 5- and 10-day-old rats but not in 1-day-old rats; clonidine (150 µg sc, twice daily) injected from postnatal day 5 to postnatal day 9 increased plasma GH 14 h after the last clonidine injection and it also increased pituitary GH content; clonidine was ineffective in pups treated from postnatal day 1 to postnatal day 5; clonidine failed to induce GH release from AP fragments incubated in vitro

Table 2. Neurotransmitters and GHRH release.

Neurotransmitter or drug	Action on GHRH release	Rat animal preparation or in vitro system	Ref. No.
Epinephrine icv	↑	Urethane anesthetized treated with SRIH-antiserum	
Norepinephrine icv	↑	" " "	
Dopamine icv	→	" " "	(16)
Acetylcholine icv	→	" " "	
Serotonin icv	→	" " "	
Serotonin icv	↑	Freely moving treated with GHRH antiserum	(18)
γ-Aminobutyric acid icv	↑	" " "	(19)
Phenylephrine	↓	Urethane-anesthetized pretreated with SRIH-antiserum	(16)
Clonidine icv	→	" " "	
Clonidine	↑	Freely moving reserpinized pretreated with SRIH-antiserum	(20)
Clonidine	↑	Perifused hypothalamus*	(21)
Clonidine	→	Freely moving monosodium glutamate pretreated	(22)
Clonidine	→	Freely moving pretreated with GHRH-antiserum	(23)

Key to symbols: ↑, stimulation; ↓, inhibition; →, no effect. When not indicated, drugs were administered systemically or added in vitro.
*In the same system, propranolol was ineffective but potentiated the effect of clonidine.

and its GH-releasing effect was completely suppressed by pretreatment with a GHRH-antiserum (7). In summary, these data support the idea that under these experimental conditions, clonidine stimulated GH release and syn-thesis. This view is supported by the finding that similar to clonidine, acute short-term administration of GHRH (20 ng/100 g sc, twice daily) to 5-day-old rats induced changes in GH secretion superimposable to those elicited by clonidine (24).

More cogent proof that both GHRH and clonidine stimulate GH release and synthesis in infant rats was provided by showing that either compound increased incorporation of ^{3}H-leucine into the electrophoretic band of GH in the pituitary from 10-day-old rats, pretreated in vivo for 5 days (25).

Galanin. From the reported data it appears that clonidine-induced activation of α_2-adrenoceptors is a potent stimulus of GH release in the rat; clonidine also is a GH secretagogue in other animal species (4), including man (26). In rodents, the GH releasing effect of clonidine is a postsynaptic event because pretreatment with inhibitors of CA biosynthesis (10) or depletion of CA stores by reserpine (20) does not suppress the ability of the drug to release GH. Whether the effect of clonidine is due to activation of adrenergic receptors normally occupied by NE or E is presently unknown.

Another way through which CAs may contribute to activation of the GHRH-secreting structures is as mediators of the neuroendocrine effect of CNS peptides. Galanin, a 29 amino acid peptide named for the presence of N-terminal glycine and C-terminal alanine residues, was isolated and characterized from extracts of porcine intestine (27) during the purification process of the peptides PHI and PYY. Subsequently, galanin immunoreactivity has been localized to cell bodies of several hypothalamic nuclei and to nerve terminals in the external layer of the ME (28). Recent data have shown that galanin (50-200 pmole) injected icv into freely moving adult rats induced a brisk, dose-dependent GH rise, while it failed to significantly alter either GH or prolactin release in doses ranging from 10^{-9} to 10^{-6} M from dispersed perifused AP cells (29). In a study by our group, galanin (5-25 µg/kg sc) induced a dose-dependent rise in plasma GH levels in 10-day-old rats (data not shown). Apparently the GH-releasing effect of galanin occurs via activation of CA, namely E, neurotransmission. As shown in Figure 2 (panel A), both an inhibitor of DA-β-hydroxylase and a selective inhibitor of phenylethanolamine methyltransferase, the enzyme that converts NE to E, were effective in suppressing the GH-releasing effect of galanin. Pretreatment of infant rats with GHRH antiserum completely prevented the effect of galanin, while galanin was hardly able to increase GH levels in rats pretreated with a SRIH-antiserum (data not shown). It is worth noting that inhibition of E biosynthesis induced per se a clear-cut reduction of plasma GH levels, demonstrating the influence exerted by E neurotransmission on tonic GH secretion in the infant rats (Fig. 2, panels A and B).

It is expected that galanin-like peptides may be further studied to increase our understanding about the role of E on GH release and on the interaction(s) between epinephrinergic neurons and GHRH secretory structures.

The presynaptic action of galanin on CA neurons occurs in contrast to the postsynaptic mechanism of clonidine (Fig. 2, panel B), at least in rodents, and holds promise that testing with galanin and clonidine, both potent GH secretagogues in humans (26,30), may unravel discrete alterations of CA neurotransmission in subjects with growth disorders (31).

CHOLINERGIC NEUROTRANSMISSION

The hypothalamic cholinergic system plays an important role in GH release mechanisms. In addition to a stimulatory effect on GH release by activation of cholinergic muscarinic receptors (32,33), antagonists of cholinergic receptors have been shown to abolish the rise in plasma GH elicited by different GH secretagogues in humans (34,35). It has also been demonstrated that cholinergic blockade with pirenzepine and atropine can reduce the sleep-related GH release in normal adults and children (36-38).

A breakthrough of the understanding of the major role played by ACh neurotransmission on GH secretion came from the observation of Massara and

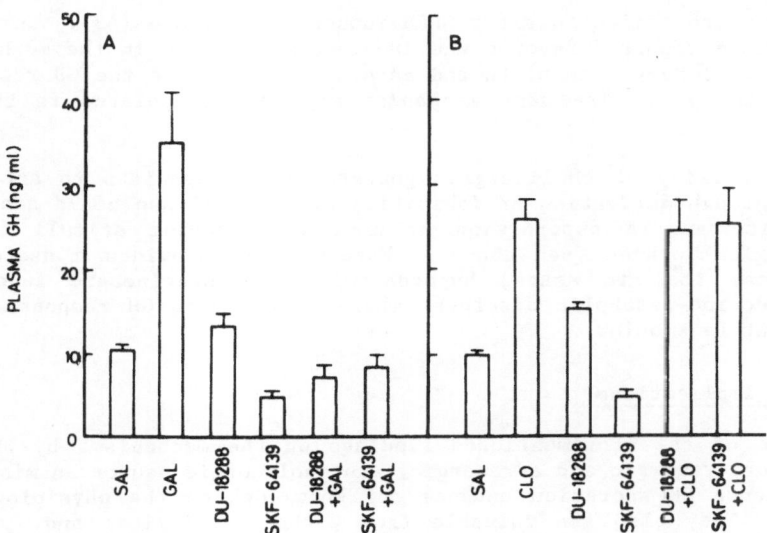

Fig. 2. Effect of synthetic porcine galanin (Gal, 25 µg/kg sc) (panel A) or clonidine (CLO, 150 µg/kg sc) (panel B) on plasma GH levels in 10-day-old rats pretreated or not with inhibitors of norepinephrine (DO-18288, 6 mg/kg ip) or epinephrine (SKF 64139, 50 mg/kg ip) synthesis. Each bar and vertical line represents the mean and SEM of 9-20 determinations made in duplicate. For clarity, differences statistically significant among groups have been omitted (SKF 64139 vs. saline, P<0.01; SKF 64139 plus clonidine vs. clonidine, P<0.01).

associates (39). They demonstrated that pirenzepine and atropine completely abolished the GHRH-induced GH rise. Complementary to this observation was the finding that pyridostigmine, an inhibitor of ACh-cholinesterase, was capable of potentiating the GHRH-induced GH rise (39). The effectiveness of pirenzepine and atropine ruled out the possibility that cholinergic influences for GH release were directly acting on GHRH-secreting structures and favored, instead, an action via SRIH, or directly on the pituitary, where in rodents muscarinic ACh receptors have been located (40).

We have recently faced this problem. We studied in a rat model characterized by depletion of hypothalamic SRIH the modulatory effect of cholinergic agonists and antagonists on the GHRH-induced GH rise. Briefly, our data can be summarized as follows: in freely moving rats, as in humans, atropine (0.5 mg/kg iv), pirenzepine (0.5 mg/kg iv), and the direct cholinergic agonist pilocarpine (3 mg/kg iv) blunted or enhanced, respectively, the rise in plasma GH induced by GHRH (2 µg/kg iv); in rats with hypothalamic SRIH depletion, i.e., rats with anterolateral deafferentation of the MBH (41) or rats treated with cysteamine (42), the modulatory action of cholinergic drugs on the neuroendocrine effect of GHRH was completely absent; in these two experimental models, an antiserum raised against SRIH failed to increase plasma GH and measurement of hypothalamic SRIH content revealed a clear-cut reduction of the neuropeptide; atropine (1 µmol/1) and pilocarpine (1 µl/1) added to pituitary cells in vitro failed to alter GHRH-induced GH release (43). In summary, the evidence reported favored the involvement of SRIH in the mechanism(s) by which cholinergic agonists and antagonists modulate the GH response to GHRH in the rat. The same mechanism may be extrapolated to the human findings.

The ability of cholinergic agonists and antagonists to act respectively through activation or inhibition of SRIH release could account for the indiscriminate suppression of most GH-releasing stimuli following cholinergic blockade (see above). Moreover, it provides a useful pharmacological tool to assess hypothalamic somatostatinergic function in neuroendocrine-metabolic disorders where a defective GH response to GHRH is present (see below).

Clinical Implications

Some of the aforementioned findings on the mechanisms by which CA, namely noradrenergic and adrenergic, and cholinergic neurotransmission act to influence GH secretion enhance our knowledge on the physiology of GH control. They also are valuable from pathophysiological and, possibly, diagnostic and therapeutic points of view.

The observation that cholinergic drugs modulate, likely via SRIH, somatotroph responsiveness to GHRH, may indicate that, ultimately, the existence of increased or decreased hypothalamic cholinergic tone contributes to the extent of pituitary responsiveness to GHRH-mediated stimuli. Furthermore, it can be hypothesized that the blunted response to GHRH of some children with different kinds of short stature (44,45) or metabolic disorders (44) suggests defective cholinergic tone in the hypothalamus. Figure 3 shows that enhancement of the cholinergic tone by pyridostigmine clearly increased the GH response to GHRH in children with familial short stature (FSS), constitutional growth delay (CGD), and, although not so markedly, in children with GH deficiency. In addition, pyridostigmine alone induced a GH response that in many children with FSS and CGD was greater than after insulin hypoglycemia or GHRH. Similarly, in children with simple obesity, pretreatment with pyridostigmine completely counteracted the blunted GH response to GHRH (Loche et al., unpublished observations).

Thus, it is apparent that a combination of pyridostigmine and GHRH may represent the best provocative test to evaluate the secretory capacity of the somatotrophic cell. In addition, the same combination of drugs may find its place as therapy in patients in whom GHRH replacement is recommended, but unresponsiveness to GHRH ensues during treatment (46).

The ability of α_2-receptor agonists to trigger GH release and synthesis via GHRH may be used to treat children with growth disorders, likely due to deficiency of GHRH release but not synthesis. In a preliminary study, we reported that a 2-month period of clonidine therapy (100 $\mu g/m^2$ daily) was competent to stimulate linear growth in 2/4 children with GH deficiency and 4/4 with CGD (31). As an extension of these studies, we have given clonidine to 34 children with CGD for a 6-month period and 22 for 12 months. In 21 children, the height velocity increased by more than 2 cm/yr during the first 6 months of clonidine treatment. Of the 22 who were treated for 12 months, the increment in height velocity was maintained in 13. Clonidine did not induce noticeable side effects (47). These data confirm the view that in some children with CGD, enforcement of "sluggish" α_2-adrenergic function is capable of accelerating linear growth and that clonidine may be a useful form of therapy.

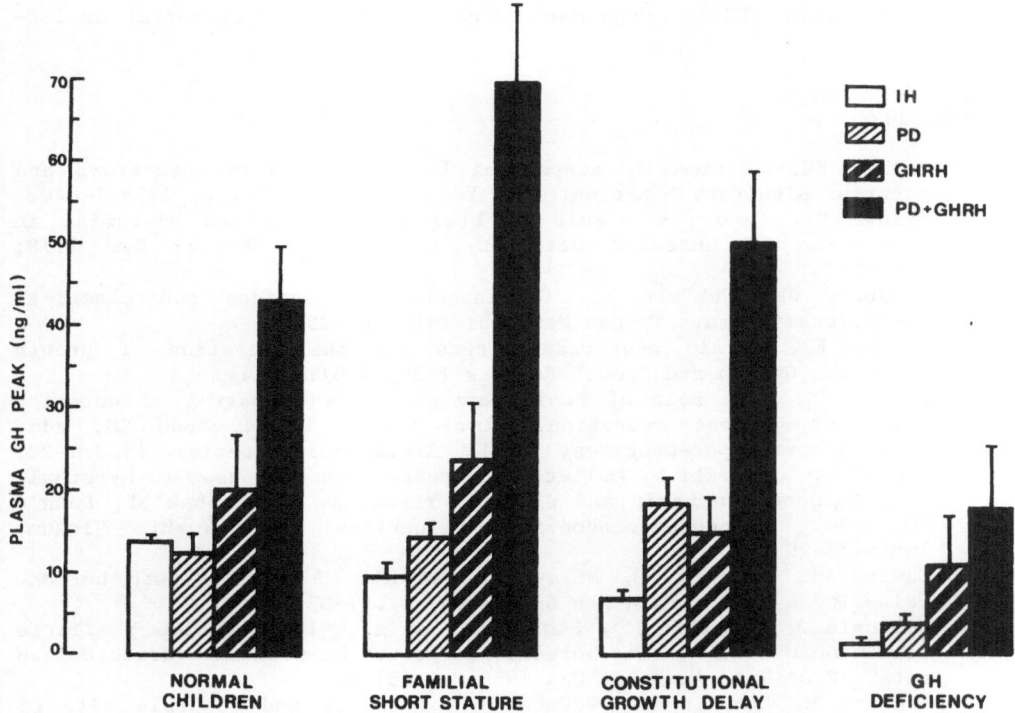

Fig. 3. Peak plasma GH responses (mean and SEM) after insulin-induced hypoglycemia (0.15 IU/kg iv), pyridostigmine (PD, 60 mg/kg po), GHRH (1 µg/kg iv) and PD plus GHRH in normal children, children with familial short stature, children with constitutional growth delay and children with GH deficiency. Each point is the mean of 5-10 determinations in 5-10-year-old subjects.

CONCLUSIONS

Though slow to be introduced into endocrine physiology, the concept of the neural regulation of GH secretion is now undisputably established and the complex mechanisms subserving this function are being clarified. It is now apparent that a cohort of neurotransmitters and neuropeptides affects somatotroph function modulating GHRH and/or SRIH release. Although a physiologic role of such compounds is still controversial, comprehension of their mechanism of action, and hence function, is gradually increasing. Aside from the well-studied CAs, an important role in both animals and humans is now emerging for the once overlooked cholinergic neurons.

New knowledge about neurotransmitter mechanisms of action and the increasing awareness that some disorders of growth and metabolism may result from a CNS and not pituitary deficiency add a new dimension to the diagnostic and therapeutic applications of neuroactive compounds in these illnesses.

ACKNOWLEDGMENTS

The original studies of the authors were supported by grants from the M.P.I. (FC) and special research project "Oncology," no. 86.00499.44, from the C.N.R., Rome (EEM). Miss Maria Lupo contributed secretarial assistance.

REFERENCES

1. Muller EE, Nistico G, Scapagnini U. Brain neurotransmitters and anterior pituitary function. New York: Academic Press, 1978:1-440.
2. Weiner RI, Ganong W. Role of brain monoamines and histamine in regulation of anterior pituitary secretion. Physiol Rev 1978; 58:905-7.
3. Lundberg JM, Hokfelt T. Coexistence of peptides and classical neurotransmitters. Trends Neurosci 1983; 6:325-31.
4. Muller EE. Brain neurotransmitters and the secretion of growth hormone. Growth and Growth Factors 1986; 1(3):65-74.
5. McCann SM. The role of brain peptides in the control of anterior pituitary hormone secretion. In: Muller EE, MacLeod RM, eds. Neuroendocrine perspectives; vol 1. Amsterdam: Elsevier, 1982:1-22.
6. Cocchi D, Locatelli V, Muller EE. Nonspecific responses to hypothalamic hormones in basic and clinical research. In: Shah NS, Donald AG, eds. Psychoneuroendocrine dysfunction. New York: Plenum, 1984:173-208.
7. Samson WK, Lumpkin MD, Nilaver G, et al. A novel growth hormone releasing agent. Brain Res Bull 1984; 12:57-62.
8. McDonald JK, Lumpkin MD, Samson WK, et al. Neuropeptide Y affects secretion of luteinizing hormone and growth hormone in ovariectomized rats. Proc Natl Acad Sci USA 1985; 82:561-4.
9. Samson WK, Lumpkin MD, McCann SM. Presence and possible site of action of secretin in the rat pituitary and hypothalamus. Life Sci 1984; 34:155-63.
10. Katakami H, Kato Y, Matsushita N, et al. Involvement of alpha-adrenergic mechanisms in growth hormone release induced by opioid peptide in conscious rats. Neuroendocrinology 1981; 33:129-35.
11. Meister B, Hokfelt T, Vale WW, et al. Coexistence of tyrosine hydroxylase and growth hormone-releasing factor in a subpopulation of tuberoinfundibular neurons of the rat. Neuroendocrinology 1986; 42:237-47.
12. Sawcenko PE, Swanson LW, Rivier J, et al. The distribution of growth hormone releasing factor (GRF)-immunoreactivity in the central nervous system of the rat: an immunohistochemical study using antisera directed against rat hypothalamic GRF. J Comp Neurol 1985; 257:100-15.
13. Hokfelt T, Everitt BJ, Theodorsson-Norheim E, et al. Occurrence of neurotensin like immunoreactivity in subpopulations of hypothalamic mesencephalic and medullary catecholamine neurons. J Comp Neurol 1984; 222:543-59.
14. Everitt BJ, Hokfelt T, Wu SY, et al. Coexistence of tyrosine hydroxylase-like and gamma-aminobutyric acid-like immunoreactivities in neurons of the arcuate nucleus. Neuroendocrinology 1984; 39:189-91.
15. Ciofi P, Croix D, Tramu D. Coexistence of hGHRF and NPY immunoreactivities in neurons of the arcuate nucleus of the rat. Neuroendocrinology 1984; 45:425-8.
16. Arimura A, Merchenthaler I, Culler MD, Iwasaki K. Distribution and release of GRF. In: Labrie F, Proulx F, eds. Endocrinology. Amsterdam: Excerpta Medica, 1984:827-30.
17. Cella SG, Locatelli V, De Gennaro V, et al. Pharmacological manipulations of α-adrenoceptors in the infant rat and effects on growth hormone secretion. Study of the underlying mechanisms of action. Endocrinology 1987; 120:1639-44.
18. Murakami Y, Kato Y, Kabayama T, et al. Involvement of growth hormone-releasing factor in growth hormone secretion induced by seroto-

ninergic mechanisms. Endocrinology 1986; 119:1089-92.

19. Murakami Y, Kato Y, Kabayama Y, et al. Involvement of growth hormone-releasing factor in growth hormone secretion induced by gamma-aminobutyric acid in conscious rats. Endocrinology 1985; 117:787-9.

20. Eden S, Eriksson E, Martin JB, et al. Evidence for a growth hormone releasing factor mediating alpha-adrenergic influence on growth hormone secretion in the rat. Neuroendocrinology 1981; 33:24-7.

21. Kabayama Y, Kato Y, Murakami Y, et al. Stimulation by alpha-adrenergic mechanisms of the secretion of growth-hormone releasing factor (GRF) from perifused rat hypothalamus. Endocrinology 1986; 119:432-4.

22. Katakami H, Kato Y, Matsushita N, et al. Effect of neonatal treatment with monosodium glutamate on growth hormone release induced by clonidine and prostaglandin E_1 in conscious male rats. Neuroendocrinology 1984; 38:1-5.

23. Miki N, Ono M, Shizume K. Evidence that opiatergic and α-adrenergic mechanisms stimulate rat growth hormone release via growth hormone-releasing factor. Endocrinology 1984; 114:1950-2.

24. Cella SG, Locatelli V, De Gennaro V, et al. In vivo studies with growth hormone (GH)-releasing factor and clonidine in rat pups: ontogenetic development of their effect on GH release and synthesis. Endocrinology 1986; 119:1164-70.

25. Cozzi MG, Zanini A, Locatelli V, et al. Growth hormone-releasing hormone and clonidine stimulate biosynthesis of growth hormone in neonatal pituitaries. Biochem Biophys Res Commun 1986; 138:1223-30.

26. Gil-Ad I, Topper E, Laron Z. Oral clonidine as a growth hormone stimulant test. Lancet 1978; 2:278-80.

27. Tatemoto K, Rokaeus A, Jornvall H, et al. Galanin-a novel biologically active peptide from porcine intestine. FEBS Lett 1983; 164:124-8.

28. Rakaeus A, Melander T, Hokfelt T, et al. A galanin-like peptide in the central nervous system and intestine of the rat. Neurosci Lett 1984; 47:161-6.

29. Ottlecz A, Samson WK, McCann SM. Galanin: evidence for a hypothalamic site to release growth hormone. Peptides 1986; 7:51-3.

30. Bauer FE, Venetikou M, Burrin JM, et al. Growth hormone release in man induced by galanin, a new hypothalamic peptide. Lancet 1986; 2:192-4.

31. Pintor C, Cella SG, Corda R, et al. Clonidine accelerates growth in children with impaired growth hormone secretion. Lancet 1985; i:1482-4.

32. Bruni JF, Meites J. Effects of cholinergic drugs on growth hormone release. Life Sci 1978; 23:1351-7.

33. Casanueva FF, Betti R, Cella SG, et al. Effects of agonists and antagonists of cholinergic neurotransmission on growth hormone release in the dog. Acta Endocrinol (Copenh) 1983; 103:15-20.

34. Casanueva FF, Villanueva L, Cabranes JA, et al. Cholinergic mediation of growth hormone secretion elicited by arginine, clonidine and physical exercise in man. J Clin Endocrinol Metab 1984; 59:526-30.

35. Delitala G, Frulio T, Pacifico A, et al. Participation of cholinergic muscarinic receptors in glucagon- and arginine-mediated growth hormone secretion in man. J Clin Endocrinol Metab 1982; 55:1231-3.

36. Delitala G, Giusti M, Monachesi M, et al. Cholinergic receptor control mechanism in spontaneous and sleep-related growth hormone secretion in man. In: Molinatti GM, Martini L, eds. Endocrinology 85. Amsterdam: Excerpta Medica; 163-6.

37. Peters JR, Evans PJ, Page MD, et al. Cholinergic muscarinic receptor blockade with pirenzepine abolishes slow wave sleep-related growth hormone release in normal adult man. Clin Endocrinol 1986; 25:213-7.

38. Taylor BJ, Smith PJ, Brook CGD. Inhibition of physiological growth hormone secretion by atropine. Clin Endocrinol 1985; 22:497-501.

39. Massara F, Ghigo E, Demislis K, et al. Cholinergic involvement in the growth hormone releasing hormone-induced growth hormone release: studies in normal and acromegalic subjects. Neuroendocrinology 1986; 43:670–5.

40. Mukherjee A, Snyder G, McCann SM. Characterization of muscarinic cholinergic receptors on intact rat anterior pituitary cells. Life Sci 1980; 27:475–82.

41. Brownstein M, Arimura A, Fernandez-Durango R, et al. The effect of hypothalamic deafferentation on somatostatin-like activity in the rat brain. Endocrinology 1977; 100:246–9.

42. Szabo S, Reichlin S. Somatostatin in rat tissue is depleted by cysteamine administration. Endocrinology 1981; 109:2255–7.

43. Locatelli V, Torsello A, Redaelli M, et al. Cholinergic agonist and antagonist drugs modulate the growth hormone response to growth hormone-releasing hormone in the rat: evidence for mediation by somatostatin. J Endocrinol 1986; 111:271–8.

44. Pintor C, Loche S, Puggioni R, et al. Growth hormone response to hpGRF-40 in different forms of growth retardation and endocrine-metabolic disease. Eur J Pediatr 1986; 144:475–81.

45. Gelato M, Malazowski CS, Caruso-Nicoletti M, et al. Growth hormone (GH) responses to GH-releasing hormone during pubertal development in normal boys and girls: comparison to idiopathic short stature and GH deficiency. J Clin Endocrinol Metab 1986; 63:174–9.

46. Ross JM, Tsagarakis S, Grossman A, et al. Treatment of growth-hormone deficiency with growth-hormone release hormone. Lancet 1987; i:5–8.

47. Pintor C, Cella SG, Loche S, et al. Clonidine treatment for short stature. Lancet 1987; i:1626–9.

9

ACROMEGALY

Hiroo Imura, M.D., Yuzuru Kato, M.D.,* and
Naoki Hattori, M.D.

Department of Medicine, Kyoto University Faculty of
Medicine, Sakyo-ku, Kyoto 606; *Department of Medicine,
Shimane Medical University, Izumo, Shimane 693, Japan

INTRODUCTION

A unique disfigurement of acromegaly was seen in ancient paintings or statues, but the association of pituitary enlargement with this disease was first noted by Pierre Marie. Its association with growth hormone (GH) hypersecretion was suggested by Cushing and later confirmed by bioassay and radioimmunoassay (RIA). Since then, RIA has been extensively used in the diagnosis and evaluation of treatment of acromegaly.

In the past decade, some progress has been made in the etiology, diagnosis and treatment of this disease. In this manuscript, we first refer to the etiology of acromegaly briefly, and then discuss new diagnostic approaches and therapeutic means.

ETIOLOGY OF ACROMEGALY

Acromegaly is usually caused by GH hypersecretion from GH-producing pituitary adenoma. In recent years, however, production of GH-releasing hormone (GHRH) by hypothalamic or ectopic tumors is known to cause acromegaly (1,2). Pituitary lesions in these patients are usually GH cell hyperplasia but adenomas are also found (3). GHRH-producing tumors seem to be very uncommon as shown in a multi-institutional study performed in Japan. Of 401 randomly collected acromegalic patients, there were 267 patients with eosinophilic adenoma, 71 with chromophobe adenoma and 63 with mixed adenoma of the pituitary gland (4). None had GH cell hyperplasia suggestive of GHRH-producing tumors. Thus, most patients with acromegaly have pituitary adenoma.

The pathogenesis of pituitary adenoma is unknown. It is still unknown whether overstimulation by the hypothalamus produces adenoma in the pituitary. As discussed in the next section, most patients with acromegaly respond to exogenous GHRH. In addition, insulin-induced hypoglycemia and arginine elicit GH increases in approximately half of the patients studied (5). These results suggest that adenoma cells retain an ability to respond to endogenous GHRH or other stimulatory influences. Cerebrospinal fluid levels of GHRH were reported not to be suppressed in patients with acromegaly (6). The latter observation is difficult to interpret, however, because (1) the origin and metabolism of GHRH in cerebrospinal fluid is not known; (2) there is technical difficulty in RIA measurement of GHRH; and, (3) the regulatory mechanism of GH secretion is complex and not fully understood. Clinical observations on the course of acromegaly after transsphenoidal adenomectomy provide no definite evidence indicating that there is a form of GH cell adenoma caused by hypothalamic overstimulation.

DIAGNOSIS OF ACROMEGALY

The diagnosis of acromegaly is usually not difficult and is based on clinical manifestations and X-ray findings. The measurement of plasma GH levels confirms the diagnosis and is essential for diagnosing mild or atypical cases. Conventional RIA for GH is usually sufficient, since most of the patients have values of more than 5 ng/ml. In a series of 657 patients studied in Japan (7), however, the minimum level in repeated plasma GH determinations was below 5 ng/ml in 7% and they required further evaluations. Computed tomography and magnetic resonance imaging are useful in the diagnosis of pituitary microadenoma. In this manuscript, we discuss some relatively new diagnostic tests.

Plasma GH Responses to Provocative Tests

Plasma GH responses to glucose load are abnormal in acromegalic patients and this study is still an important diagnostic test. In our series (5), 89% of the patients showed either a paradoxical rise or no significant change in response to glucose loading (Table 1). In the remaining patients, plasma GH decreased from basal level but did not reach a level below 5 ng/ml. Plasma GH levels increased in response to thyrotropin-releasing hormone (TRH), luteinizing hormone releasing hormone (LHRH) and vasoactive intestinal polypeptide (VIP) in 64%, 13% and 33% of the patients in our series, respectively (5). Such paradoxical responses are clues to the diagnosis of acromegaly and are also used for evaluating the completeness of treatment. Plasma GH levels also increased in response to GHRH injection in 80% of acromegalic patients (5). In certain patients, this response is useful as a marker of residual tumor following surgery.

Dopaminergic agents increase plasma GH levels in normal subjects but lower plasma GH in more than half of acromegalic patients. Such paradox-

Table 1. Plasma GH responses to various agents which are potentially useful for diagnosis or management.

Agent	Response	Percent
Glucose	No change or increase	89
TRH	Increase	64
LHRH	Increase	13
VIP	Increase	33
GHRH	Increase	80
L-dopa	Decrease	29
Bromocriptine	Decrease	34
Dopamine	Decrease and rebound rise	69

ical responses suggest the presence of acromegaly and predict the effectiveness of bromocriptine treatment. However, an oral L-dopa or bromocriptine test often give equivocal results because of the fluctuation of basal GH levels in acromegaly. We, therefore, use the intravenous dopamine test. In this test, plasma GH decreases to less than 50% of the basal level, followed by a rebound rise after the cessation of dopamine infusion in responders (74% of the cases), as shown in Figure 1 (5). Such responses to dopamine disappeared following successful pituitary surgery. Since the response to dopamine can be evaluated both by a decrease of plasma GH during the infusion and by a rebound rise following the end of infusion, it is the most reliable test to evaluate plasma GH responsiveness to dopaminergic agents and to predict the efficacy of bromocriptine treatment. The site of action of dopamine appears to be at the pituitary level, since dopamine does not cross the blood-brain barrier and since dopamine inhibits GH release from perifused pituitary adenoma cells in vitro (8,9).

Plasma Somatomedin-C/Insulin-like Growth Factor I (SmC/IGF-I) Levels in Acromegaly

A simplified RIA procedure for measuring plasma SmC/IGF-I levels is now available and is extensively used in the diagnosis of GH secretory disorders. In our experience, patients with acromegaly have values more than 2 U/ml, significantly higher than in normal subjects. Clemmons et al. (10) reported that there was no overlap in plasma SmC/IGF-I levels between normal subjects and acromegalic patients. They also showed that acromegalic patients who had plasma GH levels below 5 ng/ml still had high plasma SmC/IGF-I levels, indicating that the elevation of plasma SmC/IGF-I alone might be sufficient to justify therapy. Such a discrepancy may be caused by the limitation in sensitivity of the conventional RIA. Although plasma SmC/IGF-I level is a useful marker in the diagnosis of active acromegaly, it must be kept in mind that plasma SmC/IGF-I levels decrease even in acromegalic patients during starvation or severe illnesses.

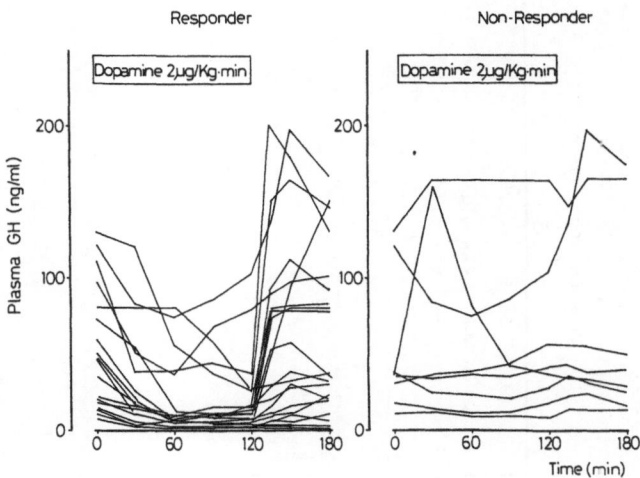

Fig. 1. Plasma GH changes during and after the intravenous infusion of dopamine (2 μg/kg body weight/min) on plasma GH levels in acromegalic patients. In responders (left) plasma GH was lowered during the infusion with a rebound rise whereas the change was not significant in nonresponders (right).

Measurement of Plasma and Urinary GH by Highly Sensitive Enzyme Immunoassay (EIA)

Conventional RIA for GH is usually satisfactory in diagnosing acromegaly, but a few patients have values below 5 ng/ml which are usually considered to be normal range. We have developed a highly sensitive sandwich EIA according to the method of Hashida et al. (10,11). In this EIA, a polyclonal antibody for GH is bound to beads and its Fab' fragment is labeled with horseradish peroxidase. The minimal detectable quantity of this method is 30 fg/tube or 1.5 pg/ml. Plasma GH levels after an overnight fast and in resting state were between 50 pg/ml to 2 ng/ml (5). Repeated blood samplings over a period of 4 h showed considerable fluctuation in plasma GH levels in normal subjects (13). In our experience, all patients with acromegaly have plasma GH values higher than 8 ng/ml. Plasma GH levels were significantly decreased following successful treatment but still slightly elevated than in normal subjects (5). Although we have not used this to measure plasma GH levels which were less than 5 ng/ml by conventional RIA, we assume that this highly sensitive EIA can discriminate mildly elevated GH values from normal values in a few acromegalics.

The highly sensitive EIA enabled us to measure urinary GH excretion. Urine was dialyzed overnight and subjected to EIA without any concentration procedure (unpublished observation). The normal range of urinary GH was 0.4 to 15 ng/g creatinine. In untreated acromegalic subjects, it was more than 40 ng/g creatinine, significantly higher than in normal subjects (Fig. 2). Those who had hypopituitarism or pituitary dwarfism had low values. Thus, urinary GH excretion reflects integrated plasma GH levels during the period of urine collection.

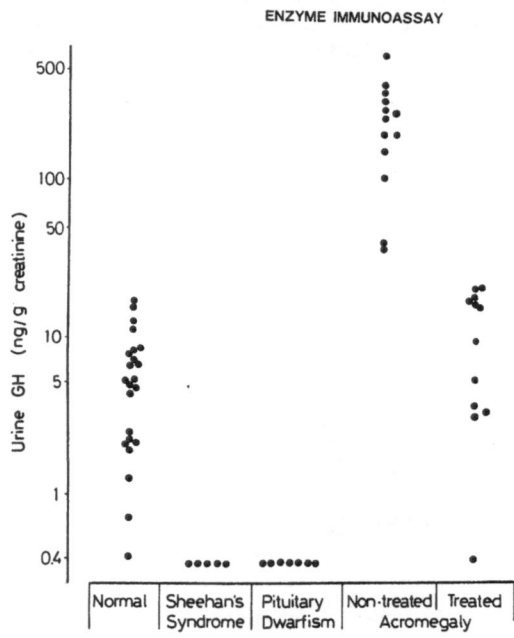

Fig. 2. Urinary GH excretion in normal subject and patients with Sheehan's syndrome, pituitary dwarfism, nontreated and successfully treated acromegaly. Twenty-four h urine was subjected to EIA for GH and the value is expressed as ng/g creatinine.

To confirm the validity of urinary GH measurement, we compared plasma and urinary GH levels during provocative testing. There was a linear correlation between plasma and urinary GH levels when plasma GH exceeded 1 ng/ml. We also examined the gel filtration profile of plasma and urinary GH in acromegalic patients. As shown in Figure 3, the major immunoreactive GH in urine eluted at the position of authentic GH with some high molecular weight forms. The major peak of plasma GH also emerged at the position of authentic GH with certain amounts of high molecular weight forms. These results support the validity of urinary GH measurement. One must be cautious, however, about interpretation of urinary GH in the presence of renal dysfunction, since patients with renal disease had high urinary GH levels (unpublished observation). There was a positive correlation between urinary GH and urinary β_2-microglobulin concentrations. Those patients with serum creatinine levels greater than 1.6 mg/dl all had elevated urinary GH excretion. In the absence of renal disease, however, urinary GH excretion reflects GH secretion. Spot urine collected early in the morning demonstrated GH values comparable to 24-h urinary GH excretion when expressed as ng/g creatinine. It can be concluded, therefore, that a single GH measurement in a morning spot urine is of diagnostic value.

TREATMENT OF ACROMEGALY

The management of acromegaly includes surgical, radiological and medical treatments. The first treatment of choice is in most cases transsphenoidal adenomectomy and, if patients have encapsulated microadenoma, the results of surgery are usually satisfactory. In invasive adenoma or macroadenoma, normalization of plasma GH following surgery is usually difficult. External radiation therapy also causes a decrease in plasma GH levels, although the decrease is slow and, in many cases, incomplete. Moreover, unwanted effects, such as hypopituitarism and brain tumors, may occur. Therefore, medical treatment is now more extensively used.

Bromocriptine

Although many dopaminergic agents have been attempted in the treatment of acromegaly, bromocriptine has been the most extensively used. Results of multi-institutional study in Japan are shown in Table 2. More than two-thirds of the patients studied responded to bromocriptine with clinical improvements, although normalization of plasma GH was seen in only 28%. Depot bromocriptine is now available (13), but our experience is still preliminary to draw any conclusions. When bromocriptine is not effective or cannot be used because of side effects, the following drugs are available: cyproheptadine, SMS 201-995.

Cyproheptadine

Cyproheptadine lowers plasma GH in only 25% of the patients. We have experienced, however, two patients who did not respond to bromocriptine but responded well to cyproheptadine (5). Clinical improvements were seen as well as improvements in glucose intolerance and hand volume were noted. Although these patients were previously treated with radiotherapy, the efficacy of cyproheptadine was confirmed by transient interruptions of the treatment which was associated with a sharp rise in plasma GH. As a side effect, increased appetite with weight gain was observed. The site of action of cyproheptadine appears to be at the pituitary level, since cyproheptadine is known to inhibit GH secretion from dispersed adenoma cells in vitro (14).

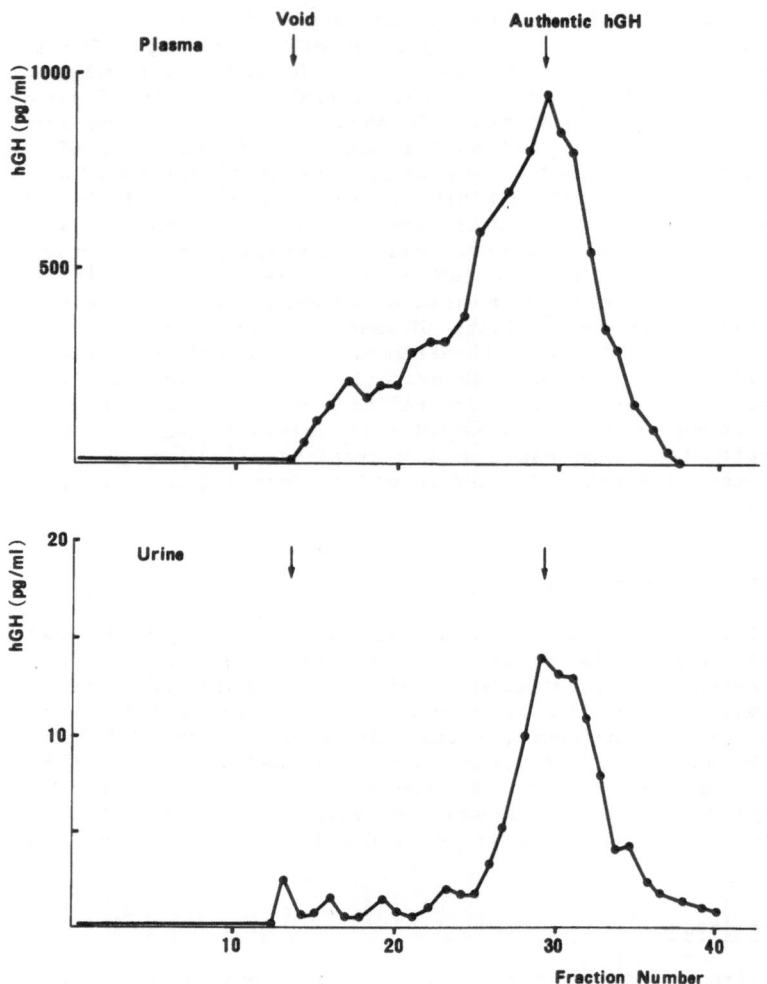

Fig. 3. Gel filtration profiles of immunoreactive GH in plasma (upper) and urine (lower) on Sephadex G-100 column in an acromegalic patient.

Table 2. Effect of bromocriptine treatment on plasma GH levels in acromegalic patients.

Plasma GH	No. of Patients (%)	Clinical Improvement
<5 ng/ml	42 (28)	+
5 - 10	25 (17)	+
11 - 20	35 (24)	+
>21 or No change	23 (15)	+
>21 or No change	24 (16)	−
Total	149	

Study group on hypothalamo-pituitary diseases in Japan (4).

A long-acting analog of somatostatin, SMS 201-995, is now available and its effectiveness in acromegaly was confirmed in several studies (15-17). In our experience, a single injection of 50 µg of SMS 201-995 decreased plasma GH; the nadir was attained between 1 and 4 h following injection. A significant fall of plasma GH was noted up to 6 h. Plasma GH fell in all 19 patients studied, although 8 of them did not respond to bromocriptine. Repeated injections of 50 µg SMS 201-995, 3 times a day, lowered morning plasma GH levels in 12 of 19 patients, whereas GH concentrations were not significantly decreased in the remaining 7 patients. In the latter group, a daily dose of 300 µg or more was required to significantly lower morning plasma GH levels. Barnard et al. (17) reported that some patients required up to 1500 µg/day of SMS 201-995 to significantly lower plasma GH. Plasma SmC/IGF-I levels decreased by continuous treatment with SMS 201-995 in 10 of 12 of our patients. Improvements of clinical manifestations, such as sweating, headache, and paresthesia of extremities, were also noted in the responsive group. As to the side effects, epigastric discomfort, diarrhea, nausea, and constipation were noted in only a few patients. Plasma cholesterol and albumin levels were not significantly changed during the treatment, although plasma glucose levels only slightly and transiently changed in some subjects. These results suggest that SMS 201-995 is an effective and safe drug to lower plasma GH in acromegaly.

One of the problems of SMS 201-995 treatment is the duration of action which is short in some patients. In such patients, 3 injections per day were not sufficient to continuously lower plasma GH levels. We therefore injected 10-22.5 µg of SMS 201-995 every 2 h using a pulsatile infusion pump. In all 5 patients, a daily profile of plasma GH during the pulsatile treatment showed significantly lower levels than those on control days or during the treatment with SMS 201-995, three times a day. Figure 4 shows plasma GH levels in a representative patient which were consistently low throughout the day. It is concluded, therefore, that pulsatile treatment with SMS 201-995 using an infusion pump is an effective means to treat patients who did not respond well to three injections per day of SMS 201-995.

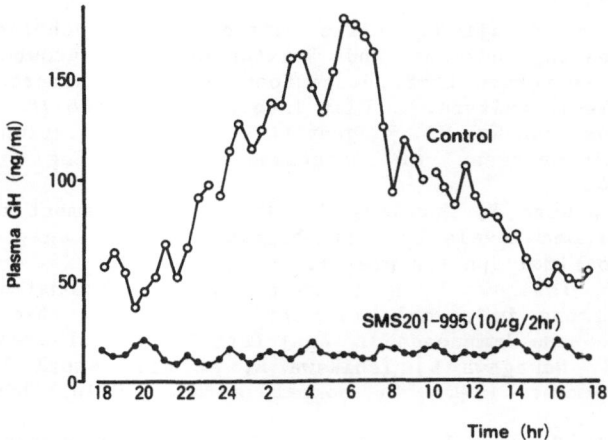

Fig. 4. Twenty-four h profile of plasma GH levels in a patient with acromegaly before and during a pulsatile treatment with SMS 201-995, 10 µg every 2 h.

SUMMARY

New approaches in the diagnosis and treatment of acromegaly are discussed. Urinary GH excretion and plasma SmC/IGF-I levels are of diagnostic value, especially in patients whose plasma GH concentrations are borderline. These tests, as well as plasma GH responses to provocative tests, can be used also for evaluating the results of treatment, especially for detecting residual tumors after surgery. In regard to medical treatment, SMS 201-995, a long-acting analog of somatostatin, is effective even in bromocriptine-resistant cases. Repeated injections of 50 to 100 µg or even more, 3 times a day, are usually required to lower morning plasma GH levels. If 3 injections are not satisfactory, pulsatile administrations of 10-22.5 µg of SMS 201-995 every 2 h by using an intermittent infusion pump are useful to effectively lower plasma GH levels. Cyproheptadine is also effective in some patients.

REFERENCES

1. Beck C, Larkins RG, Martin TJ, et al. Stimulation of growth hormone release from superfused rat pituitary by extracts of hypothalamus and of human lung tumours. J Endocrinol 1973; 59:325-33.
2. Asa SL, Scheithauer BW, Bilbao JM, et al. A case for hypothalamic acromegaly: a clinicopathological study of six patients with hypothalamic gangliocytomas producing growth hormone-releasing factor. J Clin Endocrinol Metab 1984; 58:796-803.
3. Scheithauer BW, Kovacs K, Randall RV, et al. Pathology of excessive production of growth hormone. Clin Endocrinol Metab 1986; 15:665-81.
4. 1980 Annual Report of Study Group on Hypothalamopituitary Diseases supported by Ministry of Health and Welfare, 1980:15-24.
5. Imura H, Kato Y, Ishikawa E. Growth hormone secretion in acromegaly. In: Robbins R, Melmed S, eds. Acromegaly: a century of scientific and clinical progress. New York: Plenum Press, 1987:83-95.
6. Kashio Y, Chihara K, Kaji H, et al. Presence of growth hormone-releasing factor-like immunoreactivity in human cerebrospinal fluid. J Clin Endocrinol Metab 1985; 60:396-8.
7. Matsushita N, Kato Y, Katakami H, et al. Stimulation of growth hormone release by vasoactive intestinal polypeptide from human pituitary adenoma in vitro. J Clin Endocrinol Metab 1981; 53:1297-300.
8. Ishibashi M, Yamaji T. Direct effects of catecholamines, thyrotropin-releasing hormone and somatostatin on growth hormone and prolactin secretion from adenomatous and nonadenomatous human pituitary cells in culture. J Clin Invest 1984; 73:66-78.
9. Clemmons DR, Van Wyk JJ, Ridgway EC, et al. Evaluation of acromegaly by radioimmunoassay of somatomedin-C. N Engl J Med 1979; 301:1138-42.
10. Hattori N, Kato Y, Murakami Y, et al. Measurement of urine human growth hormone levels by ultra-highly sensitive enzyme immunoassay. Folia Endocrinol Jpn (in press).
11. Hashida S, Ishikawa E, Nakagawa K, et al. Demonstration of human growth hormone in normal urine by a highly specific and sensitive sandwich enzyme immunoassay. Anal Lett 1985; 18:1623-34
12. Hashida S, Nakagawa K, Ishikawa E, et al. Basal level of human growth hormone (hGH) in normal serum. Clin Chim Acta 1985; 151:185-6.
13. Grossman A, Ross R, Wass JAH, et al. Depot-bromocriptine treatment for prolactinomas and acromegaly. Clin Endocrinol 1986; 24:231-8.
14. Ishibashi M, Fukushima I, Yamaji T. Cyproheptadine-mediated inhibition of growth hormone and prolactin release from pituitary adenoma cells of acromegaly and gigantism in culture. Acta Endocrinol

(Copenh) 1985; 109:474-80.

15. Lamberts SWJ, Uilterlinden P, Verschoor L, et al. Long-term treatment of acromegaly with the somatostatin analogue SMS 201-995. N Engl J Med 1985; 313:1576-80.

16. Tolis G, Yotis A, del Pozo E, et al. Therapeutic efficacy of somatostatin analogue (SMS 201-995) in active acromegaly. J Neurosurg 1986; 65:37-40.

17. Barnard LB, Grantham WG, Lamberton P, et al. Treatment of resistant acromegaly with a long-acting somatostatin. Ann Intern Med 1986; 105:856-61.

10

SUMMARY OF SESSION II

NEUROENDOCRINE REGULATION OF GROWTH HORMONE SECRETION

John S. Parks, M.D., Ph.D.

Professor of Pediatrics
Emory University School of Medicine
Atlanta, GA 30322

OVERVIEW

The presentations on neuroendocrine regulation of growth hormone (GH) secretion raised several new issues of great interest to basic scientists and clinicians. These were: (1) reciprocal rhythms of growth hormone releasing factor (GHRH) and somatostatin (SRIH) secretion; (2) strategies for chronic, therapeutic modulation of GH release; (3) the potential role of galanin; and, (4) new capabilities for the measurement of extremely low concentrations of GH in serum and urine.

RECIPROCAL RHYTHMS OF GHRH AND SRIH SECRETION

Dr. Tannenbaum's elegant studies in the rat show a 3.3-h ultradian rhythm of GH secretion. The GH spikes represent coincidence of a peak of GHRH secretion and a nadir of SRIH secretion. When GHRH is given at 13:00 h, in the face of maximum SRIH secretion, the GH response is markedly attenuated. Administration of anti-SRIH antibody raises the resting level of GH and permits a maximal response to GHRH. Short loop feedback by GH and long loop feedback by IGF-I appear to involve both an inhibition of GHRH and an enhancement of SRIH secretion.

THERAPEUTIC MODULATION OF GH RELEASE

Similar mechanisms are operative in humans, though the detailed responses to neurotransmitter and environmental stimuli differ. Deficiencies in GH secretion may reflect excess SRIH levels or enhanced pituitary responsiveness to SRIH, as well as deficient generation or activity of GHRH. The varying GH responses to GHRH in normal humans may be due to the timing of the stimulus in relation to peaks of SRIH secretion. Dr. Muller pointed out that more attention needs to be paid to the cholinergic system in regulation of GH release. Pyridostigmine, a cholinesterase inhibitor, enhances responses to GHRH and it appears to do so by inhibiting SRIH release or activity. Episodic release of GH is enhanced and growth rate is improved in some short children by the chronic administration of clonidine, an alpha 2 agonist. Specific pharmacologic probes may prove to be of value in choosing the most effective stimulant to restoration of normal growth in an individual child.

GALANIN

Dr. Martin's account of the galanin story was new to many of us. This 29 amino acid peptide is found in the same hypothalamic neurons as is GHRH. Peak GH responses to galanin are similar in magnitude to those following GHRH, though their onset is delayed. Several questions about the physiologic role of galanin remain to be answered. Dr. Muller observed that GH responses to galanin in the rat require an intact noradrenergic system. Dr. Martin showed that galanin as well as GHRH has a direct effect on GH release by dispersed rat pituitary cells. Furthermore, the effects of the two peptides are additive. Dr. Brazeau questioned the importance of galanin in pointing out that peak responses to galanin required a molar concentration 10,000 times that of GHRH. It remains to be seen whether peptides related to galanin will be useful in the characterization or correction of defective GH secretion.

AN ULTRASENSITIVE ASSAY FOR GH IN SERUM AND URINE

Dr. Imura shed new light into the old disease called acromegaly. An ultrasensitive immunoassay for GH highlights the difference between normal and excessive GH secretion. A greater than one hundredfold increase in sensitivity, to 3 pg/ml, is achieved by coupling a polyclonal antibody to a bead and detecting bound GH with horseradish peroxidase linked to Fab fragments of the same antibody. The normal 50 to 1,000 pg/ml resting GH levels detected with this assay correspond to the levels estimated by Dr. Baumann following immunoaffinity concentration of GH from massive quantities of serum. Measurement of GH in serial blood samples from acromegalics permits a clear differentiation from normals. Furthermore, the assay can be used to measure the extremely small quantities of GH excreted in urine. There is promise that a single morning urinary GH to creatinine ratio will be useful in the diagnosis and posttreatment follow-up of acromegaly. If so, this will be a breakthrough in assessing the effectiveness of surgery or second-line medical management with bromocriptine or the SRIH analog SMS 201-995.

III. ASSESSMENT OF GROWTH HORMONE SECRETION IN CHILDREN

11

DYNAMICS OF GH SECRETION IN CHILDREN

Kerstin Albertsson-Wikland and Sten Rosberg

Departments of Pediatrics II and Physiology
University of Goteborg
Goteborg, Sweden

INTRODUCTION

Growth and development during fetal and early postnatal life proceeds at a normal or near normal rate in the absence of growth hormone (GH) both in experimental animals and in man. Later on, somatic growth progressively becomes dependent upon GH. In contrast to other hormones, GH is the only hormone known to produce a dose-dependent stimulation of proportional body growth: in man, excess of growth hormone (GH) is known to cause gigantism and deficiency of GH leads to hypophyseal dwarfism. However, it is not known whether differences in growth rates among normal children are due to differences in endogenous secretion of GH. There is also insufficient knowledge about the influence of age and sex during the prepubertal period, as well as the influence of puberty on spontaneous GH secretion in children. In normal humans, serum levels of GH fluctuate in a pulsatile pattern, with great inter-individual variations in terms of pulse height and pulse frequency. Surges of GH secretion from the pituitary are spontaneous, with no apparent relationship to external stimuli. The release of pituitary GH is controlled by growth hormone releasing factor (GHRH) and growth hormone inhibitory factor, somatostatin. Each secretory episode of GH is initiated by changes in the concentration of these two hypothalamic peptides in the hypophyseal portal blood. The hypothalamic neuronal cell bodies producing GHRH or somatostatin interact with suprahypothalamic brain regions. Clearly, higher brain centers are involved in the control of GH secretion and, consequently, by affecting the secretory pattern of GH, the brain participates in the regulation of body growth.

Since GH is secreted in bursts (1-3), it is impossible to estimate the amount of secreted GH in children with single blood samples. Moreover, it has been shown that both the total amount of secreted GH and the pattern of GH secretion are of importance for the growth rate in animals (4,5). A pump withdrawal method has been described for measuring GH over a longer period of time (6). Frequent integrated sampling of blood over a 24-h period with this method may thus be a convenient way of getting information on both the total amount of secreted GH and the pattern of GH secretion. In the present study, we have investigated the relationship between age, sex, growth and stage of puberty in normal children versus spontaneous secretion of endogenous GH.

MATERIALS AND METHODS

Study Group

One hundred twelve children of different growth rates were investigated at the Children's Hospital, Goteborg. All children were considered healthy, well nourished and were not under medical treatment at the
time of investigation. All children below -2 SD in height had a normal GH
response to the insulin-arginine test, and had a normal biopsy of the
intestine to exclude celiac disease.

Seventy-six of the children, 54 boys and 22 girls, were prepubertal
(for age and sex distribution, see Figure 1). Their chronologic ages
ranged from 3-16 years, with the same age distribution for boys and girls,
and their bone ages were, at most, 2 years delayed and ranged from 2-14
years. Thirty-six of the children, aged 10-16 years, were in puberty.
Their bone ages ranged from 11-16 years. Their pubertal stages were
estimated according to Tanner (14 children were in stage 2, 13 in stage 3,
and 9 in stage 4). The growth of all the children has been followed since
birth at the Swedish Pediatric Health Care Centers, and after the age of 7
at school. All children followed their "growth channel." The heights at
the time of the investigation were expressed in standard deviation (SD)
scores, in comparison with normal Swedish children (7).

The study was approved by the Ethical Committee of the Medical
Faculty, University of Goteborg. Informed consent was obtained from
parents and patients.

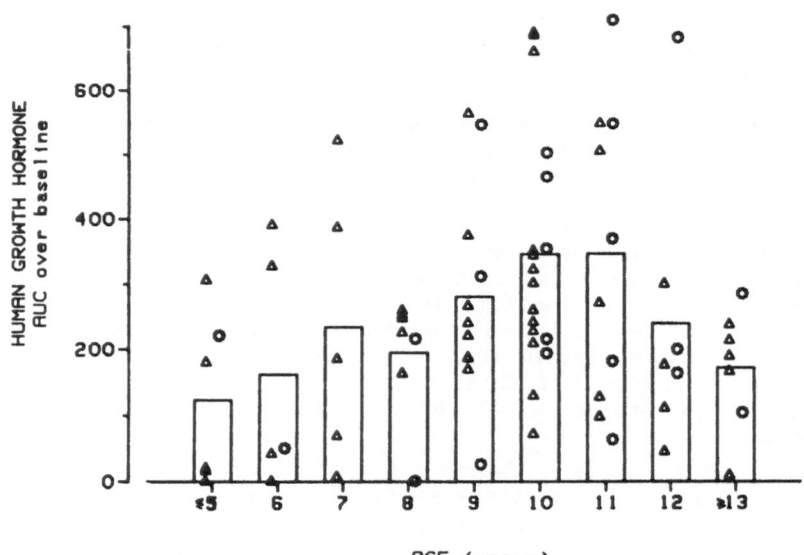

Fig. 1. Age and GH distribution of all prepubertal
children in the study. The GH secretion, estimated
as area under the curve above the calculated baseline (AUC_b), is plotted as a function of age of
prepubertal boys (Δ) or girls (o). The bars indicate the mean AUC_b, boys and girls together, for
each age group.

Study Protocol

The children stayed at the hospital for at least 2 days. They received a normal diet, with breakfast at 8:00, lunch at 12:00, dinner at 5:00, and they were allowed normal activity and sleep. A heparinized needle (Viggo AB, Helsingborg, Sweden) was inserted the first evening. The following morning, at 8:00-9:00, the blood withdrawal began. A Sigma motor constant withdrawal pump with a nonthrombogenic catheter (Viggo AB, Helsingborg, Sweden; Hepcote®, LKB, Stockholm, Sweden) was used, according to the Cormed-Kowarski method (6). The heparinized tubes were changed every 20 min for 24 h; therefore, there were 72 samples.

Treatment of Samples and hGH Measurements

The heparinized tubes of blood were kept at room temperature, and centrifuged within 24 h. After centrifugation, the plasma samples were frozen and stored until assayed. We found that repeated freezing-thawing cycles did not detrimentally affect the plasma GH levels. Generally, the assays were performed 1-3 weeks after sampling. However, assays repeated up to 4 years after the first assay gave virtually identical results.

Measurement of GH was performed by a double antibody radioimmunoassay, using goat polyclonal antibodies. The WHO first IRP hGH 66217 was used as standard, with levels expressed in mU/l (2 mU/l = 1 ng/ml). Duplicate samples were assayed and the intra-assay coefficients of variation were 29%, 19%, 13% and 8% at 2, 5, 15 and 50 mU/l, respectively. The inter-assay coefficients of variation were 33%, 30%, 11% and 8% at 2, 5, 15 and 50 mU/l, respectively. Diluted samples paralleled the standard curve, and the recovery was approximately 100%. The minimal detectable concentration, estimated according to Rodbard (8), averaged 1 mU/l (at P<0.01 confidence level) for 20 µl samples. All samples in a 24-h GH profile were run in the same assay.

Analysis of 24-h GH Profiles

The pattern of pulses in the 24-h GH profiles were analyzed with the Pulsar program of Merriam and Wachter (9). The calculations were performed on a desktop computer (Hewlett Packard 9845B) with the Pulsar program translated to HP-Basic (SR). The standard deviation coefficients of the assay were calculated from the duplicates of the 24-h GH curve.

The parameters $G(1)$ to $G(5)$ of the Pulsar program were set to: $G(1)=3.98$, $G(2)=2.4$, $G(3)=1.7$, $G(4)=1.2$, $G(5)=0.9$. The smoothing time was set at half of the total profile time, i.e., 12 h (36 points) for the 24-h GH profiles. The splitting cutoff parameter was set at 2.7, and the weight assigned to peaks was 0.05. The program did not, with these settings, detect any peaks in 72 consecutive samples in each of three different plasma pools.

From the Pulsar analyses of the 24-h GH curves, the following values were extracted: the overall mean, the maximal value, the minimal value, the mean of the baseline, the number of peaks, the mean inter-peak interval, the mean height of peaks, the mean length of peaks, the mean peak amplitude, and the peak area. The area under the curve (AUC) was estimated above the zero level (AUC_t) as well as above the calculated baseline (AUC_b).

Statistics

The correlation coefficient (r) for linear correlation of the second kind, with 95% tolerance limits (ellipse), are given (11). Two-way analysis of variance was used to test the influence of sex and age, respectively, on the distribution of AUC_b in Figure 1.

RESULTS

Twenty-four-hour GH Profiles versus Age and Sex in Prepubertal Children

The age distribution of the prepubertal children, as well as the AUC above the calculated baseline, AUC_b, for the different ages is shown in Figure 1. As can be seen from the figure, there was no sex difference in the AUC_b (P=0.2 with two-way ANOVA), nor was there any correlation between the AUC_b and the age of the children (r=0.2, P>0.1).

Twenty-four-hour GH Profiles versus Height

Typical 24-h GH profiles of a prepubertal child of short stature (height below -2 SD), of normal stature (height within ± 2 SD) and of tall stature (height above +2 SD) are shown in Figure 2.

The height expressed in standard deviation (SD) scores of the 76 prepubertal children was found to be highly correlated (r=0.65; P<0.001) with the total amount of measured GH, expressed as AUC_b over the 24-h period (Fig. 3). A significant correlation of AUC_b was also found versus height expressed in cm, and versus height velocity in SD score. No difference was seen, in these respects, between girls and boys. The correlation was less prominent when AUC above zero line was used as an estimate of the total amount of GH. Correlations between the heights of the children, expressed in SD scores, and other estimates from the 24-h GH profiles were also found, i.e., with the amplitude, the length, and the area of the peaks.

Twenty-four-hour GH Profiles versus Stage of Puberty

The result of a cross-sectional study in children of different pubertal stages is shown in Figure 4. Estimation of spontaneously secreted GH over a 24-h period, AUC_b, is plotted versus the pubertal stage of 36 pubertal children. A marked increase in GH secretion was seen at pubertal stage 3 and 4. The mean value, the AUC over zero level, the AUC_b, the peak maximum, the peak height and the peak area, respectively, all increased in pubertal stage 3 and 4 (data not shown). However, the number of peaks and the length of the peaks did not differ with the pubertal stage.

Typical 24-h GH profiles of 3 children in puberty, in pubertal stage 2, 3, and 4, respectively, are shown in Figure 5.

DISCUSSION

In the present study, we have analyzed the 24-h GH profiles of prepubertal and pubertal boys and girls of different ages and heights. The measured GH secretion was not obviously influenced by the age of the

Fig. 2 (opposite page). Twenty-four-hour GH profiles of prepubertal children of different heights. In the top part of the figure, a short (≤2 SD) child is shown (12.5-year-old boy, -2.0 SD); in the middle part of the figure, a normal child (± 1 SD) is shown (6-year-old boy, 0.8 SD); and in the bottom part of the figure, a tall child (≥2 SD) is shown (10-year-old boy, 4.5 SD).

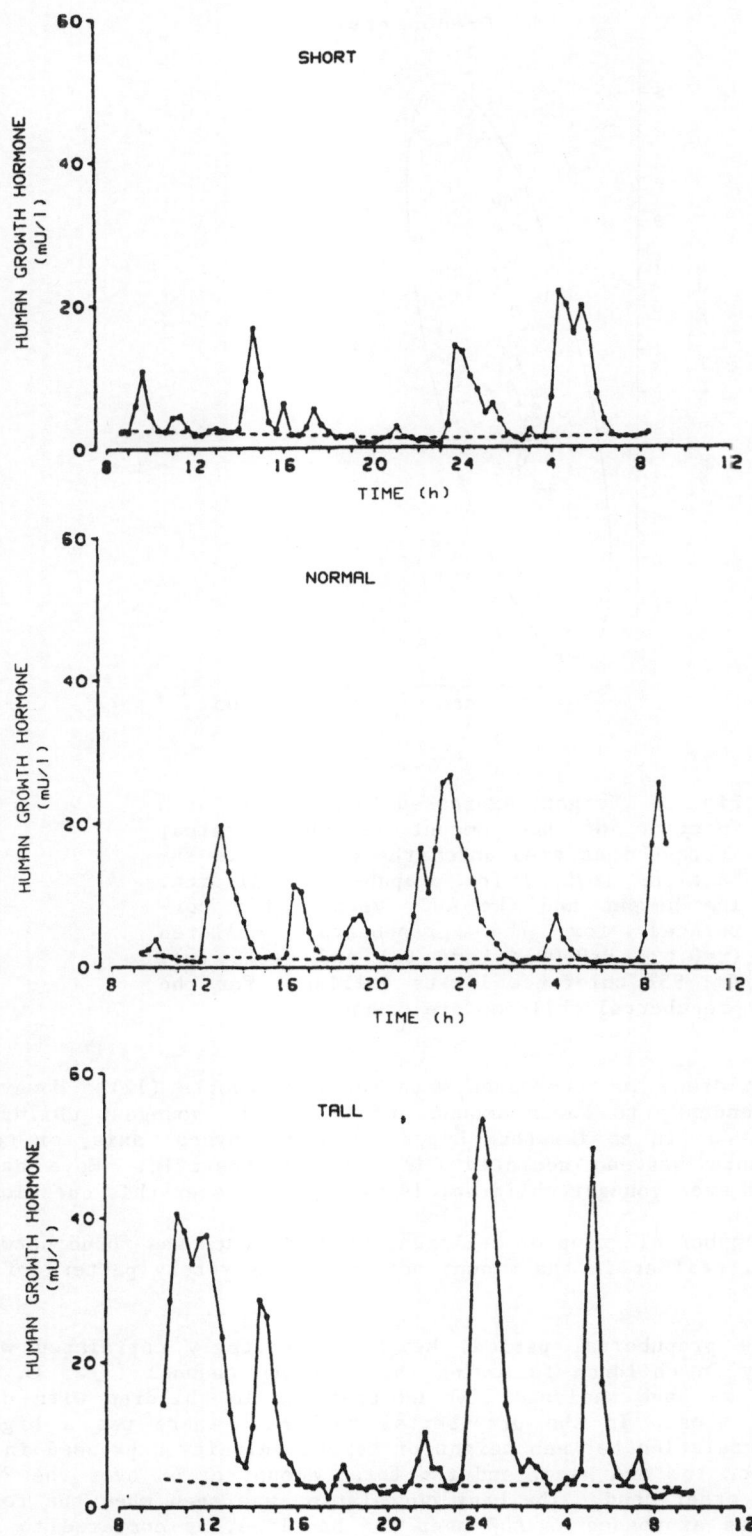

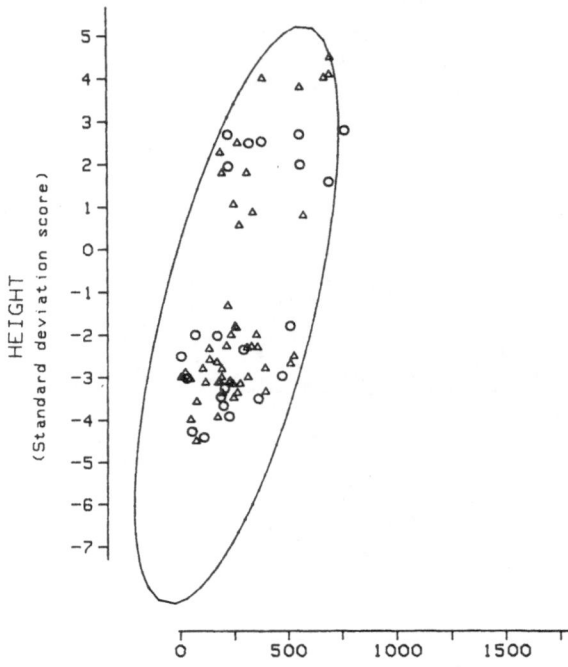

Fig. 3. Height, expressed in SD score, as a
function of the amount of GH secreted,
expressed as area under the curve above the
baseline (AUC$_b$), for prepubertal children.
The height and the AUC$_b$ were highly correlated for the prepubertal children
(r=0.63; P<0.001; boys (Δ) and girls (o).
The 95% tolerance limits (ellipse) for the
prepubertal children are drawn.

prepubertal children, in accordance with earlier reports (12). However,
there was a tendency to lower amounts of GH in the youngest children,
which might be due to an immature hypothalamo-hypophyseal axis, or to a
different balance between secreted GHRH and somatostatin. More data,
preferably from even younger children, is needed to answer this question.

In the prepubertal group of children, no difference was found between
boys and girls, neither in the amount nor in the secretory pattern of GH
secretion.

During the prepubertal period, height is strongly correlated with
height velocity in children following their growth channel (7). In the
present study, we have analyzed 24-h GH profiles in children with different growth rates. In the prepubertal children, there was a highly
significant correlation between height or height velocity expressed in SD
scores or cm, on the one hand, and the total amount of GH over the 24-h
period, on the other hand. The best correlation was seen when the total
amount of GH was expressed as AUC over the baseline, as compared to AUC
over the zero line. The reason for this difference might be that the

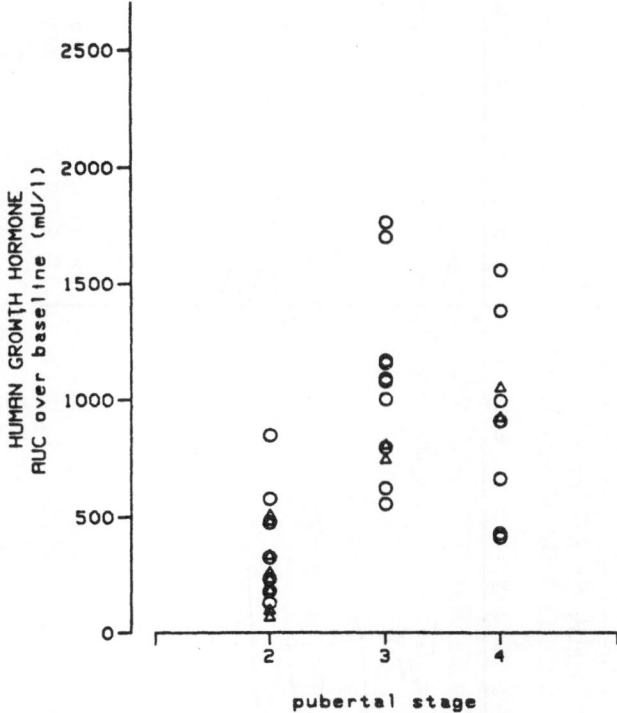

Fig. 4. The pubertal stage as a function of the
GH secreted, expressed as area under the curve
above the baseline (AUC$_b$) for boys (Δ) and girls
(o). The AUC$_b$ at stage 3 and 4 are both significantly higher than that at stage 2 (P<0.01).

influence of the inter- and intra-assay variation in the lower part of the
standard curve is minimized by subtracting the calculated baseline. It is
also possible that the peak pattern and peak amplitude of GH is the dominant factor determining growth rate, and that the AUC cver the baseline
is a better estimate of this factor. In fact, the height, length and area
of the peaks all gave highly significant correlations with the growth of
the children.

The finding that height correlates with the secretec amount of GH is
not surprising, since there is a well-known dose-respcnse relationship
between GH and somatic growth. In general, short children secrete less
amount of GH compared to taller children. However, the ranges of the
secreted GH within the groups are large and overlapping, thereby making it
difficult to estimate a cutoff limit for diagnostic purposes.

The results presented in this study clearly show that a correlation
exists between growth and the amount of spontaneously secreted GH in
normal prepubertal children, over a wide range of growth rates, including
the normal range. Thus, in a certain fraction of short children, a low
secretion rate of GH may be the limiting factor for height velocity
(13-15). In fact, children with the lowest amount of secreted GH have
been given exogenous GH, despite normal responses to provocative tests;
and the results from this treatment indicate that these children benefit
from the GH treatment. Moreover, there was an inverse relationship
between growth response to therapy and spontaneously secreted GH (16).

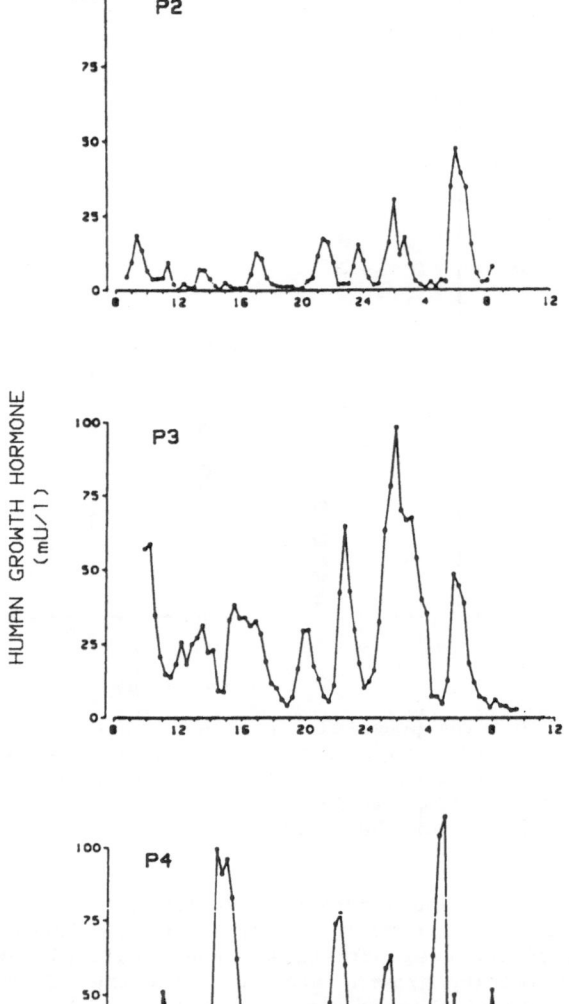

Fig. 5. Spontaneous GH secretory pattern
in 3 girls of pubertal stage 2 (top),
stage 3 (middle), and stage 4 (bottom).

In the pubertal group, there was also a correlation between growth
and GH secretion. In this group, height velocity correlated much better
than the height of the child.

During puberty, there was a marked increase in GH secretion in both
boys and girls. However, the GH secretion in girls seems to increase at

an earlier pubertal stage than in boys. Interestingly, this parallels the pubertal growth spurt which occurs earlier in girls than in boys. There are recent reports indicating the influence of estrogen, but not testosterone, on GH secretion (17,18). The rise of estrogen early in puberty in girls may account for increased GH secretion and, ultimately, the growth spurt. However, longitudinal studies are needed to explore the dynamics of GH secretion during puberty.

ACKNOWLEDGMENTS

We would like to thank Ms. Marianne Svensson for her excellent technical help; the staff at ward 34, Children's Hospital, Goteborg, for taking care of the children; Dr. Johan Karlberg for carrying out the growth analyses; and Dr. Olle Isaksson and Dr. Otto Westphal for their stimulating discussions. The Pulsar program was kindly provided by Dr. George Merriam.

This work was supported by grants from the Swedish Medical Research Council (6465, 7509, 27), the Swedish Society of Medical Sciences, Jeansson's Foundation, Lundgren's Foundation, Tore Nilsson's Foundation and KabiVitrum AB.

REFERENCES

1. Finkelstein JW, Roffwarg HP, Boyar RM, Kream J, Hellman L. Age related change in the twenty-four-hour spontaneous secretion of growth hormone. J Clin Endocrinol Metab 1972; 35:665-70.
2. Plotnick LP, Thompson RG, Kowarski A, de Lacerda L, Migeon CJ, Blizzard RM. Circadian variation of integrated concentration of growth hormone in children and adults. J Clin Endocrinol Metab 1975; 40:240-6.
3. Miller JD, Tannenbaum GS, Colle E, Guyda HJ. Daytime pulsatile growth hormone secretion during childhood and adolescence. J Clin Endocrinol Metab 1982; 55:989-94.
4. Jansson JO, Albertsson-Wikland K, Eden S, Thorngren K-G, Isaksson O. Circumstantial evidence for a role of the secretory pattern of growth hormone in control of body growth. Acta Endocrinol (Copenh) 1982; 99:24-30.
5. Clark RG, Jansson JO, Isaksson O, Robinson ICAF. Intravenous growth hormone: growth responses to patterned infusions in hypophysectomized rats. J Endocrinol 1985; 104:53-61.
6. Kowarski A, Thompson RG, Migeon CJ, Blizzard RM. Determination of integrated concentration of true secretion rate of human growth hormone. J Clin Endocrinol Metab 1971a; 32:356-60.
7. Karlberg P, Taranger J, Engstrom I, Lichtenstein H, Svennberg-Redegren I. The somatic development of children in a Swedish urban community. Acta Paediatr Scand (suppl) 1976; 258:1.
8. Rodbard D. Statistical estimation of the minimal detectable concentration ("sensitivity") for radioligand assays. Anal Biochem 1978; 90:1-12.
9. Merriam GR, Wachter KW. Algorithms for the study of episodic hormone secretion. Am J Physiol 1982; 243:E310-8.
10. Veldhuis JD, Rogol AD, Johnson ML. Minimizing false-positive errors in hormonal pulse detection. Am J Physiol 1985; 248:E475-81.
11. Scientific tables. Diem K, Lentner C, eds. Basel, Switzerland: Ciba-Geigy Ltd., 1970.
12. Zadik Z, Chalew SA, McCarter RJ, Meistas M, Kowarski AA. The influence of age on the 24-hour integrated concentration of growth hormone in normal individuals. J Clin Endocrinol Metab 1985;

      60:513-6.
13.   Bierich JR.   Constitutionally low growth hormone secretion.   In:
      Ranke M, Bierich JR, eds.   Workshop on growth hormone deficiency,
      Tubingen, 1981.   Munich, Vienna, Baltimore: Urban & Schwarzenberg,
      1984.
14.   Spiliotis BE, August GP, Hung W, Sonis W, Mendelson W, Bercu BB.
      Growth hormone neurosecretory dysfunction.   A treatable cause of
      short stature.   JAMA 1984; 251:2223-30.
15.   Zadik Z, Chalew SA, Raiti S, Kowarski AA.   Do short children secrete
      insufficient growth hormone?   Pediatrics 1985b; 76:355-60.
16.   Albertsson-Wikland K.   Growth hormone treatment in short children.
      Acta Paediatr Scand (suppl) 1986; 325:64-70.
17.   Ho KY, Evans WS, Blizzard RM, et al.   Effects of sex and age on the
      24 hour secretory profile of GH secretion in man: importance of
      endogenous estradiol concentrations.   J Clin Endocrinol Metab 1987;
      64:51-8
18.   Link K, Blizzard RM, Evans WS, Kaiser DL, Parker MW, Rogol AD.   The
      effect of androgens on the pulsatile release and the twenty-four-hour
      mean concentration of growth hormone in peripubertal males.   J Clin
      Endocrinol Metab 1986; 62:159-64.

12

GROWTH HORMONE NEUROSECRETORY DYSFUNCTION: UPDATE

Barry B. Bercu, M.D.

Department of Pediatrics, University of South Florida
College of Medicine, Tampa, and All Children's Hospital,
St. Petersburg, Florida 33731

INTRODUCTION

The neuroregulation of GH secretion is complex involving the dual regulatory control of a GH releasing hormone (GHRH) and GH inhibiting hormone (somatostatin or SRIH) (see Figures 1 and 2). These neurohormones are further regulated by neurotransmitters (Fig. 1). Experimental evidence (animal and human) for anatomic distribution and the possible role of neurotransmitters (dopaminergic, catecholaminergic, cholinergic, serotonergic, histaminergic, gama-aminobutyric acidergic) are reviewed in greater detail elsewhere (1,2). We hypothesize that defects in the neuro-regulatory control of GH secretion results in decreased or disordered GH secretion which is, ultimately, expressed as poor growth velocity and short stature.

The time-honored definition of GH deficiency has been based on blunted provocative GH testing in the appropriate clinical setting (poor growth velocity, delayed skeletal age). However, it had been suspected that some children may have disturbances in GH secretion not detected by conventional provocative testing. Insight into a treatable cause of short stature, we termed GH neurosecretory (GHND) (significantly short children with one or more normal GH provocative tests, poor growth velocity, delayed skeletal age), comes from a series of studies and observations which are briefly summarized here.

Reduced growth rate is frequently associated with cranial irradiation. Classical GH deficiency occurs after high-dose cranial irradiation involving the hypothalamic-pituitary area (3,4). Lesser doses of cranial irradiation cause variable results in standard provocative GH testing (4-15). Clinical (9,10) and animal (15) studies done in parallel by our group led to the conclusion that there was a defect in neurosecretion of GH in leukemic children who received prophylactic cranial irradiation (see reviews, references 1 and 2). Figure 3 shows an example of endogenous GH secretion in a child who previously received central nervous system irradiation. Such children frequently have normal GH secretion following standard provocative GH testing. In summary, these studies demonstrated: (1) correlation of anatomic (brain computerized axial tomography) abnormalities to endogenous GH secretion; (2) lack of correlation of endogenous GH secretion with provocative GH testing; and, (3) differential interpretation of previously considered "standard" provocative GH testing

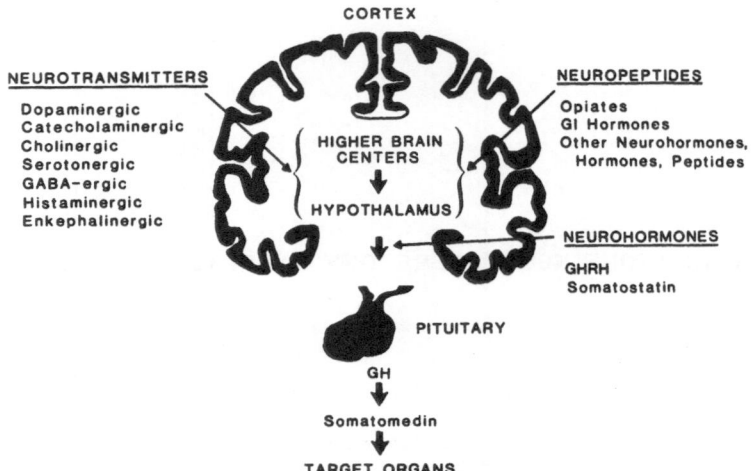

CORTEX

NEUROTRANSMITTERS

Dopaminergic
Catecholaminergic
Cholinergic
Serotonergic
GABA-ergic
Histaminergic
Enkephalinergic

HIGHER BRAIN
CENTERS

HYPOTHALAMUS

NEUROPEPTIDES

Opiates
GI Hormones
Other Neurohormones,
Hormones, Peptides

NEUROHORMONES

GHRH
Somatostatin

PITUITARY

GH

Somatomedin

TARGET ORGANS

Fig. 1. Diagrammatic representation of neurotransmitters, neurohormones and neuropeptides which regulate GH secretion. Reprinted with permission (1).

(e.g., the response of GH to L-dopa and insulin-induced hypoglycemia stimulation may be different, depending on the underlying etiologic problem).

Exogenous hGH treatment has been used effectively in a variety of children without classical GH deficiency. Various terminologies have been used to describe this heterogenous group: "normal variant short stature" (19), "biologically inactive GH molecule" (20-24), "GH-dependent growth failure" (25), and "idiopathic short stature." On the other hand, approximately 40% of short (<first percentile) prepubertal children will have a short-term increase in growth rate (mean increase 3.2 cm/yr) after hGH therapy (26). Other investigators have demonstrated short-term growth velocity acceleration in short children without classical GH deficiency (27,28). Our approach had been to examine the GH neurosecretory axis. We subsequently described a subgroup of short-statured children (GHND), who had decreased endogenous GH secretion and responded to exogenous hGH (29,30).

Here we present our cumulative experience at All Children's Hospital (University of South Florida) on GHND, classical GH deficient and control children.

Fig. 2 (opposite page). Diagrammatic representation of GHRH and somatostatin in the human adult hypothalamus. (a), (b) and (c) are frontal sections from anterior to posterior planes redrawn with kind permission from Daniel and Prichard (16); with permission, GHRH is represented by dots and redrawn from Bloch et al. (17). Somatostatin is represented by diagonal lines; these are taken from the written description by Cooper et al. (18). The GHRH cell bodies around the inferior portion of a more anterior view and the somatostatin cell bodies in the suprachiasmatic nucleus are not shown. Abbreviations: ARC = arcuate nucleus; AC = anterior commissure; D = nucleus of diagonal band; DM = dorsomedial nucleus; F = fornix; IR = infundibular recess; LV = lateral ventricle; ME = median eminence; MF = midline fissure; OT = optic tract; PO = preoptic nucleus; PV = paraventricular nucleus; S = pituitary stalk; SO = supraoptic nucleus; T = lateral tuber nucleus; V3 = third ventricle; VM = ventromedial nucleus.

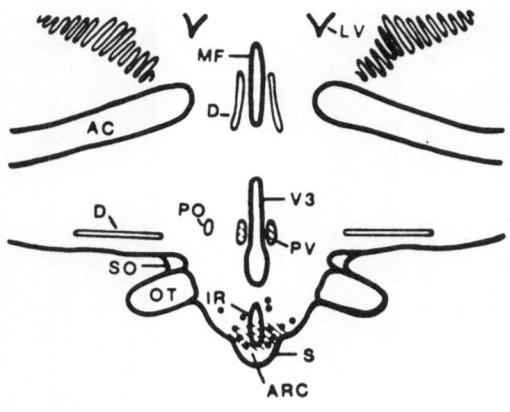

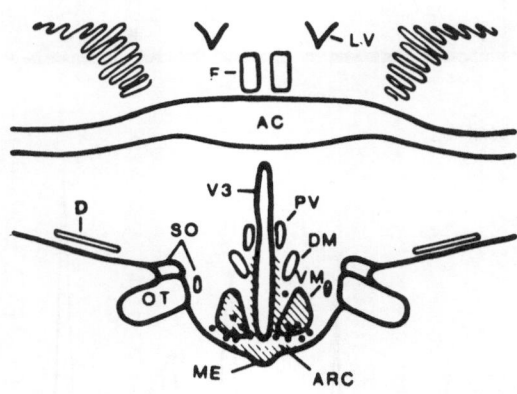

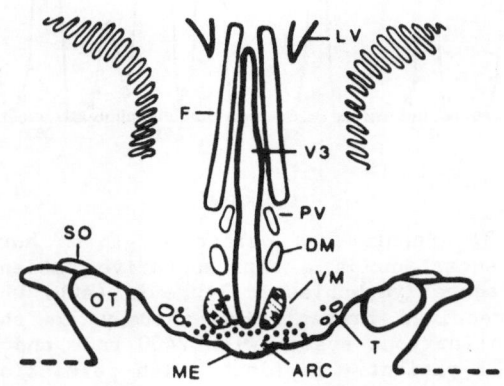

(See Figure 2 legend on opposite page.)

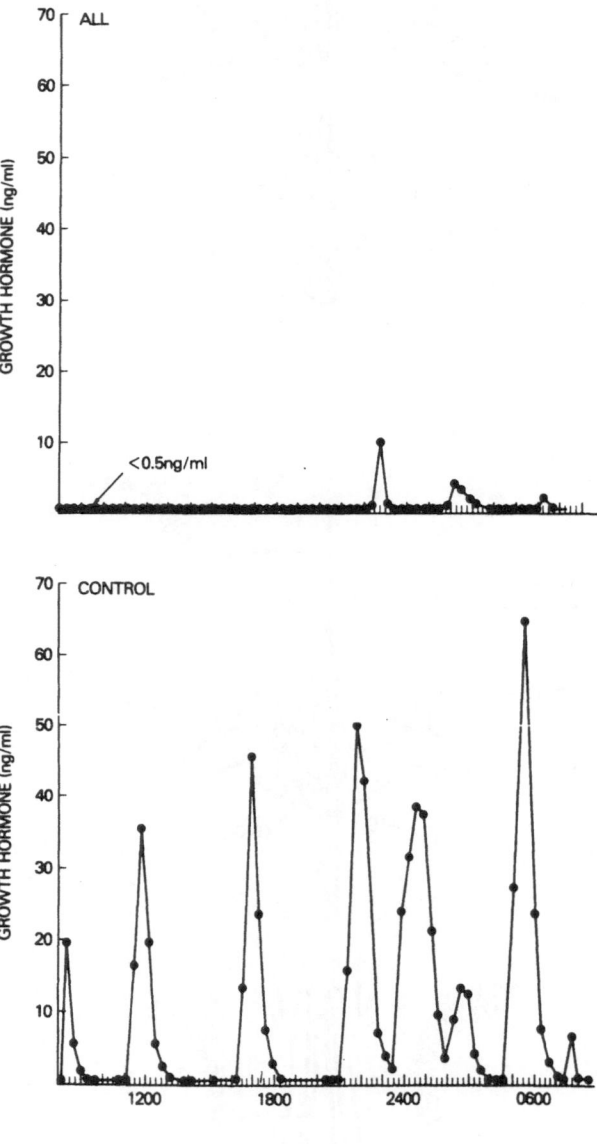

CLOCK TIME

Fig. 3. Spontaneous pulsatile growth hormone secretion in a representative patient with acute lymphoblastic leukemia (ALL) who had received preventative therapy to the central nervous system with 2400 rads and a control patient. Reprinted with permission (13).

MATERIALS AND METHODS

Patient Groups and Study Protocol

Seventy-one children were referred for evaluation of short stature. One additional child was referred for tall stature and is included in the control group. All children underwent provocative testing with two or more pharmacological stimuli (arginine 0.5 g IV; insulin 0.1 U/kg IV; L-dopa 250-500 mg orally; and clonidine 0.15 mg/m2 orally). The GH secretory response to GHRH 1-40 (1 µg/kg IV) was also measured in most children. The GH responses after GHRH were considered separately from assessment of the peak GH responses to other provocative stimuli. GHRH was kindly provided by Dr. Michael Thorner of the University of Virginia (Charlottesville, VA) and Drs. Wylie Vale and Jean Rivier of the Salk Institute (La Jolla, CA). All children underwent a 24-h study of endogenous GH secretion. Plasma somatomedin-C (SmC)/insulin-like growth factor-I (IGF-I) concentrations were determined at 0900 and 2100 h during the 24-h study. Clinical data including chronologic age, bone age, growth velocity and Tanner staging are presented in Table 1. Breast and genital stages were defined according to the method of Tanner (31). Bone age was determined by the method of Greulich and Pyle (32). No child had hypothyroidism or malnutrition.

For the 24-h study, all children were fasted after 2400 h. The following morning prior to 0800 h, an indwelling catheter was placed in a forearm vein. One ml blood samples were obtained every 20 min for 24 h. During this time, children ate standard hospital meals and were encouraged to continue normal activity. Based on the mean concentration of GH in the 73 samples and the peak responses to provocative testing, patients were categorized into three major groups: classical GH deficiency (n=22 [10 organic, 12 idiopathic]; peak GH response to provocative testing ≤10 ng/ml); GHND (n=22 [9 organic, 13 idiopathic], peak GH response to any single provocative test ≥10 ng/ml, mean 24-h GH <2.6 ng/ml); and control (n=26; peak GH response to provocative testing ≥10 ng/ml, mean 24-h GH concentration ≥2.6 ng/ml). Children in the classical GH deficient and GHND groups with the exception of 10 patients (6 classical GH deficient, 4 GHND) were growing at a rate of ≤4.0 cm/yr during a minimum of 6 months of observation; of these 10 children, 8 were pubertal. One prepubertal child with classical GH deficiency had microphallus, TSH and ACTH deficiencies. He grew at a rate of 6.4 cm/yr. All but 5 patients in the control group were growing at a rate of >4.0 cm/yr during a similar period of observation.

Assays

Serum GH concentrations were measured by a double antibody radioimmunoassay (33). All 73 GH samples from an individual child were measured in a single assay. Intra- and interassay coefficients of variation for GH were less than 12.5% for values above 5 ng/ml and less than 4.0% for values between 0.5 and 2 ng/ml. The sensitivity of the GH assay varied between 0.5 and 1.0 ng/ml. Samples measuring below the sensitivity of the assay were assigned the value of the lowest standard. SmC/IGF-I was measured using a kit from Nichols Institute. Serum prolactin was measured by double antibody radioimmunoassay (34).

Statistical Analysis

Pulsatile GH secretory data were analyzed at the University of Virginia with a computer program referred to as cluster analysis (35). Mean peak GH pulse was defined as the arithmetic mean of significant GH pulses. Highest nocturnal GH pulse was defined as the peak GH hormone level meas-

Table 1. Summary of clinical information on classical GH deficient, GHND and control children.

	Age Range (years)	Tanner Stage		Bone Age Delay	Growth Velocity cm/yr	SmC/IGH-I U/ml
		Breast(♀)/Genit(♂)	Pubic Hair			
I. Classical GH deficiency (n=22)						
Female(7)	10.8-17.3 (14.0±0.9)*	I(4)[a] III(2)	I(4) III(2) V(1)	5.0-0.0 (3.3±0.9) V(1)	1.0-3.7 (2.3±0.5)	0.16-1.37 (0.58±0.20)
Male(15)	8.1-17.3 (13.3±0.8)	I(5) II(6)	I(9) II(2) III(3)	5.5-1.3 (2.7±0.3) III(3) IV(1)	0.0-6.4 (3.1±0.5)	0.17-1.26 (0.59±0.11)
II. GHND (n=22)						
Female(9)	7.1-17.0 (12.3±0.9)	I(7) II(1)	I(8) V(1) III(1)	5.4-0.0[b] (2.4±0.6)	1.0-4.0 (3.2±0.8)	0.16-3.69 (0.98±0.36)
Male(13)	7.2-16.3 (12.0±0.7)	I(7) II(5)	I(11) II(2) IV(1)	4.3-1.7 (2.5±0.2)	2.7-4.8 (3.5±0.2)	0.36-1.00 (0.58±0.06)
III. Control (Endogenous GH Sufficient; n=26)						
Female(7)	5.8-12.6 (10.5±1.0)	I(6) II(1)	I(6) II(1)	3.5-1.4 (2.0±0.3)	3.2-6.5 (5.1±0.4)	0.74-2.64 (1.33±0.26)
Male(19)	4.0-16.8 (11.4±0.8)	I(12) II(6)	I(16) II(3) III(1)	4.5(+2.0) (2.1±0.3)	2.7-8.8 (4.8±0.2)	0.08-2.40 (0.77±0.13)

*mean ± SE
[a] number of children in each stage of puberty in parentheses.
[b] includes child with septo-optic dysplasia treated for 8 years with exogenous GH.
Genit = genitalia

ured between 2200 and 0600 h. The nurse drawing the blood specimens also noted the time at which the patient first fell asleep; this allowed for identification of the first GH peak following onset of sleep. In addition to calculating the mean of the 73 GH specimens, daytime (0800-1600 h), and nighttime pools (2200 to 0600 h) were assessed for GH concentration. Analysis of variance and Scheffe's test were also used to analyze the data. Data are expressed as mean ± standard error. A P value of <0.05 was considered statistically significant.

RESULTS

Endogenous and Provocative GH Secretion

Endogenous pulsatile GH data and peak GH responses to provocative testing (excluding GHRH) are shown in Table 2 and Figures 4 and 5. Mean 24-h GH concentrations were similar for the classical GH deficient (1.7 ± 0.4 ng/ml) and GHND (2.0 ± 0.3 ng/ml) children. Both groups had significantly lower mean 24-h GH levels compared to control children (4.4 ± 0.3 ng/ml) (P<0.001). Peak GH concentration after provocative testing was higher in control (23.5 ± 2.2 ng/ml) and GHND groups (18.5 ± 1.5 ng/ml) than in the classical GH deficient group (5.6 ± 0.7 ng/ml) (P<0.01). The peak GH response of the GHND group was intermediate between classical GH deficient and control but not statistically different from control children.

Mean peak GH responses and percent of individuals with a GH response of ≥10 ng/ml to specific provocative agents including GHRH are shown in Table 3 and Figures 6 to 8. Mean peak GH responses (except for L-dopa test) for the GHND group were intermediate between the control and classical GH deficient groups. Only 39% of the GHND group responded to insulin-induced hypoglycemia with a peak GH concentration ≥10 ng/ml compared to 78% of control children. GHND children responded best to clonidine (59% vs. 82% of controls) and GHRH (75% vs. 93% of controls).

Fifty percent of classical GH deficient children also responded to one injection of GHRH. The mean GH secretory response (area under the curve) to GHRH was decreased for classical GH deficient compared to control children (P<0.01); the GHND group was intermediate (Fig. 9). Although GHND children had an intermediate GH secretory response to insulin-induced hypoglycemia (mean for group was 9.7 ± 1.3 ng/ml), Figure 10 demonstrates a young girl with idiopathic empty sella syndrome in whom a normal GH response to insulin-induced hypoglycemia was evident, and yet 24-h endogenous GH secretion was extremely low. This child's growth velocity increased from 3.6 to 7.6 cm/yr during GH therapy.

The number and magnitude of GH peaks within each group are shown in Figure 11. Control children had the highest total number of peaks as well as the most peaks measuring 5 ng/ml or greater compared to the other two groups. Interestingly, the classical GH deficient group had the greatest number of small peaks (<5 ng/ml) (P<0.05 vs. control group). Few GH peaks >20 ng/ml were observed in either the GHND (2 patients) or the classical GH deficient (1 patient) groups. Mean peak GH pulse was significantly greater in the control group compared to other groups (P<0.01) (Table 2). The importance of pulsatile GH activity in stimulating growth is exemplified in Figure 12. This patient (included in the classical GH deficient group) had TSH and ACTH deficiency following surgery and radiation therapy for a cerebellar astrocytoma. Although her mean GH concentration was 3.3 ng/ml which was in the normal range, no distinct GH pulses were observed over an 18-h sampling period.

Table 2. Summary of pulsatile and peak provocative data.

	Mean 24-h G ng/ml	Highest Peak GH After Provocative Testing ng/ml	Pool GH Day/Night ng/m.	Mean Peak GH Pulse ng/ml	Peak GH After First Asleep ng/ml	Highest Nocturnal GH Pulse ng/ml
I. Classical GH Deficiency (n=22)						
Mean±SE	1.7±0.2	5.6±0.7	1.2±0.1/2.2±0.3	3.6±0.4	5.5±1.0	6.5±1.2
Range	0.7-3.3	1.0-9.8	0.5-3.7/0.5-4.2	1.0-8.9	1.0-12.1	1.0-21.5
II. GHND (n=22)						
Mean±SE	2.0±0.1	18.5±1.5	1.2±0.1/3.0±0.2	6.1±0.6	10.4±1.3	11.2±1.2
Range	1.0-2.6	10.6-29.2	0.5-2.2/1.0-4.8	1.0-14.2	1.0-21.1	1.0-24.8
III. Control (n=26)						
Mean±SE	4.4±0.3	23.5±2.2	2.5±0.2/7.0±0.7	12.1±1.1	22.1±2.6	25.2±2.3
Range	2.0-7.7	9.7-45.9	0.5-4.2/1.9-18.6	4.9-24.5	8.3-44.4	10.7-54.8

See appropriate figures for results of statistical analyses.

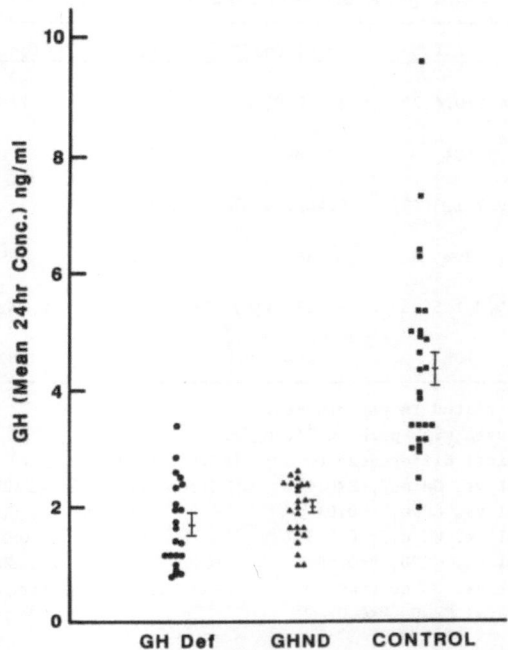

Fig. 4. Mean 24-h GH concentrations in classical GH deficient, GHND and control groups.

Pooled Data and Circadian Patterns

The first GH peak after sleep and the highest nocturnal pulse was of intermediate magnitude in GHND children compared to control and classical GH deficient groups (Table 2 and Figure 13). While 23 out of 24 (96%)

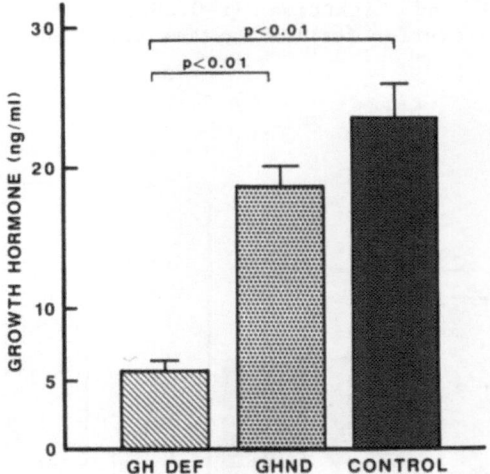

Fig. 5. Highest peak GH concentration following GH provocative stimulation (excluding GHRH) in the three groups of children.

Table 3. Mean peak GH response to provocative testing.

	ITT	Arginine	L-dopa	Clonidine	GHRH
I. GH Deficiency	4.2±0.6(23)[a]	3.2±0.9(16)	3.0±0.5(17)	4.7±0.6(20)	12.2±3.2(18)
	0%[b]	0%	0%	0%	50%
II. GHND	9.7±1.3(18)	9.4±1.3(13)	9.7±1.3(18)	14.2±2.3(17)	26.2±6.2(12)
	39%	38%	50%	59%	75%
III. Control	14.0±1.5(23)	16.2±3.0(14)	14.0±1.5(23)	21.3±2.3(22)	35.6±5.2(15)
	78%	64%	33%	82%	93%

[a] number of patients tested in parentheses.
[b] percent of individuals with peak GH ≥10 ng/ml.
Summary of statistical differences below: (ANOVA:Scheffe's test)

ITT: Control vs. GH def, P<0.001   Clon: Control vs. GH def, P<0.001
     Control vs. GHND, P<0.01   Control vs. GHND, P<0.05
Arg: Control vs. GH def, P<0.001   GH def vs. GHND, P<0.01
     Control vs. GHND, P<0.05   GHRH: Control vs. GH def, P<0.01
L-dopa: Control vs. GH def, P<0.001   ITT = insulin tolerance test
        GH def vs. GHND, P<0.01

control children had a peak GH level of >10 ng/ml after the child first went to sleep, 9 of 19 (47%) GHND children and 4 of 23 (17%) classical GH deficient children had a similar response. All control children had a nocturnal pulse of >10 ng/ml, whereas 13 of 21 (62%) GHND and 5 of 23 (22%) classical GH deficient children had a nocturnal pulse of this magnitude or greater.

The correlation of the single pooled 24-h GH concentration was very high compared to the mean 24-h concentration (mean of 73 samples) (r=0.97, P<0.001). Mean 24-h GH concentration correlated positively with daytime (r=0.70, P<0.001) and nighttime (r=0.88, P<0.001) pools. There was significantly more overlap for the daytime vs. 24-h GH concentration.

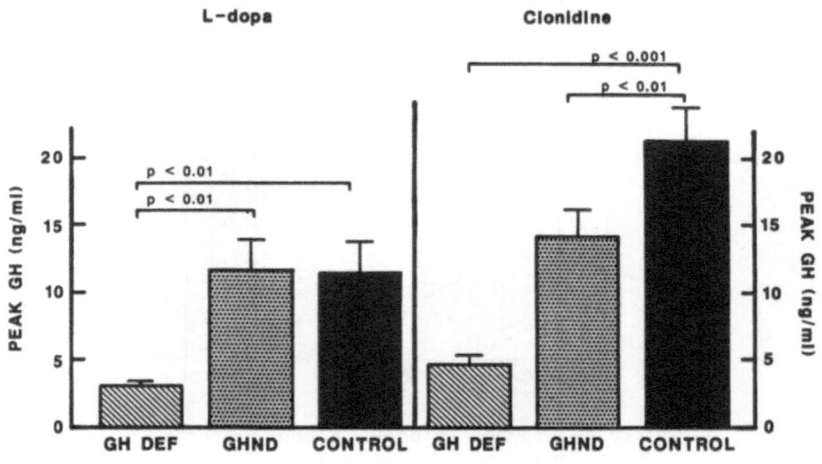

Fig. 6. Peak GH after arginine and insulin-induced hypo-glycemia in the three groups.

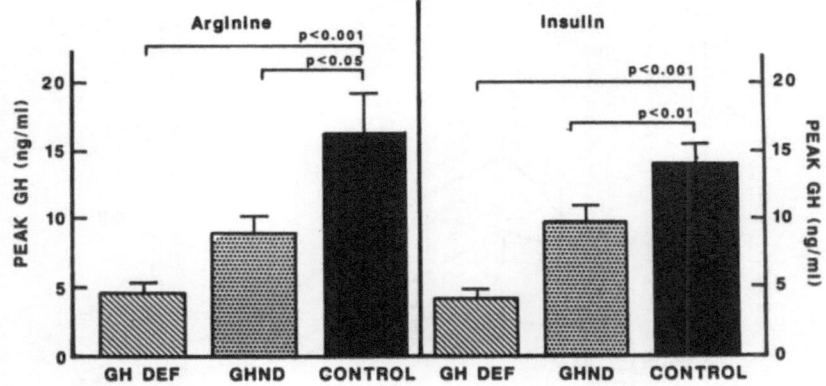

Fig. 7. Peak GH after L—dopa and clonidine stimulation in the three groups.

Mean 24—h GH concentration correlated with the mean of morning and evening SmC/IGF—I concentrations (r=0.36, P<0.01) (Fig. 14). For SmC/IGF—I concentrations, there was overlap and no statistical differences for all three groups (Table 1).

Daytime and nighttime pooled GH concentrations were significantly lower in both classical GH deficient and GHND compared to control children (P<0.01) (Table 2, Fig. 15). While daytime and nighttime pooled GH concentrations were also significantly lower in GHND children compared to controls (P<0.01), there was overlap between groups, particularly with

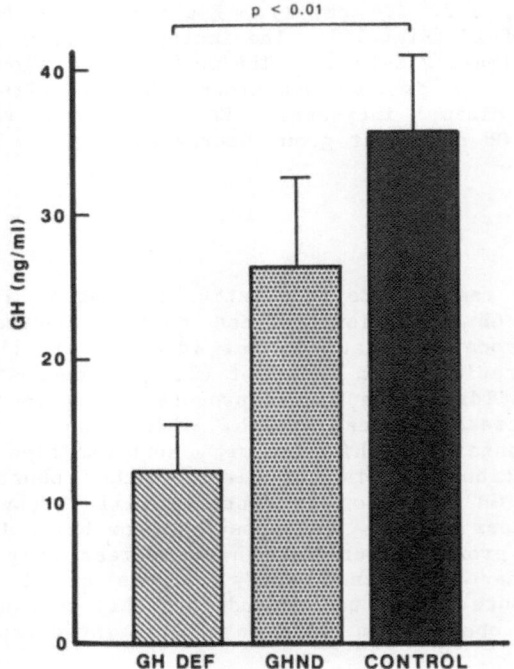

Fig. 8. Peak GH concentration after GHRH stimulation in the three groups of children.

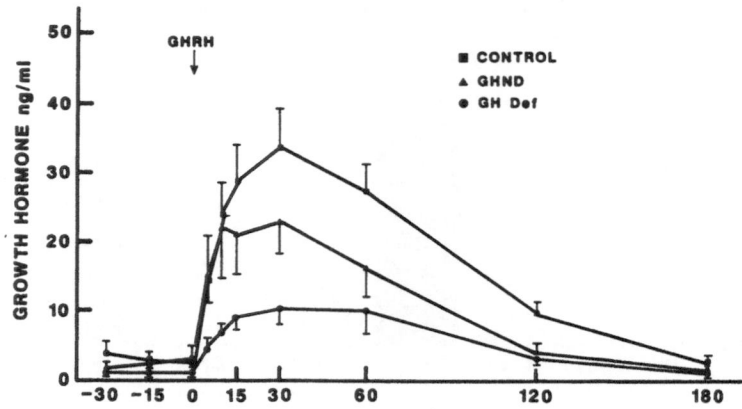

Fig. 9. GH secretory response following GHRH stimulation
in classical GH deficient, GHND and control children.

regard to the daytime pools. Diurnal secretion was relatively preserved
in both GHND (78%) and classical GH deficient (71%) groups.

Response to Exogenous GH Therapy

Eleven children in the GHND group have received 3 to 8 months of
therapy with methionyl hGH 0.1-0.2 U/kg/dose three times weekly. In all
children, there was an increase in growth velocity; in three children, it
was minimal (1.2, 1.2, 1.4 cm/yr). Eight children had an increase of
greater than 1.8-fold (Fig. 16). The increase in growth velocity was from
1.3- to 8.5-fold (mean 2.8-fold). The mean growth velocity was from 3.1 ±
0.4 to 7.7 ± 0.7 cm/yr in the GHND group; these results include the three
children who had minimal increases. For comparison, the growth velocity
of the classical GH deficient group increased from 2.4 ± 0.3 to 8.9 ± 0.6
cm/yr.

DISCUSSION

GH secretory response to provocative testing is a poor predictor of
endogenous 24-h GH secretion. These data demonstrate that abnormal
responses to provocative tests do not identify all children with deficiency in GH secretion. Van Vliet et al. (26) demonstrated that 40% of
selected short children with normal provocative tests responded to exogenous GH with increased linear growth. This group of children is likely
heterogeneous, containing children with abnormalities of GH synthesis,
secretion and action. It is not clear whether short children without
abnormalities of GH secretion or function will respond to exogenous GH
with improved linear growth. This issue is now being investigated by our
group and other groups. Our data here address only that subgroup of
children which have decreased daily outputs of GH secretion. These
children may be more likely to respond favorably to exogenous replacement
GH therapy. This observation has been substantiated recently (37).

The secretion of GH is influenced by a variety of neurohormones,
neuropeptides and neurotransmitters (1,2). We hypothesize that defects in
neurotransmitter secretion, resulting in decreased GHRH and/or increased

130

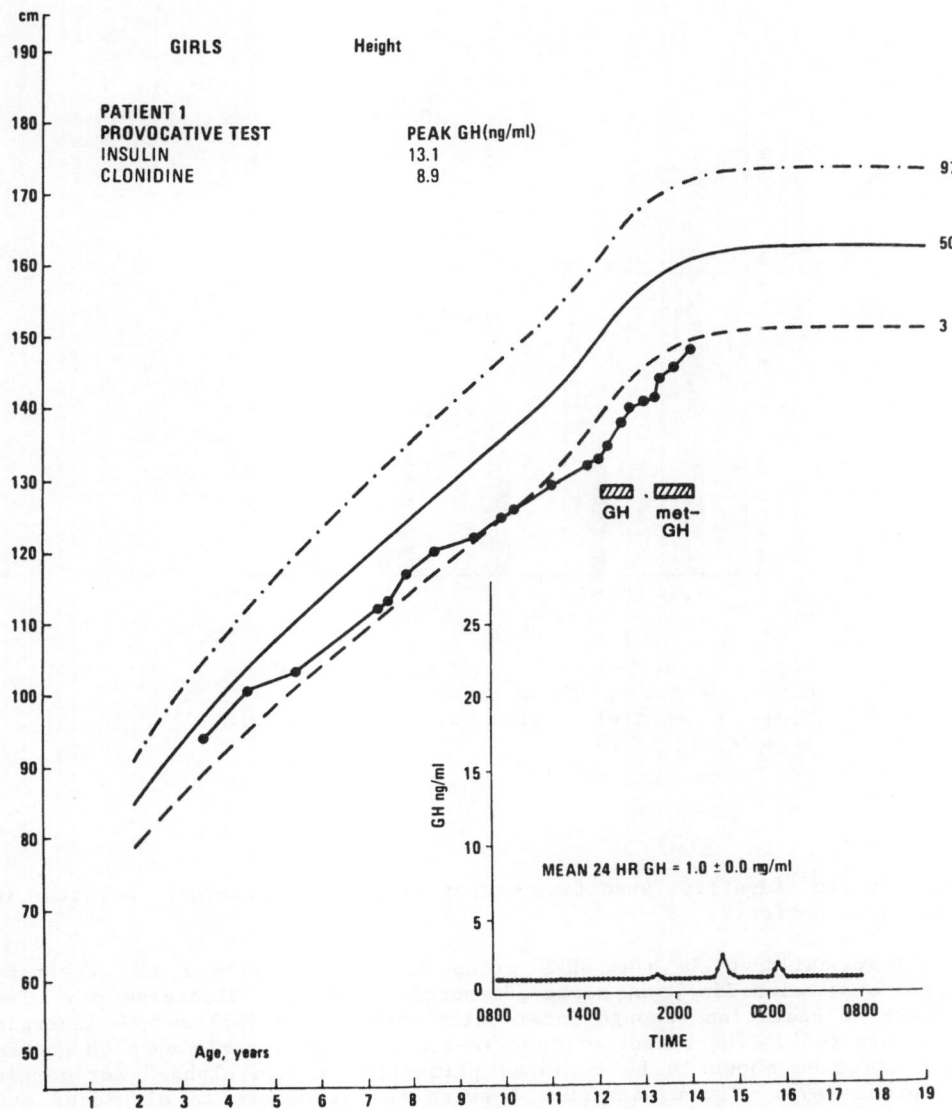

Fig. 10. Growth chart, peak GH responses to provocative testing, and endogenous 24-h GH secretion in a girl with idiopathic
empty sella syndrome. Reprinted with permission (36).

somatostatin secretion, are responsible for GHND and frequently classical
GH deficiency. Several investigators have demonstrated short-term
improvement in growth velocity in various groups of children (GH deficiency, intrauterine growth retardation, constitutional delay of growth
and adolescent development, short stature) following treatment with
dopaminergic and alpha-adrenergic stimulatory drugs (38-43). Long-term
studies have not yet been reported. On the basis of a single provocative
test, our studies here show preservation of dopaminergic and partial
preservation of alpha-adrenergic function in the GHND group compared to
the classical GH deficient group (44). It is important to emphasize that
there is overlap between the GHND and classical GH deficient groups.
Using more specific and improved technology in the future, it may be

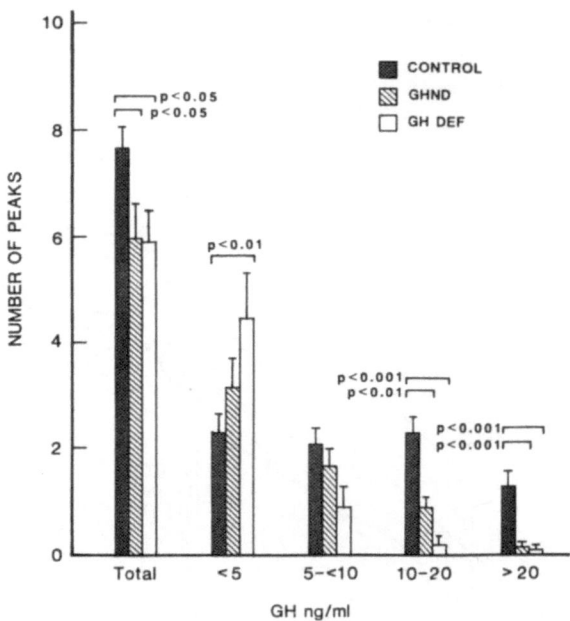

Fig. 11. Number and magnitude of GH peaks
during 24-h sampling of serum GH concentration in control, GHND and classical GH
deficient children.

possible to identify specific neurotransmitter secretory defects in
individual patients.

Most children in the GHND group also had a normal GH secretory
response to clonidine, an alpha-adrenergic agonist. Clonidine may also
mediate GH secretion through interaction with opioid (45) and cholinergic
receptors (46). The effect of insulin-induced hypoglycemia upon GH secretion has been shown to be mediated primarily through alpha-2 adrenergic
receptors (47). The discordance between the responses to clonidine and
insulin hypoglycemia in the GHND group suggests that these stimuli act
through different neuronal pathways.

In the present studies, we have assessed indirectly other neurotransmitter secretory pathways including serotonergic and/or cholinergic
secretion by measuring GH levels after the onset of clinical sleep. The
data show that the GHND group has intermediate sleep GH concentrations
between control and classical GH deficient subjects, suggesting that there
may be some compromise of serotonergic and/or cholinergic secretion for
the GHND group. However, for individual patients there is considerable
overlap. Further investigation is necessary to better define these
possible neurotransmitter secretory abnormalities.

Our pulsatile GH secretory data demonstrate that amplitude and total
GH secretory output (expressed as mean 24-h GH secretion) are the most
important criteria in predicting decreased GH secretion. However, the one
classical GH deficient patient with elevated endogenous GH secretion
appears exceptional. This patient may have had both reduced pulsatile

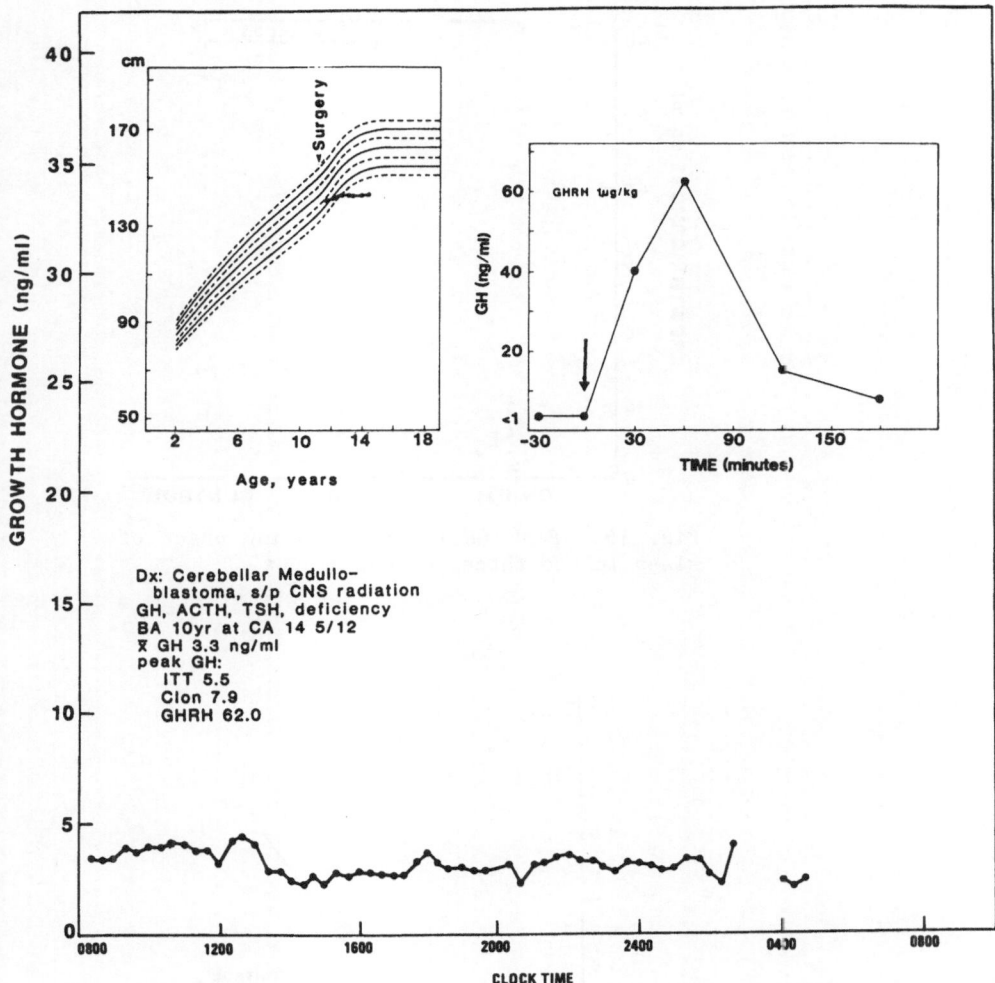

Fig. 12. Growth chart, peak GH responses to provocative testing, and endogenous GH secretion over a 24-h sampling period in
a girl with a cerebellar astrocytoma, status postsurgery and
radiation therapy. No GH peaks were observed. Technical
difficulties prevented the completion of 24-h GH sampling.
Reprinted with permission (36).

GHRH secretion (lack of GH pulses) and diminished somatostatin secretion
(elevated basal GH levels). The elevated basal GH secretion is reminis-
cent of the observed role of somatostatin secretion on basal GH secretion
in the rat (48). It is possible that the high dose radiation therapy
impaired both GHRH and somatostatin secretion, perhaps through a common
neurotransmitter secretory pathway, e.g., dopamine.

The relative preservation of GH response to GHRH in both the classical GH deficient and GHND groups is consistent with the observations of
others and supports current evidence that most GH deficient children have

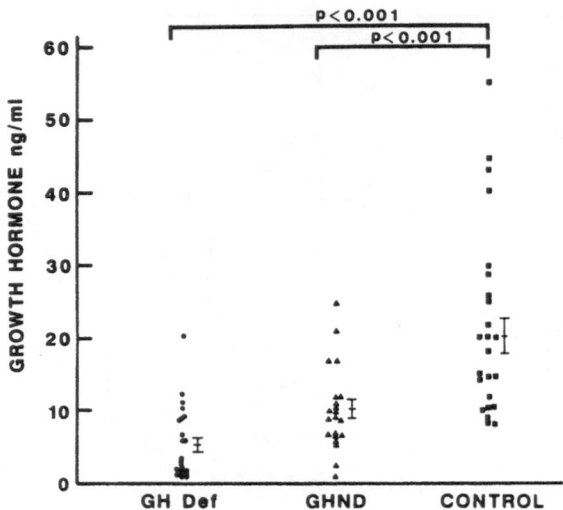

Fig. 13. Peak GH pulse following onset of sleep in the three patient groups.

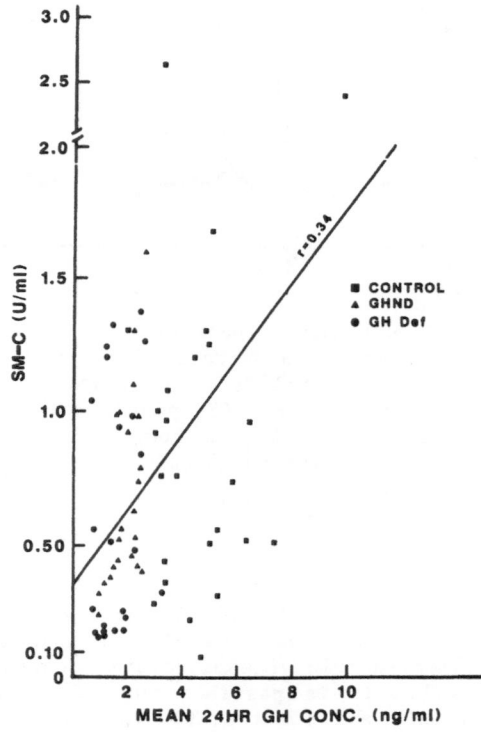

Fig. 14. Correlation of plasma SmC/IGF-I and mean 24-h GH concentration in GH deficient, GHND, and control children. The SmC/IGF-I concentration represents the mean of 2 samples (0900 h and 2100 h).

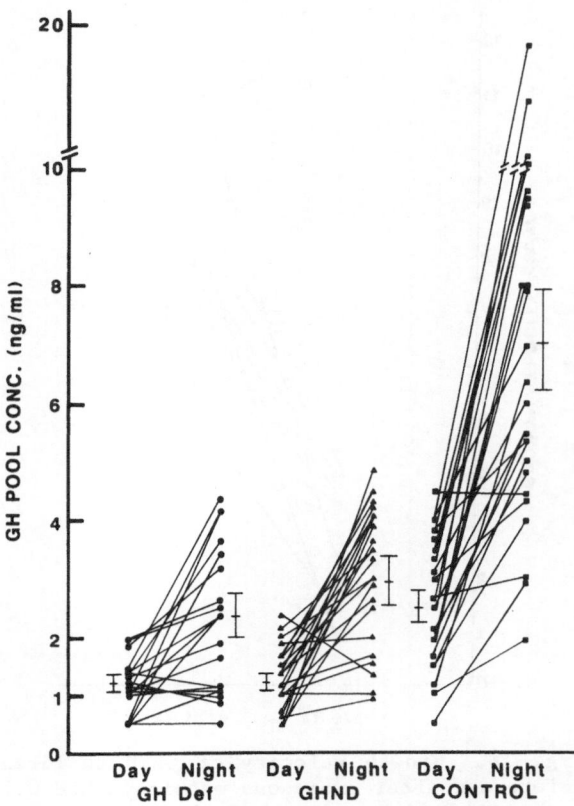

Fig. 15. Circadian pattern of GH secretion
in the three patient groups. Daytime pool
(0800-1600 h); nocturnal pool (2200-0600 h).

an abnormality in the control of GH secretion above the level of the
pituitary gland (49-52). All but one of our control children had peak GH
secretory responses to GHRH 10 ng/ml. Studies are now in progress to
assess the other side of neurohormonal-pituitary axis, i.e., somatostatin
inhibitory secretion.

Circadian GH secretory rhythm was assessed in the three patient
groups. The pattern was relatively preserved, but at a lower amplitude
for both GHND and GH deficient compared to control children. In the GHND
group, except for one patient, mean 24-h pooled and circadian prolactin
secretory patterns were normal (52A); however, in that GHND patient, a
higher nocturnal prolactin secretory pattern was preserved. Further
studies are necessary to ascertain defects in specific neurotransmitter
secretion (and hypothalamic GHRH/SRIH) and the relationship to the circadian secretory patterns of GH and prolactin.

Endogenous pulsatile GH secretion appears to be slightly increased
during pubertal development (53,54). This is also suggested by studies in
children with precocious puberty (55). Our control group is still too
small to directly assess this question. Ultimately, longitudinal studies
in both sexes are necessary.

In our study, the correlation between mean 24-h GH concentration and
SmC/IGF-I is positive; however, there is significant overlap among groups.

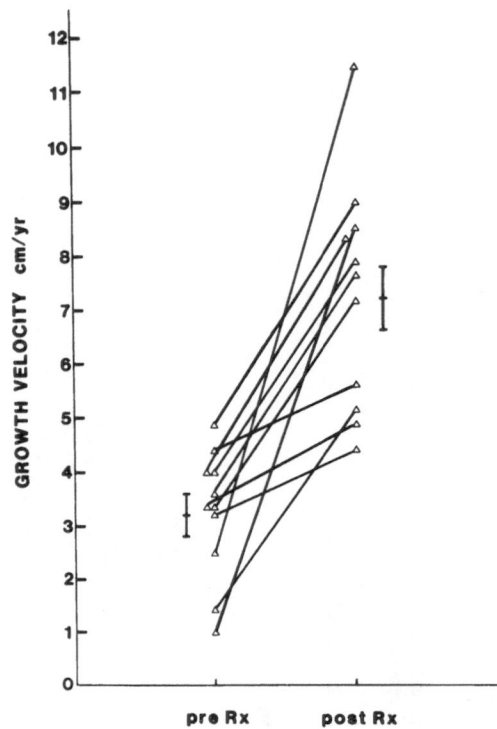

Fig. 16. Growth velocity of GHND children
before and after exogenous methionyl hGH 0.1
to 0.2 U/kg three times a week.

This is especially seen in children who are pubertal even if they have
markedly reduced endogenous (and/or also provocative) GH secretion.

Because 24-h studies to determine endogenous GH secretion are not
practical in all clinical settings, we examined mean GH secretion at
shorter intervals (30). For groups of patients, the nighttime or daytime
12-h intervals and 6-h daytime intervals are long enough to determine
whether the output of endogenous GH is subnormal. However, for individual
children, there was considerable overlap for the 6- and 12-h daytime
interval analyses compared to the 24-h study.

Normal growth is dependent on multiple factors including nutrition,
genetic factors, metabolic milieu, hormonal influences and as yet
unexplained factors. Although here we have demonstrated normal GH secretion and SmC/IGF-I concentration in short-statured control children, it is
of interest that, at the other end of the spectrum, in tall-statured girls
there is increased endogenous GH secretion (56). Very tall children and
adults often have increased SmC/IGF-I concentrations (57), and short children have decreased levels (58) when compared with appropriate age-matched
control groups. Zadik et al. have demonstrated that 40% of short children
have decreased endogenous GH (59). Reports comparing different size
species of dogs suggest that body size is related to SmC/IGF-1 concentrations in blood (60,61), suggesting that the SmC/IGF-I concentration
increase in the larger species may be due to elevated GH secretion. More
studies, including longitudinal ones, are necessary to better understand
these complex relationships.

In our series, 65% of children with GHND had perinatal complications (62), and a few others had obvious causes for hypothalamic-pituitary dysfunction as a result of injury in later childhood. Thus, because there are children who do not have either identifiable perinatal or childhood medical problems, there may be overlap between GH neurosecretory dysfunction and constitutional delay of growth and adolescence. Bierich has suggested that endogenous GH is decreased (based on 5-h nocturnal studies) (63), whereas more recently Lanes et al. (64) have shown no abnormality in nighttime (9-h) endogenous GH secretion.

In our first report of GHND (29), 6 of 7 children with GHND studies at the NIH were observed to grow at an increased rate following initiation of hGH therapy. In the present study, 11 additional children from All Children's Hospital have received hGH therapy. All except 3 children, one who was admittedly noncompliant, demonstrated a very significant increase in growth velocity over a brief period of observation. Increased linear growth in response to exogenous GH therapy should be included in the definition of any subgroup of GH deficiency. We suggest that the 24-h study identifies a larger group of GH deficient subjects not previously identified by provocative testing who may benefit from growth hormone therapy. Long-term studies are necessary to ultimately assess whether endogenous GH secretory studies are useful predictors of the response to exogenous GH therapy. Such studies should include treatment of short children with "normal" endogenous secretion of GH. Moreover, control studies should further examine the pulsatile GH secretory pattern of normal-statured children before and during the course of pubertal development. The clinician must still consider growth velocity as a critical criterion in the decision-making process.

ACKNOWLEDGMENTS

Supported in part by March of Dimes Birth Defects Foundation Grant 6-427 and Eleanor Naylor Dana Charitable Trust.

I thank Dr. Alan Rogol, Dr. Johannes Veldhuis and Mr. Cheng-Shih Hu for their invaluable help in the statistical analysis of the data, and I also thank Ms. Cheryl A. Cooper for her competent secretarial assistance.

REFERENCES

1. Bercu BB, Diamond F. A determinant of stature: regulation of growth hormone secretion. In: Barness L, ed. Advances in pediatrics. Chicago: Yearbook Medical Publishers, Inc, 1986:331-80.
2. Bercu BB, Diamond F. Growth hormone neurosecretory dysfunction. In: Savage M, Randall R, eds. Growth disorders. Clin Endocrinol Metab 1986; 15:537-90.
3. Richards GE, Wara WM, Grumbach MM, et al. Delayed onset of hypopituitarism: sequelae of therapeutic irradiation of central nervous system, eye and middle ear tumors. J Pediatr 1976; 89:553.
4. Shalet SM. Disorders of the endocrine system due to radiation and cytotoxic chemotherapy. Clin Endocrinol (Oxf) 1983; 18:637-59.
5. Shalet SM, Beardwell CG, Morris-Jones PH, Pearson D. Growth hormone deficiency after treatment of acute leukemia in children. Arch Dis Child 1976; 51:489-93.
6. Shalet SM, Beardwell CG, Pearson D, Morris-Jones PH. The effect of varying doses of cerebral irradiation on growth hormone production in childhood. Clin Endocrinol (Oxf) 1976; 5:287-90.
7. Dacou-Vaitekakis C, Xypolyta A, Haidas ST, et al. Irradiation of the

head: immediate effect on growth hormone secretion in children. J Clin Endocrinol Metab 1977; 44:791-4.

8. Swift PGF, Kearney PJ, Dalton RG, et al. Growth hormonal status of children treated for acute lymphoblastic leukemia. Arch Dis Child 1978; 53:890-4.

9. Oliff A, Bode U, Bercu BB, et al. Hypothalamic-pituitary dysfunction following CNS prophylaxis in acute lymphocytic leukemia, correlation with CT scan abnormalities. Med Pediatr Oncol 1979; 7:141-51.

10. Bode U, Oliff A, Bercu BB, DiChiro G, Glaubiger D, Poplack D. Absence of CT brain scan abnormalities with less intensive CNS prophylaxis. Am J Pediatr Hematol Oncol 1980; 2:21-4.

11. Romche CA, Zipf WB, Miser A, et al. Evaluation of growth hormone release and human growth hormone treatment in children with cranial irradiation-associated short stature. J Pediatr 1984; 104:177-81.

12. Dickinson WP, Berry DH, Dickinson L, et al. Differential effects of cranial radiation on growth hormone response to arginine and insulin infusion. J Pediatr 1978; 92:754-7.

13. Blatt J, Bercu BB, Gillin JC, Mendelson WB, Poplack D. Reduced pulsatile growth hormone secretion in children after therapy for acute lymphoblastic leukemia. J Pediatr 1984; 104:182-6.

14. Muhlendahl KEV, Gadner H, Riehm H, et al. Endocrine function after antineoplastic therapy in 22 children with acute lymphoblastic leukemia. Helv Paediatr Acta 1976; 31:463-71.

15. Chrousos GP, Poplack D, Brown T, O'Neill D, Schwade JG, Bercu BB. Effects of cranial radiation on hypothalamic-adenohypophyseal function: abnormal growth hormone secretory dynamics. J Clin Endocrinol Metab 1982; 54:1135-9.

16. Daniel PM, Prichard ML. Studies of the hypothalamus and the pituitary with special reference to the effects of transsection of the pituitary stalk. Acta Endocrinol [suppl] (Copenh) 1978; 201:1-216.

17. Bloch B, Brazeau P, Esch F, et al. Immunohistochemical detection of growth hormone-releasing factor in brain. Nature 1983; 301:607-8.

18. Cooper PE, Fernstrom MH, Rorstad OP. Leeman SE, Martin JB. The regional distribution of somatostatin, substance P and neurotensin in human brain. Brain Res 1981; 218:219-32.

19. Rudman D, Kutner MH, Blackston RD, Jansen RD, Patterson JH. Normal variant short stature: subclassification based on responses to exogenous human growth hormone. J Clin Endocrinol Metab 1979; 49:92-9.

20. Kowarski AA, Schneider J, Ben-Galim E, Weldon VV, Daughaday WH. Growth failure with normal serum RIA-GH and low somatomedin activity: somatomedin restoration and growth acceleration after exogenous GH. J Clin Endocrinol Metab 1978; 47:461-4.

21. Lanes P, Plotnick LP, Spencer ME, Daughaday WE, Kowarski AA. Dwarfism associated with normal serum growth hormone and increased bioassayable, receptorassayable, and immunoassayable somatomedin. J Clin Endocrinol Metab 1980; 50:485-8.

22. Lanes P, Plotnick LP, Spencer ME, Daughaday WE, Kowarski AA. Dwarfism associated with normal serum growth hormone and increased bioassayable, receptorassayable, and immunoassayable somatomedin. J Clin Endocrinol Metab 1980; 50:485-8.

23. Hayek A, Peake GT. Growth and somatomedin-C responses to growth hormone in dwarfed children. J Pediatr 1981; 99:868-72.

24. Valenta LH, Siegel MB, Lesniak MA, et al. Pituitary dwarfism in a patient with circulating abnormal growth hormone polymers. N Engl J Med 1985; 312:214-7.

25. Frazer TE, Gavin VR, Daughaday WH, Hillman RE, Weldon VV. Growth hormone-dependent growth failure. J Pediatr 1982; 101:12-5.

26. Van Vliet G, Styne DM, Kaplan SL, Grumbach MM. Growth hormone treatment for short stature. N Engl J Med 1983; 309:1016-22.

27. Gertner JM, Genel M, Gianfredi SP, et al. Prospective clinical trial

of human growth hormone in short children without growth hormone deficiency. J Pediatr 1984; 104:172-6.

28. Grunt JA, Howard C, Daughaday WH. Comparison of growth and somatomedin C responses following growth hormone treatment in children with small-for-date short stature, significant idiopathic short stature and hypopituitarism. Acta Endocrinol (Copenh) 1984; 106:168-74.

29. Spiliotis B, August G, Hung W, Sonis W, Mendelson W, Bercu BB. Growth hormone neurosecretory dysfunction: a treatable cause of short stature. JAMA 1984; 251:2223-30.

30. Bercu BB, Shulman D, Root AW, Spiliotis BE. Growth hormone provocative testing frequently does not reflect endogenous growth hormone secretion. J Clin Endocrinol Metab 1986; 63:709-16.

31. Tanner JM. Growth at adolescence. Springfield: Charles C. Thomas, 1962.

32. Greulich WW, Pyle SJ. Radiographic atlas of skeletal development of the hand and wrist. Palo Alto: Stanford University Press, 1973.

33. Root AW, Rosenfield RL, Bongiovanni AM, Eberlein WR. The plasma growth hormone response to insulin-induced hypoglycemia in children with retardation of growth. Pediatrics 1967; 39:884-52.

34. Reiter EO, Root AW. The effect of pyridoxine on pituitary release of growth hormone and prolactin in childhood and adolescence. J Clin Endocrinol Metab 1978; 47:689-90.

35. Veldhuis JD, Johnson ML. Cluster analysis: a simple, versatile, and robust algorithm for endocrine pulse detection. Am J Physiol 1986; E486-93.

36. Shulman DI, Bercu BB. The evaluation of growth hormone secretion: provocative testing vs endogenous 24 hour growth hormone profile. Acta Paediatr Scand (in press).

37. Costin G, Kaufman FR. Growth hormone secretory patterns in children with short stature. J Pediatr 1987; 110:362-8.

38. Huseman CA, Hassing JM. Evidence for dopaminergic stimulation of growth velocity in some hypopituitary children. J Clin Endocrinol Metab 1984; 58:419-25.

39. Huseman CA. Growth enhancement by dopaminergic therapy in children with intrauterine growth retardation. J Clin Endocrinol Metab 1985; 61:514-9.

40. Huseman CA, Hassing JM, Sibilia MG. Endogenous dopaminergic dysfunction: a novel form of human growth hormone deficiency and short stature. J Clin Endocrinol Metab 1986; 62:484-90.

41. Castro-Magana M, Angulo M, Fuentes B, et al. Effect of prolonged clonidine administration on growth hormone concentrations and rate of linear growth in children with constitutional growth delay. J Pediatr 1986; 109:784.

42. Pintor C, Cella SG, Corda R, et al. Clonidine accelerates growth in children with impaired growth hormone secretion. Lancet 1985; 1:1482-5.

43. Loche S, Pintor C, Puggioni R, et al. Treatment of short stature with clonidine: stimulatory effect in children with constitutional growth delay (CGD) [Abstract]. Presented at the 68th Annual Meeting of the Endocrine Society, Anaheim, California, 1986.

44. Bercu BB, Root AW, Shulman DI. Preservation of dopaminergic and alpha adrenergic function in children with growth hormone neurosecretory dysfunction. J Clin Endocrinol Metab 1986; 63:968-73.

45. Brammert M, Hokfelt B. Partial blockage by naloxone of clonidine-induced increase in plasma growth hormone in hypertensive patients. J Clin Endocrinol Metab 1984; 58:374-7.

46. Delitala G, Maioli M, Pacifico A, et al. Cholinergic receptor control mechanisms for L-dopa, apomorphine, and clonidine-induced growth hormone secretion in man. J Clin Endocrinol Metab 1983; 57:1145-9.

47. Tater P, Vigas M. Role of alpha 1 and alpha 2 adrenergic receptors in the growth hormone and prolactin response to insulin induced

hypoglycemia in man. Neuroendocrinology 1984; 39:275-80.

48. Tannenbaum GH, Ling N. The interrelationship of growth hormone (GH)-releasing factor and somatostatin in generation of the ultradian rhythm of GH secretion. Endocrinology 1984; 115:1952-7.

49. Thorner MO, Speiss J, Vance ML, et al. Human pancreatic growth hormone releasing factor selectively stimulates growth hormone secretion in man. Lancet 1983; 1:24-8.

50. Chalew S, Armour KM, Levin PA, Thorner MO, Kowarski AA. Growth hormone response to GH-releasing hormone in children with subnormal integrated concentrations of GH. J Clin Endocrinol Metab 1986; 62:1110-5.

51. Gelato MC, Malozowski S, Caruso-Nicoletti M, et al. Growth hormone (GH) responses to GH-releasing hormone during pubertal development in normal boys and girls: comparison to idiopathic short stature and GH deficiency. J Clin Endocrinol Metab 1986; 174:174-9.

52. Schrioch EA, Lustig RH, Rosenthal SM, Kaplan SL, Grumbach MM. Effect of growth hormone (GH)-releasing hormone (GRH) on plasma GH in relation to magnitude and duration of GH deficiency in 26 children and adults with isolated GH deficiency or multiple pituitary hormone deficiencies: evidence for hypothalamic GRH deficiency. J Clin Endocrinol Metab 1984; 58:1043-9.

52A Shulman DI, Root AW, Hu CS, Bercu BB. 24 hour prolactin secretion in short normal, classical growth hormone deficient and growth hormone neurosecretory dysfunction children [Abstract 790]. 69th Annual Endocrine Society Meeting, Indianapolis, Indiana, 1987:218.

53. Mauras N, Blizzard RM, Link K, Johnson ML, Rogol AD, Veldhuis JD. Augmentation of growth hormone secretion during puberty: evidence for a pulse amplitude-modulated phenomenon. J Clin Endocrinol Metab 1987; 64:596-601.

54. Zadik Z, Chalew SA, McCarter J Jr, Meistas M, Kowarski AA. The influence of age on the 24 hour integrated concentration of growth hormone in normal individuals. J Clin Endocrinol Metab 1985; 60:513-6.

55. Ross JL, Pescovitz OH, Barnes K, Loriaux DL, Cutler GB Jr. Growth hormone secretory dynamics in children with precocious puberty. J Pediatr 1987; 110:369-72.

56. Albertsson-Wikland K, Isaksson O, Rosberg S, et al. Secretory pattern of growth hormone in children of different growth rates [Abstract]. Acta Endocrinol (Copenh) 1983; 103(suppl 256):72.

57. Gourmelen M, Le Bouc Y, Girard F, et al. Serum levels of insulin-like growth factor (IGF) and IGF binding protein in constitutionally tall children and adolescents. J Clin Endocrinol Metab 1984; 59:1197-203.

58. Cacciari E, Cicognani A, Pirazzoli P, et al. Differences in somatomedin-C between short-normal subjects and those of normal height. J Pediatr 1985; 106:891-4.

59. Zadik F, Chalew SA, Raiti S, Kowarski AA. Do short children secrete insufficient quantities of growth hormone? Pediatrics 1985; 76:355-60.

60. Eigenmann JE, Patterson DF, Zapf J, et al. Insulin-like growth factor I in the dog: a study in different dog breeds and in dogs with growth hormone elevation. Acta Endocrinol (Copenh) 1984; 105:294-301.

61. Eigenmann JE, Patterson DF, Froesch ER. Body size parallels insulin-like growth factor I levels but not growth hormone secretory capacity. Acta Endocrinol (Copenh) 1984; 106:448-53.

62. Bercu BB, Shulman DI, Root AW. High incidence of prenatal and perinatal complications associated with growth hormone neurosecretory dysfunction (GHND) [Abstract]. Pediatr Res 1987; 224A.

63. Bierich JR. Treatment of constitutional delay of growth and adolescence with human growth hormone. Klin Padiatr 1983; 195:309-16.

64. Lanes R, Bohorquez L, Leal V, et al. Growth hormone secretion in patients with constitutional delay of growth and pubertal development. J Pediatr 1986; 109:781-3.

13

GROWTH HORMONE SECRETION AND GROWTH IN

CENTRAL NERVOUS SYSTEM IRRADIATED CHILDREN

R. Rappaport, M. Fontoura, and R. Brauner

Unit of Pediatric Endocrinology and Diabetes
Hopital des Enfants Malades
Paris, France

External cranial irradiation is currently used in various therapeutic protocols for malignant systemic and intracranial diseases. Some patients receive spinal irradiation in addition. These therapies have significantly improved the survival rate in a number of malignant systemic or cranial diseases. The impact of radiotherapy on growth and the mechanism of growth retardation observed in these patients has generated much interest. Earlier data, although demonstrating late effects on growth, have often been difficult to interpret. In fact, several factors may contribute to growth retardation, such as age at irradiation, doses delivered to the hypothalamic-pituitary region, chemotherapy and glucocorticoids, spinal irradiation and other endocrine abnormalities involving gonadotropin secretion or thyroid dysfunction. For practical purposes it is also important to analyze the data according to the diseases, each of which involves a different treatment protocol.

GROWTH

The general pattern of growth in children since time of irradiation is presented in Figure 1 (unpublished personal data), comparing 3 groups of prepubertal children classified according to their irradiation protocol: (1) children with acute lymphoblastic leukemia (ALL) present a significant but moderate height loss during the first year following therapy, and thereafter have a normal growth rate until puberty without catch-up. They have received 24 Gy in 12 x 2 Gy fractions. (2) Children who received cranial doses ranging from 30-55 Gy have an average height loss of 1.1 SD 7 years after irradiation. (3) The growth fall-off is quite dramatic when there is additional spinal irradiation at doses in the range of 27-38 Gy as in our group of untreated patients with medulloblastoma; they have an average height loss of 3 SD 7 years after irradiation. The collection of similar data throughout puberty is in progress.

Acute Lymphoblastic Leukemia

A recent retrospective analysis of height velocity up to 8 years after diagnosis and cranial irradiation confirms that the rate of growth decreases slightly during the first years of treatment and thereafter returns to normal (1). In parallel, an excessive weight gain occurred. The impact of prophylactic cranial irradiation on growth in ALL during the

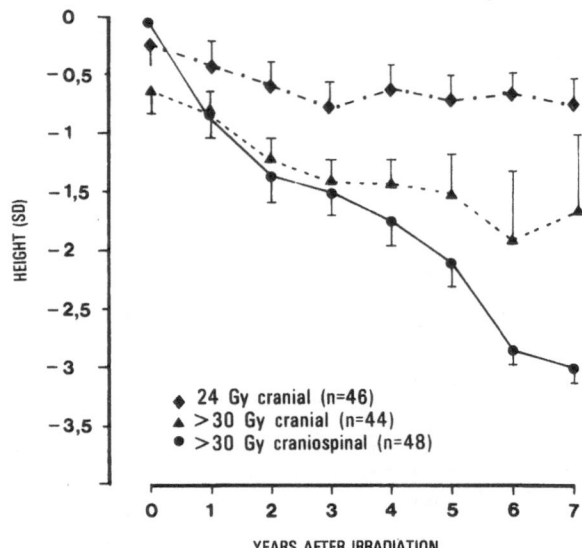

Fig. 1. Prepubertal growth of 3 groups of children followed since time of irradiation (for description, see text). 1 Gray = 100 rad.

first year following this treatment is questionable. A transient spontaneous reduction of GH secretion has been reported by Dacou-Voutetakis (2) a few weeks after completion of irradiation. However, in a prospective study (3) it was shown that bioassayable somatomedin levels were normal when children entered clinical remission and remained normal during the remainder of the first year. Presently we favor the hypothesis that this earlier impairment of growth is more likely to be due to the combined adverse effects of the acute disease, the chemotherapy and glucocorticoids rather than to a radiation-induced GH deficiency as suggested by Shalet (4). The effects on growth of 18 Gy and 20 Gy treatment were not different according to Starceski et al. (5): height percentiles among irradiated patients decreased by a mean of 12% 6 months after diagnosis and growth did not catch up. A small group of patients had a more severe fall-off which had probably begun during the first year. In a recent survey by Robison et al. (6), this shift of height following cessation of treatment was confirmed with an excess number of patients in the lower percentile categories. Intrathecal methotrexate did not appear to influence per se the height prognosis. We have also observed severe growth stunting in 2 girls with a final height at −4 SD in spite of normal GH secretion. In the group of children with ALL, the most striking finding is the apparent contrast between a rather well conserved growth rate in most cases and the lack of GH response to pharmacological stimulation after cranial irradiation.

Brain Tumors Treated with Cranial Radiation

As shown in Figure 1, the mean prepubertal height loss in this group of children who received more than 30 Gy was close to 1.1 SD 7 years after irradiation and prior to puberty. As normal GH secretion is necessary to achieve a normal pubertal growth spurt, one would expect further growth retardation and a final short stature. In a group of patients who reached adult height we observed a mean height reduction of −1.6 ± 0.2 SD (mean ± SEM).

Brain Tumors Treated with Cranial and Spinal Radiation

Spinal irradiation, at a dose of 27 Gy or more as done in children with medulloblastoma or other tumors prone to metastasize in the central nervous system, severely impairs spinal growth before and during puberty. We found a mean height of about 3 SD below the normal mean in these patients at time of onset of puberty or slightly before (Fig. 1). These patients will achieve a mean final height of −3.0 ± 0.3 SD (Fig. 2) (7). The yearly height standard deviation score (SDS) changes during the 6 years following therapy (7) indicate that a sharp and significant drop occurs during the first year (Fig. 3). This is in contrast somewhat with the lesser growth deceleration observed in children receiving only cranial irradiation. Since GH deficiency does not occur during this first year (8), we believe that early growth retardation is principally due to the immediate effect of spinal irradiation in addition to other factors such as acute disease and chemotherapy. Unfortunately, sitting height data were not available for this early period. Shalet et al. (9) showed that in adolescent or adult patients treated with craniospinal irradiation the sitting height SDS was −3.27 SD as compared to the value of −1.19 SD in the cranial irradiated group. In contrast, no difference was observed between the leg length SDS of both groups. This study also confirmed earlier data of Probert et al. (10) showing that spinal growth was considerably impaired if the spine had been irradiated before 6 years of age.

GROWTH AND ABNORMAL PUBERTAL DEVELOPMENT

There is a risk of gonadotropin deficiency and lack of spontaneous pubertal development when cranial doses above 40 Gy are used before puberty. We reported that GH deficiency was also present in these children (11). In our experience, providing the patient receives hGH therapy, a pubertal growth acceleration can be achieved with exogenous low dose testosterone or estradiol therapy. Surprisingly, true central precocious puberty may also occur in irradiated patients (12,13). We reported on a group of children that had been treated for tumors distant from the hypothalamic-pituitary region, including medulloblastoma, astrocytoma, facial tumor and ALL. The irradiation doses ranged from 24 to 45 Gy. All of them developed true precocious puberty. One could therefore speculate that different hypothalamic lesions could occur, some leading to precocious gonadotropin secretion, others with more extensive and additional destruction of gonadotropes in the pituitary, resulting in lack of

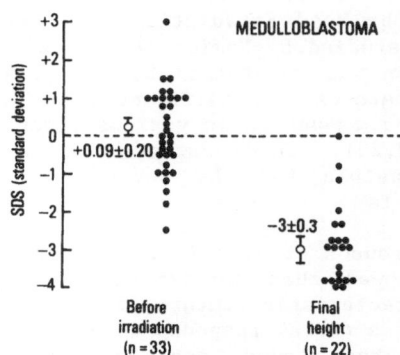

Fig. 2. Final height in children with medulloblastoma who received cranial and spinal irradiation.

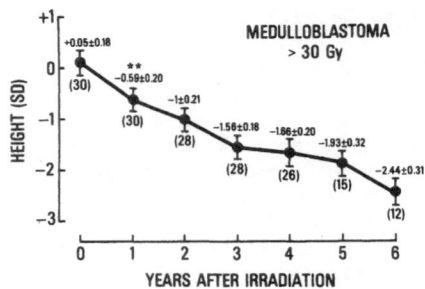

Fig. 3. Annual height changes in a prepubertal group of children with medulloblastoma who received cranial and spinal
irradiation, with permission of the authors
(7).

pubertal development. Precocious puberty leads to accelerated bone
maturation (Fig. 4) not compensated by proportional growth, thus causing
severe growth retardation. Combined gonadotropin releasing hormone analog
and hGH therapy is probably necessary in these patients to achieve the
best final height.

GROWTH HORMONE SECRETION

The occurrence of radiation-induced abnormalities of GH secretion has
been recognized over the past decade by different groups following the
early reports of Tan et al. (14) and Larkins et al. (15), and subsequently
including the more extensive studies of Shalet (16), Richards (17),
Perry-Keene (18), Czernichow (19), and Samaan (20). As the number of
reported cases and the duration of follow-up increased, it became apparent
that GH secretory dysfunction had multiple presentations depending on the
methods used to quantitate GH secretion. Discrepancies between GH
responses to pharmacological and physiological tests led to the concept of
neurosecretory dysfunction (21). Whatever interpretation is proposed for
all these data, another difficulty ensued when it became necessary, for
clinical purposes, to correlate endocrine data with growth rates. Also,
decisions need to be made regarding follow-up of these patients as well as
determining which children would benefit from hGH treatment.

Experimental animal studies have demonstrated that defects in GH
secretion are induced by head irradiation. In neonatal head-irradiated
male rats (0.6 Gy) as studied by Mosier et al. (22), the normal pulsatile
pattern of GH secretion was maintained but GH peaks and area under the
curve were reduced. There was a significant stunting of growth. However,
there was no cell number reduction in various organs as would be expected
in hypopituitarism (22,23). These authors concluded that GH deficiency
was not solely responsible for the severe stunting of growth which
occurred in these animals.

In the monkey, Chrousos et al. (24), using cranial irradiation doses
of 24 and 40 Gy, showed that impairment of GH response to insulin
hypoglycemia was a characteristic feature of radiation damage, in contrast
with the persistence of a normal response to arginine and L-dopa. Despite
this normal response, they found, one year after radiation, a marked
decrease of the 24-h physiological GH secretion. These data suggested
that pituitary somatotrophs retain their ability to secrete GH. They also
speculated that irradiation decreased the sensitivity of the hypoglyce-

146

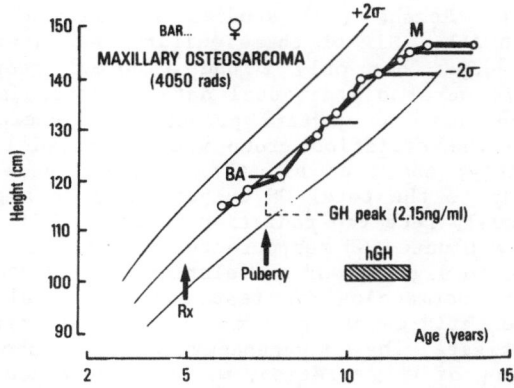

Fig. 4. Growth of a child who developed precocious puberty associated to GH deficiency after cranial irradiation. Accelerated bone maturation led to early cessation of growth and short stature.

mia-mediating area of the lateral hypothalamus and the rhythm-generating center or its connections to lower hypothalamic centers of GH secretion. It was concluded that the predominant damage occurred at the hypothalamic levels. It is likely that the site and extent of damage depends not only upon the radiation dose, but also upon the time interval since therapy as described by Brauner et al. (8) and Shalet (4). As the time interval increases, GH deficiency becomes more frequent.

Methods of Investigation

GH secretion evaluation in irradiated children is closely related to the usual methodological difficulties in assessing GH secretion. The recent interest in assessing a physiological setting such as sleep-related GH secretion or even the whole 24-h pattern of plasma GH concentration has stimulated quite a number of studies.

Several questions were asked including: (1) which pharmacological stimulation test, if any, provides the most reliable information; (2) how does physiological GH secretion correlate with the peak response to pharmacological stimulation; (3) does circulating SmC/IGF-I values provide additional information; and finally, (4) what is the correlation between biological data and growth before and during treatment with hGH.

There is some evidence that hypoglycemia-induced GH release better correlates with the abolition of pulsatile GH secretion from studies in the monkey (24) and in children generally irradiated with doses of 24 Gy or below (25-27). In some of these cases, GH peak values after arginine or L-dopa were normal or subnormal. It was concluded that the insulin tolerance test generally acted through the hypothalamus, and it was the test of choice because of the marked radiation sensitivity of the GH response to hypoglycemia (27).

Potentially the most physiologic evaluation of GH secretion is the 24-h or night GH profiles. However, because of practical difficulties in performing this technique, there are very few data showing a comparison with pharmacologic tests. Blatt et al. (28) reported on 8 children who received 24 Gy cranial radiation; these patients had reduced total basal GH output (AUC) and growth retardation. Three of them had a normal GH peak after insulin. Romshe (26) studied 9 children, 2 with medullo-blastoma and 6 with ALL. Six of these children had a normal GH response to arginine and L-dopa, but only 2 had a normal response to insulin hypoglycemia. There were no individual data reported in this study, but only the indication that the daytime pulsatile GH secretion was significantly reduced in the radiation group when compared to a short normal group. More recently, Ahmed et al. (27) compared peak GH values after arginine and insulin to the total GH output (AUC) in a group of 14 children who had previously received radiation doses of 24 Gy or greater. All 14 patients showed a blunted GH response to hypoglycemia and a low 24-h GH profile. There was no significant correlation between the maximum peak GH response to either pharmacological test and the total 24-h GH output. However, 3 of these children had a normal response to arginine. In order to further investigate the discrepancy between pharmacological and physiological testing of GH secretion, we have performed a more extensive study as part of the follow-up of 34 patients irradiated with 32-40 Gy for medulloblastoma. GH peak values after arginine-insulin tolerance test (AITT) were compared to the nocturnal sleep GH peak. Both peaks were highly and significantly correlated ($r=0.72$, $P<0.001$). However, 5 children with normal responses to AITT (>8 ng/ml) had low peaks during sleep (<10 ng/ml). This figure is similar to the reports of Blatt (28) and Ahmed (27). In addition, we found 4 children who had normal GH peaks during sleep in contrast to low responses to AITT. The results of both methods of evaluating GH secretion were concordant in 27 out of 36 irradiated children. Among the 9 children who had discrepant results, it was not possible to decide which test better reflected hypothalamic-pituitary GH function when comparing to growth rates since these patients had also received spinal radiation which was an important additional cause of growth retardation.

There are only minimal data concerning circulating SmC values in these patients (26,29). It cannot be concluded whether this is a more reliable index of GH secretion in patients with cranial irradiation.

Finally, we do not yet know how these biological criteria of GH secretion relate to growth. Ideally, low GH responses in either test would be meaningful only if accompanied by a reduced growth rate. This is difficult to assess in the craniospinal radiated patients because of the spinal growth retardation, as noted in our study and for some patients reported in other studies. A more extensive investigation is needed, in spite of methodological difficulties, to assess children who have received cranial radiation in order to decide whether there is a definite advantage in performing a physiologic test. We would suggest that in most cases pharmacological tests, and probably the insulin or arginine-insulin tests, are the most reliable. For practical purposes, sleep-related GH secretion could be performed if a normal GH response to these tests is obtained in contrast to retarded growth.

There is some indirect evidence that the hypothalamus is more sensitive to radiation than the pituitary (24,25,30), and the study of the GH response to hGHRH has provided further information. Ahmed et al. (31) reported that patients with subnormal GH responses to arginine and insulin showed a normal response to hGHRH. They suggested that this was evidence of radiation-induced hypothalamic damage leading to GHRH deficiency. In another study, a trend toward an inverse relationship between peak GH response to hGHRH and the postirradiation interval was noted (32). This might indicate that radiation induces a progressive dysfunction of GH secretion. Using hGHRH stimulation test, we have studied 18 children treated for ALL. They all had received the same cranial radiation dose of 24 Gy. Their mean GH peak response to hGHRH was significantly decreased compared to normal short stature control children. Six patients had a normal GH response to AITT. Among them, 5 had a response to hGHRH below normal. We suggested that in some patients a decreased response to hGHRH may be the only sign of hypothalamic-pituitary dysfunction (33).

The Influence of the Radiation Dose

One of the main limitations in these studies has been the difficulty of assessing retrospectively the effective radiation dose delivered to the hypothalamic-pituitary region. The effective biological dose of radiation reaching this part of the brain should ideally be calculated by a formula taking into account the total dose, the number of fractions and the duration of therapy. As this was not feasible in routine studies, we agree with Shalet (4) that most studies rely on rather approximate evaluations. In patients irradiated for retinoblastoma, we showed that radiation doses below 20 Gy were not harmful (34). Based upon the GH response to AITT, in our experience, as shown on Table 1 and Figure 5, the frequency of GH deficiency depends on the estimated radiation dose delivered to the hypothalamus and the pituitary gland. Therefore, it varies greatly with the underlying disease treated with cranial irradiation. The mean interval since radiation in this study ranged from 5-7 years. All patients had been investigated at least 2 years after irradiation. Complete GH deficiency with 2 consecutive responses to AITT below 5 ng/ml occurred in 30% of the patients with ALL (24 Gy) and reached a frequency of 75% in the group of patients irradiated with doses above 45 Gy. Partial GH responses (5-8 ng/ml) were principally observed when radiation doses remained below 45 Gy. The 8 children with radiation doses below 24 Gy had normal GH responses to AITT. Most of the children are GH deficient when radiation doses are above 45 Gy. However, we were surprised to find a few patients irradiated with such high doses had normal GH secretion and normal growth. Generally, such high radiation doses lead to multiple hormonal deficiencies. The critical issue of the minimal harmful radiation dose should be raised when alternative protocols are organized for the treatment of children with ALL or for bone marrow transplantation. In fact, these endocrine abnormalities should stimulate future protocols using less harmful doses or replacing radiotherapy with chemotherapy as presently proposed for ALL children.

The Influence of Age at Time of Radiation

Earlier data dealing with various doses of radiation suggested that the older child was less vulnerable than the younger child (35). In our group, Pomarede et al. (34) could not confirm this suggestion because of the limited age range of the patients with retinoblastoma. In a more

Table 1. Frequency of abnormal GH responses to arginine-insulin stimulation test (AITT) according to the estimated radiation dose delivered to the hypothalamus and the pituitary gland.*

Pituitary Estimated Radiation Dose (Gy)	Cases (n)	Percentage of Cases According to AITT GH Peak (ng/ml)		
		<5	5-8	>8
<24	8	0	0	100
24	86	30	22	48
25-35	11	27	0	73
35-45	40	45	25	30
>45	12	75	8	17

*Brauner et al., unpublished data.

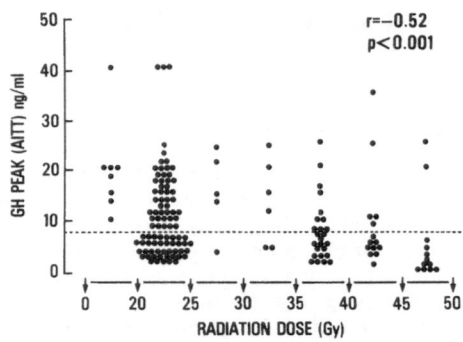

Fig. 5. GH response to the arginine-insulin tolerance test according to the calculated hypothalamic-pituitary radiation dose. The dotted line represents the lower limit of normal GH peak in prepubertal children of 8 ng/ml. All children have been studied at least 2 years after cranial radiation.

recent study (36) dealing with a well-defined group of patients similarly treated for ALL with 24 Gy (12 x 2 Gy), we demonstrated an age-related susceptibility to radiation with increased vulnerability in the younger child (Fig. 6).

The Natural Course of the Pituitary Function After Radiation

We have performed a prospective study (8) in a group of children with medulloblastoma; these children received doses of 30-45 Gy. The mean GH response to AITT evaluated every 6 months for 2 years in 9 patients decreased significantly only 18 months after irradiation. At that time, 2 out of the 9 patients were GH deficient (peak GH <5 ng/ml). Since the frequency of GHD reached 75% 5 years after this radiation dose, one can postulate that most GH deficient cases appear between the second and the fifth year following therapy. However, late occurrence of GHD is also possible (4). Our data confirm the earlier report of Shalet et al. (16). Our prospective study has also demonstrated that the poor growth observed in the first year after irradiation for brain or facial tumors was not related to early and persistent GH deficiency. We have not encountered any patient in whom GH secretion returned to normal beyond the fourth year of follow-up. Prior to that time, varying responses to repeated AITT have been observed in a few patients, which we interpreted as indicating partial GH deficiency.

SPECIFIC FEATURES RELATED TO DISEASES

Acute Lymphoblastic Leukemia

The irradiation protocol employing 24 Gy has been the most widely used. For the same total dose, the duration and fractionation are important risk factors for development of GHD (37). More recently, doses of 18 Gy have been used. However, the follow-up is too short to estimate the incidence of GHD after this lower dose. One crucial issue in this group of patients is the contrast between the relatively high frequency of low GH response to AITT and low 24-h GH secretion (peaks or integrated concentrations) and the lesser number of patients who develop overt clinical hypopituitarism and growth retardation. In our experience, only 9

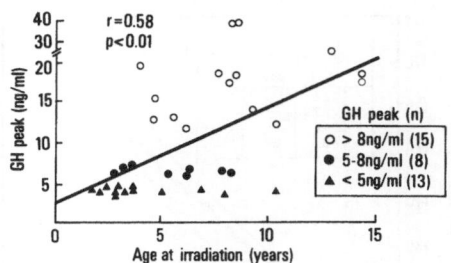

Fig. 6. GH peak response to the arginine-insulin tolerance test according to age at time of hypothalamic-pituitary radiation. The mean interval time since radiation in the 3 groups was identical. With permission of the authors (36).

out of 46 prepubertal children maintained a diminished growth rate beyond the first postirradiation year. Two of these patients had normal GH secretion; the others could be classified as GH deficient by all conventional clinical and biological criteria (29). These results suggest that in most of the ALL children physiological parameters of GH secretion were met. An intriguing observation was made in several children, as illustrated in Figure 7. In spite of a low GH response to sleep and to AITT and low plasma SmC/IGF-I values, the linear growth of these children remained normal. Some of them achieved a normal final height. A more extensive evaluation of these patients is necessary. For practical purposes, it is important to rely on both the pattern of growth and the results of GH secretion testing before making a decision to institute hGH therapy.

Medulloblastoma

Characteristic of this group of children is the addition of spinal radiation at doses superior to 27 Gy. It is well known that most of these children do end up with a very short trunk and short stature. GHD is frequent and adds to the risk of final short stature. In contrast, children receiving only cranial irradiation at similar doses appear to have reduced total height gain during puberty. We suggest that GH secretion only be studied 2 years after cranial radiation therapy in children receiving more than 25 Gy.

Total Body Irradiation

During the past several years total body irradiation (TBI) has been used in preparation for bone marrow transplantation as treatment for various diseases. A preliminary evaluation has recently been published by Saunders et al. (38). The authors addressed the question of GHD in children after various therapeutic schedules, including additional cranial irradiation. GH deficiency was present in 6 of 18 children who had not received additional cranial irradiation. However, height velocity was decreased in all patients. We have therefore selected patients who received 8-12 Gy total body irradiation. They were investigated after a mean interval time of 3 years and at least 1 year after irradiation (unpublished data). Only 1 out of the 15 patients had GH deficiency with growth retardation. Four patients were growth retarded in spite of normal GH responses to AITT. These data indicate that other causes for growth retardation must be identified in these children. This should help decide which radiation protocol carries the least risk of growth retardation.

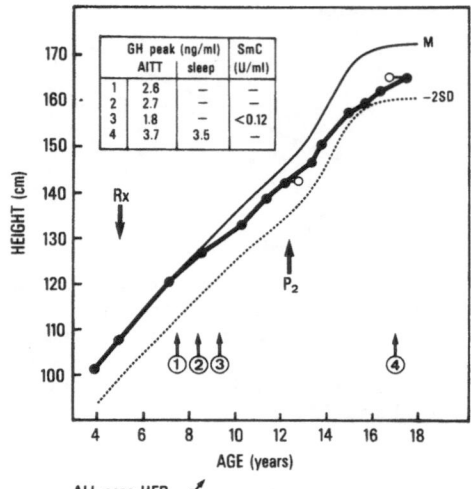

Fig. 7. Nearly normal growth pattern in a child with acute lymphoblastic leukemia treated with 2400 rads and having biological evidence of GH deficiency.

GROWTH AND GROWTH HORMONE TREATMENT

Treatment with growth hormone is now becoming an important issue in irradiated children with GH deficiency. The efficacy of hGH has been demonstrated in short-term studies (7,13,26,39). However, the analysis of these results is complicated by additional factors influencing prepubertal and pubertal growth, including damage to the spine after craniospinal irradiation, and the occurrence in some cases of early puberty or even true precocious puberty with accelerated bone maturation. Another issue is the selection of the patients to be treated by hGH. The choice of the cases to be treated is not an easy task because GH deficiency defined by biological criteria is not always accompanied by a significant reduction in growth velocity. This was observed in children treated for ALL with doses as low as 24 Gy.

Here we present our results of a 4-year follow-up in children who received more than 30 Gy for cranial or facial tumors. Before puberty, the height velocity reached a mean value of 6.5 ± 0.3 cm when treated with exogenous hGH (6 UI/w). This result is slightly lower than the height gain obtained in idiopathic GHD after similar hGH dosage. The incremental height gain decreased thereafter but remained slightly superior to the pretreatment value. The catch-up growth was about 1 SD during this period. In contrast, much lesser height increases were observed in craniospinal irradiated patients during the first year. During puberty mean height velocities in treated children were not higher as would be expected. This is partly due to large individual variation, including some children who reached 9 cm/yr at onset of therapy. These results add to the previously published data. A response comparable to that obtained in classical idiopathic GHD was reported in short-term studies by Shalet (39) and Romshe et al. (26). Others (13) reported a poor response to hGH with a skeletal maturation excessive for the increase in growth. As part of a therapeutic trial with biosynthetic methionyl-hGH, one patient who had received cranial radiotherapy developed high-titer antibodies and a decline of his growth rate (40).

From these data it can be concluded that the response to hGH is low or normal. It is likely that the response depends on the dose of hGH and the severity of GHD similar to what is observed in idiopathic GHD. The decision to treat a GH deficient child should depend primarily on his linear growth after the first year following irradiation. Since early or precocious puberty may occur and since spinal growth is more severely affected in children receiving spinal irradiation at an early age, it is also important to start hGH therapy as soon as possible before puberty. A more carefully designed prospective study would be useful in view of the natural course of growth in the different groups of patients. An alternative therapy would be hGHRH providing that the pituitary is still responsive to hGHRH.

A word of caution should be added. First, these children have undergone much stress and medical pressure during treatment of their underlying disease, and hGH therapy should only be proposed if a significant benefit can be expected. Secondly, it should be mentioned that this treatment appears to be safe in terms of tumorogenesis, as other studies in the hypopituitary population have not shown GH therapy to increase recurrence of disease nor development of malignancy (41). Since GHD is not the only consequence of cranial irradiation, one should carefully follow these children for thyroid and gonadal function which also play major roles in the control of growth.

ACKNOWLEDGMENT

We acknowledge the collaboration with the following oncology and hematology centers of Dr. C. Griscelli and J. F. Hirsch (Hopital des Enfants Malades), J. M. Zucker and P. Bataini (Institut Curie), J. Lemerle and D. Sarrazin (Institut Gustave Roussy, Villejuif), G. Schaison (Hopital St-Louis), and D. Machover (Hopital Tenon). This work was supported by a grant of the Association pour la Recherche contre le Cancer (ARC No. 415-1984) and the INSERM.

The manuscript was prepared with the skillful secretarial assistance of Mrs. M. Lacroix.

REFERENCES

1. Sainsbury CPQ, Newcombe RG, Hughes IA. Weight gain and height velocity during prolonged first remission from acute lymphoblastic leukemia. Arch Dis Child 1985; 60:832-6.
2. Dacou-Voutetakis C, Xypolyta A, Haidas S, Constantinidis M, Papavasiliou C, Zannos-Mariolea L. Irradiation of the head. Immediate effect on growth hormone secretion in children. J Clin Endocrinol Metab 1977; 44:791-4.
3. Price DA, Shalet SM, Beardwell CG, Hann IM, Jones PHM. Serum somatomedin activity (SMact) in children with acute lymphoblastic leukaemia (ALL). Pediatr Res 1978; 12:159.
4. Shalet SM. Irradiation induced growth failure. Clin Endocrinol Metab 1986; 15(3).
5. Starceski PJ, Lee PA, Blatt J, Finegold D, Brown D. Comparable effects of 1800- and 2400-rad (18- and 24-Gy) cranial irradiation on height and weight in children treated for acute lymphocytic leukemia. Am J Dis Child 1987; 141:550-2.
6. Robison LL, Nesbit ME, Sather HN, et al. Height of children successfully treated for acute lymphoblastic leukemia: a report from the late effects study committee of Children's Cancer Study Group. Med

Pediatr Oncol 1985; 13:14-21.

7. Brauner R, Czernichow P, Rappaport R. Croissance staturale apres irradiation du systeme nerveux central pour medulloblastome de la fosse posterieure. Analyse retrospective de 45 observations. Arch Fr Pediatr 1985; 42:219-23.

8. Brauner R, Czernichow P, Prevot C, Guyda HJ, Rappaport R. Longitudinal study of GH secretion, somatomedin and growth in the two years following cranial irradiation. Pediatr Res 1985; 19:613.

9. Shalet SM, Gibson B, Swindell R, Pearson D. Effect of spinal irradiation on growth. Arch Dis Child 1987; 62:461-4.

10. Probert JC, Bruce FFR, Parker R, Kaplan HS. Growth retardation in children after megavoltage irradiation of the spine. Cancer 1973; 32:634-9.

11. Rappaport R, Brauner R, Czernichow P, et al. Effect of hypothalamic and pituitary irradiation on pubertal development in children with cranial tumors. J Clin Endocrinol Metab 1982; 54:1164-8.

12. Brauner R, Czernichow P, Rappaport R. Precocious puberty after hypothalamic and pituitary irradiation in young children. N Engl J Med 1984; 311:920.

13. Winter RJ, Green OC. Irradiation-induced growth hormone deficiency: blunted growth response and accelerated skeletal maturation to growth hormone therapy. J Pediatr 1985; 106:609-12.

14. Tan BC, Kunaratnam N. Hypopituitary dwarfism following radiotherapy for nasopharyngeal carcinoma. Clin Radiol 1966; 17:302-4.

15. Larkins RG, Martin FIR. Hypopituitarism after extracranial irradiation: evidence for hypothalamic origin. Br Med J [Clin Res] 1973; i:152-3.

16. Shalet SM, Beardwell CG, Morris-Jones PH, Pearson D. Pituitary function after treatment of intracranial tumours in children. Lancet 1975; 3:104-7.

17. Richards GE, Wara WM, Grumbach MM, Kaplan SL, Sheline GE, Conte FA. Delayed onset of hypopituitarism: sequelae of therapeutic irradiation of central nervous system, eye, and middle ear tumors. J Pediatr 1976; 89:553-9.

18. Perry-Keene DA, Connelly JF, Young RA, Wettenhall HNB, Martin FIR. Hypothalamic hypopituitarism following external radiotherapy for tumours distant from the adenohypophysis. Clin Endocrinol (Oxf) 1976; 5:373-80.

19. Czernichow P, Cachin O, Rappaport R, Flamant F, Sarrazin D, Schweisguth O. Sequelles endocriniennes des irradiations de la tete et du cou pour tumeurs extracraniennes. Arch Fr Pediatr 1977; 34:CLIV-XIV.

20. Samaan NA, Bakdash MM, Caderao JB, Cangir A, Jesse RH, Ballantyne AJ. Hypopituitarism after external irradiation. Evidence for both hypothalamic and pituitary origin. Ann Intern Med 1975; 83:771-7.

21. Spiliotis BE, August GP, Hung W, Sonis W, Mendelson W, Bercu BB. Growth hormone neurosecretory dysfunction. A treatable cause of short stature. JAMA 1984; 251:2223-30.

22. Mosier HD, Jansons RA, Swingle KF, Sondhaus CA, Dearden LC, Halsall LC. Growth hormone secretion in the stunted head-irradiated rat. Pediatr Res 1985; 19:543-8.

23. Mosier HD, Jansons RA. Pituitary content of somatotropin, gonadotropin, and thyrotropin in rats with stunted linear growth following head X-irradiation. Proc Soc Exp Biol Med 1968; 128:23-6.

24. Chrousos GO, Poplack D, Brown T, et al. Effects of cranial radiation on hypothalamic-adenohypophyseal function: abnormal growth hormone secretory dynamics. J Clin Endocrinol Metab 1982; 54:1135-9.

25. Dickinson WP, Berry DH, Dickinson L, et al. Differential effects of cranial radiation on growth hormone response to arginine and insulin infusion. J Pediatr 1978; 92:754-7.

26. Romshe CA, Zipf WB, Miser A, Miser J, Sotos JF, Newton WA. Evalua-

tion of growth hormone release and human growth hormone treatment in children with cranial irradiation-associated short stature. J Pediatr 1984; 104:177-81.

27. Ahmed SR, Shalet SM, Beardwell CG. The effects of cranial irradiation on growth hormone secretion. Acta Paediatr Scand 1986; 75:255-60.

28. Blatt J, Bercu BB, Gillin JC, Mendelson WB, Poplack DG. Reduced pulsatile growth hormone secretion in children after therapy for acute lymphoblastic leukemia. J Pediatr 1984; 104:182-6.

29. Brauner R, Prevot C, Roy MP, Rappaport R. Growth, growth hormone secretion and somatomedin C after cranial irradiation for acute lymphoblastic leukemia. Acta Endocrinol (Copenh) 1986; 279(suppl):178-82.

30. Shalet SM, Price DA, Beardwell CG, Morris-Jones PH, Pearson D. Normal growth despite abnormalities of growth hormone secretion in children treated for acute leukemia. J Pediatr 1979; 94:719-22.

31. Ahmed SR, Shalet SM. Hypothalamic growth hormone releasing factor deficiency following cranial irradiation. Clin Endocrinol (Oxf) 1984; 21:483-8.

32. Lustig RH, Schriok EA, Kaplan SL, Grumbach MM. Effect of growth hormone-releasing factor on growth hormone release in children with radiation-induced growth hormone deficiency. Pediatrics 1985; 76:274-9.

33. Crosnier H, Brauner R, Prevot C, Rappaport R. GH response to hGRF as a sensitive index of GH neurosecretory dysfunction after cranial irradiation. Pediatr Res 1986; 20:1189.

34. Pomarede R, Czernichow P, Zucker JM, et al. Incidence of anterior pituitary deficiency after radiotherapy at an early age: study in retinoblastoma. Acta Paediatr Scand 1984; 73:115-9.

35. Shalet SM, Beardwell CG, Pearson D, Morris-Jones PH. The effect of varying doses of cerebral irradiation on growth hormone production in childhood. Clin Endocrinol (Oxf) 1976; 5:287-90.

36. Brauner R, Czernichow P, Rappaport R. Greater susceptibility to hypothalamopituitary irradiation in younger children with acute lymphoblastic leukemia. J Pediatr 1986; 108:332.

37. Shalet SM, Beardwell CG, Morris-Jones PH, Pearson D. Growth hormone deficiency after treatment of acute leukaemia in children. Arch Dis Child 1976; 51:489-93.

38. Saunders JE, Pritchard S, Mahoney P, et al. Growth and development following marrow transplantation for leukemia. Blood 1986; 68:1129-35.

39. Shalet SM, Whitehead E, Chapman AJ, Beardwell CG. The effects of growth hormone therapy in children with radiation-induced growth hormone deficiency. Acta Paediatr Scand 1981: 70:81-5.

40. Kaplan SL, August GP, Blethen SL, et al. Clinical studies with recombinant-DNA-derived methionyl human growth hormone in growth hormone deficient children. Lancet 1986; 1:697-700.

41. Arslanian SA, Becker DJ, Lee PA, Drash AL, Foley TP. Growth hormone therapy and tumor recurrence. Am J Dis Child 1985; 139:347-50.

14

AGE AND SEX-RELATED NEUROSECRETION OF GROWTH HORMONE

W. S. Evans,* K. Y. Ho,* A. C. S. Faria,* R. J. Krieg,
Jr.,[3] P. M. Martha, Jr.,[2] D. A. Leong,* A. D. Rogol,[2]
J. D. Veldhuis,* R. M. Blizzard,[2] M. O. Thorner*

*Departments of Internal Medicine and [2]Pediatrics,
University of Virginia Medical School, Charlottesville, VA
22908; [3]Department of Anatomy, Medical College of Virginia,
Virginia Commonwealth University, Richmond, VA 23298

INTRODUCTION

Although it has long been recognized that the secretion of growth hormone (GH) is influenced by age and sex, the mechanisms through which these factors mediate their effects remain incompletely understood. Indeed, and as is discussed below, in addition to the major gaps in our knowledge, there are numerous inconsistencies in the literature concerning issues which would seem to lend themselves to straightforward experimental approaches. We are of the opinion that much of the confusion in the literature reflects a failure to keep one premise clearly in mind: both age and sex almost certainly have both independent and interrelated effects on GH secretion. Thus, any experimental design utilized to examine issues related to GH secretion must include proper controls to account for these combined influences; failure to do so may and almost surely has provided discordant results. In addition, and although there are many factors which have prompted extensive use of the laboratory rat to address both in vivo and in vitro questions related to the secretion of GH, it must be emphasized that certain GH secretory dynamics in the rat vary markedly from those in the human; e.g., while stress and fasting have a positive effect on GH secretion in the human, they exert strongly negative influences in the rat. With these caveats having been mentioned, we now review briefly the literature concerning the effects of age and sex on the secretion of GH in the rat and human and subsequently discuss some recent observations which have resulted from our combined clinical and basic science research efforts focused on these issues.

Growth hormone becomes detectable in the fetal rat pituitary by day 18 of gestation (with birth usually occurring on day 22), and most individual somatotropes are capable of GH release in response to growth hormone releasing hormone (GHRH) by day 20 (1,2). At the time of birth, pituitary content and circulating levels of GH are very high compared to adult values (3). During the newborn period, pituitary GH content has been reported to either continue to increase (4) or remain unchanged (5), while circulating GH levels decline throughout the first postnatal week and remain at relatively low levels during the second and third weeks of life (6).

The late prepubertal and pubertal periods (approximately days 20 through 45 of life) are times of dramatic change in both body growth and GH secretion. Not only is this true within each sex, but clear sex-related differences also emerge. Mean GH levels rise again by day 30 and become significantly elevated before the onset of puberty (7). Although sequential venous blood sampling has demonstrated episodic GH secretion in the youngest rats studied to date (22 days), no sex-related differences were present. However, by 30 days, the next age group evaluated, a clear sexually differentiated pulsatile pattern was present (7). Interestingly, the rate of body growth also increases, becomes sex dependent and reaches its maximum during the same period (5,7). Between 45 and 90 days of age, the mature sexually differentiated secretory pattern of the adult becomes fully established (7). Mature male rats exhibit periods of low or undetectable GH levels interrupted at regular 3- to 4-h intervals by large complex excursions from baseline (7,8) which commonly reach values of 200 to 400 ng/ml or higher (7-9). Although these excursions often appear to comprise more than one secretory peak, detailed pulse analysis has yet to be applied to such data. In contrast, the mature female has more frequent unpredictable pulses of lower amplitude (rarely exceeding 200 ng/ml) with interpulse levels generally measurable and, therefore, elevated in comparison to the male (7,10,11).

Once established, pulsatile GH secretion remains lifelong. With the exception of higher levels in the female during late pregnancy, parturition and the immediate puerperium (11), the GH secretory pattern is felt to remain relatively constant throughout most of adult life. With advancing age, however, further changes apparently take place. Thus, 18 to 20-month-old male rats exhibit diminished GH pulse amplitude when compared to 4- to 5-month-old males but demonstrate no differences in trough levels or pulse periodicity (9). The responsiveness of the pituitary in situ to GHRH is also attenuated in older (19- to 21-month-old) male rats when compared to the response in younger (3- to 4-month-old) animals (12). Of course, these observations must be interpreted in light of the fact that rats, in obvious contrast to humans, continue to grow throughout their entire lifetime (13).

In the human, the effects of age and sex on GH secretion are somewhat less clear. An ontogenetic study undertaken by Kaplan et al. found detectable GH in the serum of human fetuses as young as 70 days gestation. Mean levels correlated positively with increased gestational age until the mid to late second trimester when values as high as 150 ng/ml were found. After 24 weeks, a significant negative correlation between advancing gestational age and serum GH was present (14). At the time of birth and for several weeks thereafter, GH levels remain high when compared to typical adult values (14,15). In addition, it has been reported that levels in males during the newborn period are higher than those in females (15). However, these data are cross-sectional with large ranges present among the individual values and, consequently, are subject to the usual concerns which apply to such data.

Very little information exists on spontaneous GH secretion in toddlers or young school-age children. However, several studies have provided indirect evidence that GH secretion in older children is intricately related to age, sex and pubertal status. For example, there are strong correlations between rising somatomedin C (SmC) levels, pubertal stage and timing of peak height velocity (16,17). In addition, although androgen therapy alone produces some increase in growth velocity in boys who are both gonadotropin and GH deficient, this is significantly less than that observed in the normal male adolescent growth spurt. By contrast, treatment of this same group of boys using combined testosterone and GH replacement therapy in appropriate doses is capable of mimicking the normal pubertal increase in growth velocity (18,19).

Unfortunately, studies designed to investigate the precise age and sex-dependent changes in GH secretion have yielded conflicting results. Thus, mean GH levels of pubertal children are claimed to be higher (20-23) or no different (24-28) than those of prepubertal children of the same sex. Likewise, mean GH levels of pubertal boys have been found to be lower (23), higher (21) and no different (25) than girls in a similar pubertal stage. Other reports have focused on the pulsatile character of GH secretion and its relationship to age and sex. Miller et al. found that GH levels greater than or equal to 5 ng/ml during daytime hours were more frequent in boys whose pubertal development was in Tanner stages III through IV than in either less sexually mature boys or in girls at any pubertal stage (21).

Our own studies, described in detail later, indicate that an increase in GH pulse amplitude, without a change in frequency, may result from the pubertal rise in gonadal steroids in boys (22,29). These discrepant findings are likely due to the presence of numerous interstudy differences including sampling frequency, subject definition, assay sensitivity, study conditions, subject activity patterns and pulse analysis methods. Consequently, one can only state at this time that, although indirect evidence indicates it is likely that individuals experience age and sex-related changes in GH secretion throughout preadult life, this is still far from certain.

In adults, a similar line of investigation has also produced occasionally conflicting results. Thus, while certain investigators have reported that GH secretion remains unaltered in the older population (30,31), others have suggested that it diminishes (23,32). Similarly, the relationship between gender/gonadal hormone environment and GH secretion remains incompletely defined. Studies performed a number of years ago found that both serum levels of GH obtained in ambulatory subjects (33) and GH secretory rates (34) are higher in premenopausal women than in men. That estrogen may be responsible for these differences has been suggested; e.g., mean serum levels of GH are said to be higher in the periovulatory (35) and luteal phases (33) of the menstrual cycle, times when serum concentrations of estrogen are relatively increased. Moreover, premenopausal women on oral contraceptives (34) and men treated with estrogen (33) demonstrate, respectively, increased secretory rates and increased basal circulating levels of GH. In a more recent report, serum concentrations of GH were shown to be elevated in postmenopausal women treated with ethinyl estradiol for 15 days, results which are consistent with the hypothesis that estrogen modulates the secretion of GH (36).

Although these and other studies implicate both age and gender and/or the gonadal hormone environment as factors strongly influencing the secretion of GH in humans, they do not address the mechanisms involved. It is now well accepted that GH release by the somatotrope reflects an interplay of two hypothalamic hormones: GHRH and GH release inhibiting hormone (somatostatin). It has long been suggested that the pulsatile release of GH may derive from reciprocal changes in the hypothalamic secretion of GHRH and somatostatin; indeed, using the rat as a model, Plotsky and Vale have recently shown that the major episodes of GH release are associated with a simultaneous elevation in portal blood concentrations of GHRH and a decrease in somatostatin (37). Given that pulsatile GH release may well reflect hypothalamic activity as well as the activity of modulating factors on the somatotropes, we felt that it would be of interest to characterize the episodic secretion of GH in humans of differing ages and sex.

Effects of Age and Sex on Basal GH Secretion Studies in Children

In an early study in boys, we investigated the role of testosterone in the pubertal rise in SmC (38). Six prepubertal GH deficient boys were given 7-day courses of GH alone, testosterone proprionate (T) alone, or the combination of GH and T. SmC levels were determined in plasma at the start and finish of each treatment period. Both GH alone and the combination of GH plus T were associated with significant increases in SmC (mean change 0.68 μ/ml after GH and 0.63 μ/ml after GH + T), while T alone caused a change of only 0.09 μ/ml. In contrast, the same dose of T resulted in a mean increase of 1.29 μ/ml in 4 GH-sufficient boys with delayed adolescence. Thus, it was concluded that T stimulates SmC production in prepubertal boys who can secrete GH, but not in those who are GH deficient. We postulated that the effect of T in this regard is due to its effect on pituitary GH secretion. To investigate further this postulate, we next studied the effects of two growth-promoting androgens, oxandrolone (OX) and testosterone (T) on the 24-h mean concentration of GH (MCGH; ng/ml), the pattern of GH secretion and the SmC concentrations in boys with short stature and/or delayed sexual development (29). Ten such boys were treated with one or the other androgenic agent, and serum GH was measured at 20-min intervals for 24 h before and 65 ± 5 days after initiation of therapy. SmC levels were measured twice during each GH study. In the boys treated with T, there were significant increases in the 24-h MCGH (mean increase 4.3-fold) and SmC levels (0.82 ± 0.46 versus 2.3 ± 0.4 μ/ml; mean ± SD), while no significant changes occurred in boys treated with OX. Although GH pulse frequency, analyzed by then available pulse analysis techniques, indicated there was also an increase in pulse frequency with T, later reanalysis using an improved computerized algorithm which minimizes the false positive rate showed the increase in GH caused by T therapy occurred only as a result of increased GH pulse amplitude and not frequency (22).

Since both of these studies indicated an augmentation of GH secretion by testosterone, we performed a cross-sectional comparison of GH secretion in prepubertal and late pubertal boys (22). Ten boys with Tanner stages I-II genital development had significantly lower 24-h MCGH values than did five boys in Tanner stages IV-V (2.7 ± 0.5 versus 5.4 ± 0.7 ng/ml; mean ± SEM). In addition, mean pulse amplitudes were significantly lower (8.6 ± 1.7 versus 17.1 ± 2.6 ng/ml; mean ± SEM) in the less sexually mature group. It should be noted, however, that 8 of the boys in Tanner stages I-II had heights less than the 5th percentile for age, while none of the boys in Tanner stages IV-V had heights below the 25th percentile. Taken together, the data from these studies strongly suggest a GH-enhancing effect of gonadal steroids during male puberty. However, confirmation of these observations will require the completion of longitudinal studies which follow a cohort of boys as they progress through their own spontaneous puberty.

Studies in Adults

We have assessed the effects of age and gender on both integrated GH concentration (IGHC) and the number and characteristics of GH pulses in adults during a 24-h period (39). Ten younger men (18-30 years), 10 younger women (18-33 years) in the early follicular phase of their menstrual cycle, 8 older men (56-71 years) and 8 postmenopausal women (57-76 years) were studied. All individuals were healthy and none was taking any medication. Growth hormone concentrations were measured by radioimmunoassay in blood samples which were obtained at 20-min intervals during the 24-h study period. Growth hormone pulses were identified and characterized using a modification of the Santen and Bardin method of pulse analysis (40). Body mass index (calculated as weight/height^2 was not significantly correlated with age but was negatively correlated with IGHC. The IGHC and indices of pulsatile GH secretion are shown in Figure 1. As can be seen, the mean IGHC was greater in women than in men and greater in the younger than in the older subjects. When separated into four groups by age and sex, younger women were found to have a higher IGHC than younger men, and higher than both older men and older women. Analysis of pulsatile GH secretion failed to demonstrate any differences in the frequency of GH pulses among the groups studied. Similarly, there were no gender-based differences in any of the other GH pulse characteristics. There were, however, striking effects of age on GH pulse parameters. Thus, younger subjects exhibited a greater mean pulse duration, pulse amplitude, and fraction of GH secreted as pulses (FGHP) in comparison to older subjects. In addition, younger individuals secreted GH in relatively larger pulses (arbitrarily defined as 3 times the threshold criterion for a pulse). Conversely, the older subjects demonstrated a greater number of smaller pulses than did the younger subjects. As was the case for IGHC, a further difference was detected upon resolution of the subjects into four groups; i.e., younger women were found to have greater amplitude pulses than older women. The mean serum levels of T and 17-beta-estradiol (E_2) in the four groups studied are shown in Table 1. Neither T nor E_2 decreased significantly as a function of age in the men. Using linear regression, serum levels of both free and total E_2 were found to correlate significantly and positively with IGHC, pulse frequency, pulse amplitude, the number of large pulses, and FGHP. Conversely, no index of GH secretion correlated with serum T. When the separate effects of age and sex on GH secretion were reassessed with the effects of E_2 removed using analysis of covariance, IGHC was no longer affected by age or sex nor was pulse amplitude affected by age.

The influence of age and sex on serum levels of SmC were also assessed. As is shown in Figure 2, SmC concentrations were greater in younger compared to older individuals. Several indices of pulsatile GH secretion, including mean amplitude, number of large pulses and FGHP correlated with SmC concentrations. Similarly, the free E_2 concentration also correlated with SmC.

Taken as a group, these results demonstrate that age and sex have independent and interrelated effects on both total GH secretion and on certain aspects of pulsatile GH secretion. Younger but not older women secrete significantly more GH than do their age-matched male counterparts, as would be predicted by earlier studies. Thus, while there is no obvious age-related decline in GH secretion in men, such diminished release clearly occurs in women. Consistent with these observations, E_2, but not T, strongly correlated with both total GH secretion and several characteristics of pulsatile GH release. If it can be assumed that reciprocal changes in portal blood concentrations of GHRH and somatostatin result in the episodic secretion of GH and that our sampling/pulse identification techniques are adequate (see below), then neither age nor sex-related factors (presumably estrogen) exert an effect on the frequency with which GHRH and somatostatin is released. However, the present data allow no inferences with regard to the amounts of the releasing hormones secreted or the response characteristics of the somatotropes within the various clinical settings.

Impact of Sampling Frequency on Sex-Related Differences in GH Pulsatility

Recently, a number of investigators have initiated a reappraisal of the technical aspects of episodic hormone release detection and analysis. There is now general agreement that the number of pulses of luteinizing hormone (LH) detected within a defined sampling interval is highly dependent on the frequency with which blood samples are obtained (41-44).

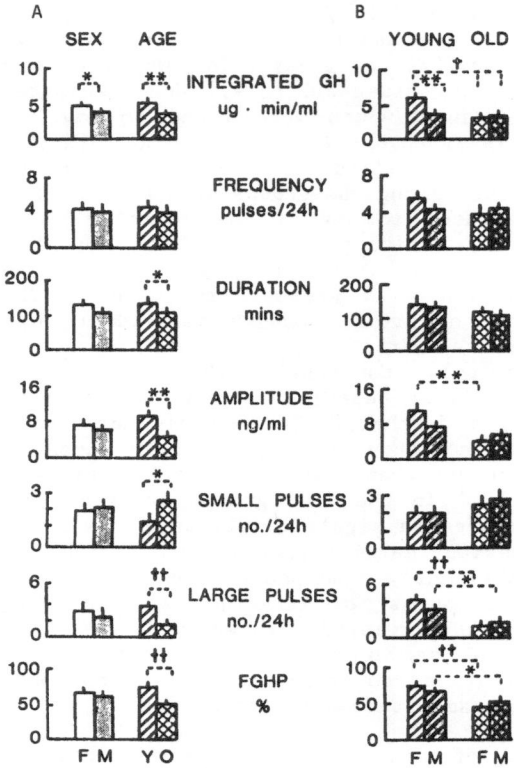

Fig. 1. Comparison of mean (± SEM) integrated GH concentration (ICHC), pulse frequency, duration, amplitude, number of small or large pulses, and fraction of GH secreted as pulses (FGHP) in study subjects grouped according to sex or age (A) or according to study subgroups of younger women, younger men, older women, and older men (B). F = women, M = men, Y = younger, O = older. *, P<0.05; **, P<0.01; , P<0,001; , P<0.0001. Reprinted with permission from Ho et al. (39).

Moreover, as the intensity of sampling is altered, appropriate statistical adjustment must be made to minimize the occurrence of false-positive (Type 1) error rates. With these concerns in mind, we questioned: (1) whether or not an every 20-min sampling paradigm as used in our initial studies and those of others is adequate to capture the majority of GH pulses; and, (2) if not, would age and/or sex-related differences in GH pulse frequency become apparent in studies utilizing a more intensive sampling schedule. To address the first issue, we combined a more rigorous sampling technique (blood obtained every 5 min for 24 h) with analysis via a novel pulse analysis algorithm (Cluster; 45) which utilizes intrinsic measurement error in the experiment series for pulse identification. In addition, this algorithm is not influenced by unstable baselines or nonuniform peak amplitudes and allows constraint of Type 1 errors to a known level (46). Seven normal young men (21-27 years) were studied in this manner. In Figure 3 is demonstrated the impact of sampling frequency on pulse detection. Both the parent 5-min data series and the constituent 10-, 15-,

Table 1. Serum free and total estradiol and testosterone concentrations in younger women, older women, younger men, and older men.

	Women		Men	
	Younger (n=10)	Older (n=8)	Younger (n=10)	Older (n=8)
Serum estradiol				
Free (pg/ml)	2.1 ± 0.3	0.32 ± 0.1	1.3 ± 0.2	0.8 ± 0.1
Total (pg/ml)	122.0 ± 19.0	18.7 ± 5.2	63.2 ± 8.5	44.1 ± 8.3
Serum testosterone				
Free (ng/dl)	1.38 ± 0.23	0.54 ± 0.13	22.6 ± 3.4	16.4 ± 2.0
Total (ng/dl)	57.8 ± 8.6	27.1 ± 7.3	874.0 ± 146.0	533.0 ± 68.0

Measurements were performed in pooled serum samples obtained from each individual's 24-h GH study samples. Values are the mean ± SEM. Reprinted with permission from Ho et al. (39).

20-, 30-, 45- and 60-min series were analyzed. The number of GH peaks detected was maximal with the 5-min sampling rate and was nearly twice that detected with 15- or 20-min sampling. Sampling at 10-min intervals resulted in a strong trend towards enhanced pulse detection but was not statistically different from the sampling frequencies. Of particular interest, mean peak height was quite stable across a number of sampling intensities (Table 2). In contrast, mean peak width varied inversely with sampling frequencies; i.e., reduced sampling frequency was associated with significantly greater mean peak duration.

With these data in mind, but restrained by the practical considerations related to blood sampling, we elected to reexamine the issue of gender-related differences in GH secretion in young adults. To this end, we sampled 15 younger men and 11 younger women at 10-min intervals for 24 h (47). In contrast to the original study in which women in both the early and late follicular phase of the menstrual cycle were studied, all women in this subsequent investigation were within the early follicular phase. When these data were analyzed with Cluster with the false positive rate set at 5%, no differences in either pulse number or pulse charac-

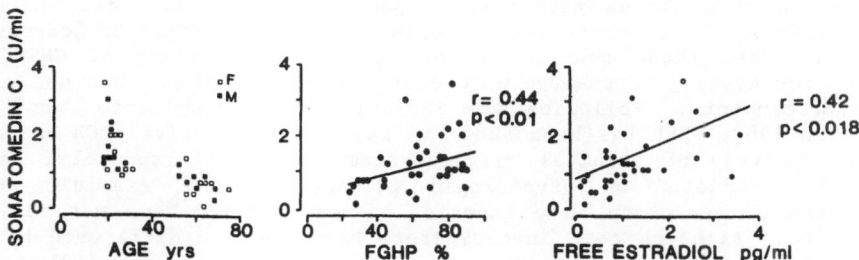

Fig. 2. Left panel, SMC concentrations in women (open) and men (closed) in relationship to age. Middle panel, correlation between SmC concentration and FGHP. Right panel, correlation between SmC and free estradiol concentrations. Reprinted with permission from Ho et al. (39).

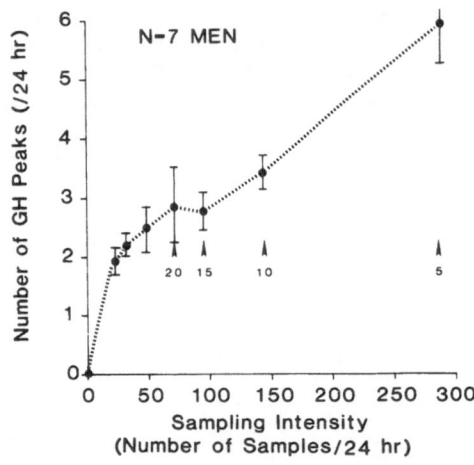

Fig. 3. Impact of sampling intensity on 24-h GH pulse frequency in normal men. The pulse frequency (mean ± SEM) was determined in the parent 5-min GH series and in the constituent 10-, 15-, 20-, 30-, 45- and 60-min series. Data obtained with certain sampling frequencies (at 5-, 10-, 15- and 20-min intervals) are denoted by the arrows for reference. Reprinted with permission from Evans et al. (46).

teristics were noted. We believe that the differences detected in the original study between young men and women may well have reflected an effect of estrogen on GH secretion in women sampled during the late follicular phase of their menstrual cycle. Proper, prospective studies performed at each stage of the cycle will be required to test this hypothesis.

Effects of Age and Sex on GHRH-Stimulated GH Secretion:
Studies in the Human

As is detailed above, characterization of total and pulsatile GH release reflects an integration of both hypothalamic input to the somato-trope and factors which modulate somatotrope function directly; i.e., such studies do not allow discrimination between the effects of age and sex at the hypothalamic versus pituitary components of the GH axis. Although direct stimulation of somatotropes would have the potential to address, at least in part, these concerns prior to the availability of GHRH, all methods for testing GH reserve were centrally mediated and thus not useful as discriminators. Following its isolation, characterization, and synthesis in 1982, GHRH has been shown to stimulate selectively GH secretion within an array of clinical circumstances (48). Unfortunately, and as might be predicted on physiologic grounds, studies examining GHRH-stimulated GH secretion as a function of age and sex have not all been consistent. Although some investigators have shown a difference between GHRH-stimulated GH secretion in young adult men versus women (49), we and others have been unable to confirm these results. Thus, Gelato and colleagues found no statistical differences in the dose of GHRH required for half maximal stimulation of GH in young men and women, nor in the midfollicular or luteal phases of the menstrual cycle (50). Likewise, in

Table 2. Relation of GH peak parameters to sampling intensity.

Sampling Frequency	Width (min)	Maximal Height (ng/ml)	Increment (ng/ml)	Area (ng/ml/min)
5	53.6 ± 4.6[a]	12.7 ± 2.9[a]	9.1 ± 2.3[a]	266.1 ± 72.4[a]
10	106.3 ± 13.4[b]	14.0 ± 3.8[a]	12.3 ± 4.0[a]	573.3 ± 183.6[ab]
15	141.4 ± 16.6[c]	17.5 ± 6.7[a]	15.8 ± 6.9[a]	769.2 ± 304[b]
20	158.3 ± 13.0[c]	13.3 ± 3.3[a]	11.6 ± 3.5[a]	667.4 ± 212.6[b]
30	217.5 ± 16.4[d]	21.4 ± 8.8[a]	20.0 ± 9.0[a]	1123.6 ± 437.8[b]
45	283.8 ± 20.5[e]	13.7 ± 3.3[a]	12.1 ± 3.4[a]	927.7 ± 318.4[b]
60	380.0 ± 65.0[f]	15.5 ± 5.8[a]	13.0 ± 6.5[a]	1280.5 ± 583.4[b]

Data are expressed as mean ± SEM. Within any column, differing superscripts are used to identify those sampling frequencies that yielded significantly different estimates of the pulse property; e.g., the mean peak width of pulses identified with a 5-min sampling frequency is smaller than those identified at all other sampling frequencies, whereas peak width associated with 15- and 20-min sampling frequencies were indistinguishable from one another but different from those identified at other sampling frequencies. Reprinted with permission from Evans et al. (46).

a second study, Gelato and co-workers found no differences in the GH response to a supramaximal dose of GHRH either between boys and girls as a group or among girls in different pubertal stages. The median response of boys in midpuberty was lower than either prepubertal boys or adult men, but statistical significance was dependent on the method of analysis (51). In our own studies, the GH response to a supramaximal dose (3.3 µg/kg) of GHRH was no different in young men compared to young women (52,53). Moreover, our data obtained during the menstrual cycle were consistent with those of Gelato mentioned above; i.e., no differences in stimulated GH release were observed during the early follicular, late follicular or midluteal phases of the menstrual cycle. Similarly, although Dawson-Hughes and colleagues were able to document an effect of ethinyl estradiol on basal GH secretion, no differences in GHRH-stimulated GH release could be found prior to or during estrogen treatment (36).

The question of whether GHRH-stimulated GH release is altered in older individuals also remains controversial. Thus, while Shibasaki and colleagues found diminished stimulated GH secretion in older versus younger men (54), Pavlov and colleagues found GHRH-stimulated GH secretion to be unchanged with aging (55). However, it cannot be overly stressed that both the failure to detect the differences in GHRH-stimulated GH secretion in certain clinical situations and the inconsistencies in results among laboratories may reflect the dynamics of the system being tested; i.e., in the human, it is not currently possible to inhibit the effects of somatostatin during GHRH administration. Thus, the release of GH by the somatotrope will reflect not only the response to exogenously administered GHRH, but also modulation by prevailing portal concentrations of somatostatin. For this reason, and in an effort to document somato-trope response characteristics as a function of age and sex, we and others have utilized in vitro techniques in which the response of isolated pituitary tissue to GHRH can be monitored. As is discussed in the introduction, the interpretation of these studies must be conducted with the understanding that the effects of the gonadal hormones may or may not be similar in the human and rat.

GHRH-Stimulated GH Secretion as a Function of Age and Sex: In Vitro Studies

In earlier work, we demonstrated that rat pituitaries, if acutely dispersed into individual cells and placed in a perifusion system, reflect the gonadal hormone milieu of the donor animal (56). Therefore, in order to define the effects of gender and the gonadal hormone environment on GHRH-stimulated GH release, we examined concentration-response relationships between GHRH and GH release in a number of groups including intact male rats, castrate male rats, castrate male rats treated with T or E_2 and female rats on diestrous day 2. The GH responses to 2.5-min pulses with 8 concentrations of GHRH are shown in Figure 4 (57). Maximal GH release occurred by cells from intact male rats and was substantially greater than that from female rats. Castration diminished GHRH-stimulated GH release and treatment with T restored the response, although not to levels seen in the intact male. Treatment of the castrate male rat with E_2 lowered stimulated GH release to a level indistinguishable from that seen in females. Although these data suggested that, in the rat, stimulated GH release is enhanced and inhibited by T and E_2 respectively, they do not address the question of the mechanisms which might subserve the differences in release potential; i.e., are there differences in the number of somatotropes and/or secretory capacity of somatotropes between the sexes?

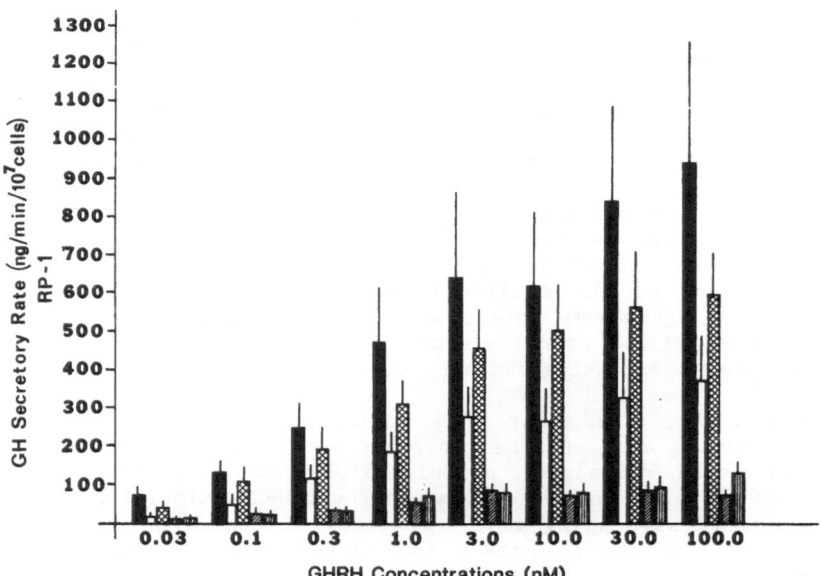

Fig. 4. Growth hormone secretion (ng/min per 10^7 cells; above basal) by perifused rat anterior pituitary cells in response to 2.5-min pulses of 8 concentrations of GHRH. Experimental groups include intact males (solid), castrate males (open), castrate males treated with testosterone (cross-hatched), castrate males treated with 17-beta-estradiol (diagonal striped), and diestrous day 2 females (vertical striped). Reprinted with permission from Evans et al. (57).

To examine these issues, we have utilized the reverse hemolytic plaque assay in which somatotropes can be identified and quantitated and hormone secretion from individual cells assessed. Our initial studies demonstrated that the percent of GH secreting cells in tissue obtained from male rats is greater than that of somatotropes in the female (Figure 5; 58) and that both sensitivity and responsivity to GHRH are greater in cells from male animals (Figure 6). That the gonadal hormone environment and not gender alone may play an important role in such sexual dimorphism has been suggested (59,60). In particular, utilizing a similar hemolytic plaque technique, Hoeffler and Frawley have demonstrated that the difference in percent of somatotropes between the sexes does not become apparent until after puberty (61). It must also be pointed out that a difference in the percent of somatotropes does not reflect a difference in absolute number since total cell yields after dispersion are consistently higher in preparations from female compared with male rats. If such yields reflect the pituitary cell population in situ, then it follows that the absolute number of somatotropes is similar, not different, between the sexes. Further more direct studies are required to resolve this question. We believe that certain gonadal hormone environments are associated with dynamic changes in the absolute number of somatotropes, raising interesting questions about the origin of these cells. Whether such changes reflect hyperplasia of existing cells or transformation from a precursor cell or other cell type remains unknown. Certainly, there is compelling evidence that certain cells within the pituitary have the ability to secrete both GH and prolactin (62,63), and there is evidence to suggest that the gonadal hormone environment may dictate the functional expression of such cells (64). The effect to which gonadal hormones influence both changes in the somatotrope population and secretory capacity and the mechanisms subserving such modulations requires intensive evaluation.

SUMMARY AND CONCLUSIONS

That GH secretion is influenced by age and sex is clear; the physiologic mechanisms which subserve these effects remain to be thoroughly defined. The interpretation of existing studies and the design of new protocols to examine these issues must be undertaken with the knowledge

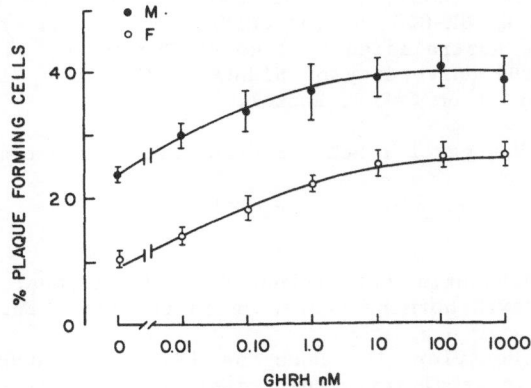

Fig. 5. Effect of log incremental concentrations of GHRH on percent of plaque-forming cells from male (solid) and female (open) rats. Values shown are means ± SEM from six experiments. Reprinted with permission from Ho et al. (58).

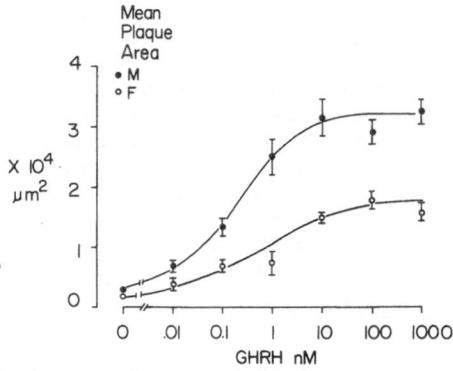

Fig. 6. Effect of log incremental concentrations of GHRH on mean plaque area of somatotropes from male (solid) and female (open) rats. Values shown are means ± SEM from six experiments. Reprinted with permission from Ho et al. (58).

that age and sex almost certainly exert both independent and interrelated effects on GH secretion. Although in vitro studies allow documentation of somatotrope numbers and secretory capacity as a function of age, gender and the gonadal hormone environment, it is highly probable that certain, if not all, somatotrope characteristics reflect input from the hypothalamus via GHRH and somatostatin in addition to or even in the absence of effects of these factors directly on the pituitary. Investigations in which hypothalamic secretion of the GH stimulating and inhibiting hormones can be monitored will be required to fully elucidate the mechanisms through which age and sex affect the secretion of GH.

ACKNOWLEDGMENTS

This work was supported by: NIH RCDA 1K04 HD0063, American Diabetes Association Feasibility Grant and University of Virginia Computer Services Grant (WSE); AG04303 (RMB); AM32632 (MOT); and USPHS General Clinical Research Center Grant RR-847 and the CLINFO Laboratory. KYH was supported by grants from the Australasian College of Physicians and the Post Graduate Foundation, the University of Sidney. ACSF is a Visiting Professor supported by a grant from CAPES, Brazil.

We thank Kay Hancock for help in preparation of the manuscript.

REFERENCES

1. Khorram O, DePalatis LR, McCann SM. Development of hypothalamic control of growth hormone secretion in the rat. Endocrinology 1983; 113:720.
2. Frawley LS, Hoeffler JP, Boockfor FR. Functional maturation of somatotropes in fetal rat pituitaries: analysis by reverse hemolytic plaque assay. Endocrinology 1985; 116:2355.
3. Rietort M. Pituitary content and plasma levels of growth hormone in foetal and weanling rats. J Endocrinol 1974; 60:261.
4. Birge CA, Peake GT, Mariz IK, Daughaday WH. Radioimmunoassayable growth hormone in the rat pituitary gland: effects of age, sex and hormonal state. Endocrinology 1967; 81:195.

5. Ojeda SR, Jameson HE. Developmental patterns of plasma and pituitary growth hormone (GH) in the female rat. Endocrinology 1977; 100:881.

6. Walker P, Dussault JH, Alvarado-Urbina G, Dupont A. The development of the hypothalamo-pituitary axis in the neonatal rat: hypothalamic somatostatin and pituitary and serum growth hormone concentrations. Endocrinology 1977; 101:782.

7. Eden S. Age- and sex-related differences in episodic growth hormone secretion in the rat. Endocrinology 1979; 105:555.

8. Tannenbaum GS, Martin JB. Evidence for an endogenous ultradian rhythm governing growth hormone secretion in the rat. Endocrinology 1976; 98:562.

9. Sonntag WE, Steger RW, Forman LJ, Meites J. Decreased pulsatile release of growth hormone in old male rats. Endocrinology 1980; 107:1875.

10. Eden S, Albertsson-Wikland K, Isaksson O. Plasma levels of growth hormone in female rats of different ages. Acta Endocrinol (Copenh) 1978; 88:676.

11. Saunders A, Terry LC, Audet J, Brazeau P, Martin JB. Dynamic studies of growth hormone and prolactin secretion in the female rat. Neuroendocrinology 1976; 21:193.

12. Sonntag WE, Hylka VW, Meites J. Impaired ability of old male rats to secrete growth hormone in vivo but not in vitro in response to hpGRF (1-44). Endocrinology 1983; 113:2305.

13. Jansson J-O, Eden S, Isaksson O. Sites of action of testosterone and estradiol on longitudinal bone growth. Am J Physiol 1983; 244:E135.

14. Kaplan SL, Grumbach MM, Shepard TH. The ontogenesis of human fetal hormones. I. Growth hormone and insulin. J Clin Invest 1972; 51:3080.

15. Cornblath M, Parker ML, Reisner SH, Forbes AE, Daughaday WH. Secretion and metabolism of growth hormone in premature and full-term infants. J Clin Endocrinol Metab 1965; 25:209.

16. Luna AM, Wilson DM, Wibblesman CJ, et al. Somatomedins in adolescence: a cross-sectional study of the effect on plasma insulin-like growth factor I and II levels. J Clin Endocrinol Metab 1983; 57:268.

17. Rosenfield RI, Furlanetto R, Bock D. Relationship of somatomedin-C concentrations to pubertal changes. J Pediatr 1983; 103:723.

18. Aynsley-Green A, Zachmann M, Prader A. Interrelation of the therapeutic effects of growth hormone and testosterone on growth in hypopituitarism. J Pediatr 1976; 89:992.

19. Tanner JM, Whitehouse RH, Hughes PCR, Carter BS. Relative importance of growth hormone and sex steroids for the growth at puberty of trunk length, limb length, and muscle width in growth hormone-deficient children. J Pediatr 1976; 89:1000.

20. Finkelstein JW, Roffwarg HP, Boyar RM, Kream J, Hellman L. Age-related change in the twenty-four-hour spontaneous secretion of growth hormone. J Clin Endocrinol Metab 1972; 35:665.

21. Miller JD, Tannenbaum GS, Colle E, Guyda HJ. Daytime pulsatile growth hormone secretion during childhood and adolescence. J Clin Endocrinol Metab 1982; 55:989.

22. Mauras N, Blizzard RM, Link K, Johnson ML, Rogol AD, Veldhuis JD. Augmentation of growth hormone secretion during puberty: evidence for a pulse amplitude-modulated phenomenon. J Clin Endocrinol Metab 1987; 64:596.

23. Zadik Z, Chalew SA, McCarter RJ, Meistas M, Kowarski AA. The influence of age on the 24-hour integrated concentration of growth hormone in normal individuals. J Clin Endocrinol Metab 1985; 60:513.

24. Thompson RG, Rodriguez A, Kowarski A, Migeon CJ, Blizzard RM. Integrated concentrations of growth hormone correlated with plasma testosterone and bone age in preadolescent and adolescent males. J Clin Endocrinol Metab 1972; 35:334.

25. Plotnick LP, Thompson RG, Beitins I, Blizzard RM. Integrated con-

centrations of growth hormone correlated with stage of puberty and estrogen levels in girls. J Clin Endocrinol Metab 1974; 38:436.

26. Zadik Z, Chalew SA, Raiti S, Kowarski AA. Do short children secrete insufficient growth hormone? Pediatrics 1985; 76:355.

27. Spiliotis BE, August GP, Hung W, Sonis W, Mendelson W, Bercu BB. Growth hormone neurosecretory dysfunction: a treatable cause of short stature. JAMA 1984; 251:2223.

28. Butenandt O, Eder R, Wohlfarth K, Bidlingmaier F, Knorr D. Mean 24-hour growth hormone and testosterone concentrations in relation to pubertal growth spurt in boys with normal or delayed puberty. Eur J Pediatr 1976; 122:85.

29. Link K, Blizzard RM, Evans WS, Kaiser DL, Parker MW, Rogol AD. The effect of androgens on the pulsatile release and the twenty-four-hour mean concentration of growth hormone in peripubertal males. J Clin Endocrinol Metab 1986; 62:159.

30. Dudl RJ, Ensinck JW, Palmer HE, Williams RH. Effect of age on growth hormone secretion in man. J Clin Endocrinol Metab 1973; 37:11.

31. Prinz PN, Weitzman ED, Cunningham GR, Karacan I. Plasma growth hormone during sleep in young and aged men. J Gerontol 1983; 38:519.

32. Rudman D, Kutner MH, Rogers M, Lubin MF, Fleming GA, Bain RP. Impaired growth hormone secretion in the adult population: relation to age and adiposity. J Clin Invest 1981; 67:1361.

33. Frantz AG, Rabkin MT. Effects of estrogen and sex difference on secretion of human growth hormone. J Clin Endocrinol Metab 1965; 25:1470.

34. Thompson RG, Rodriguez A, Kowarski A, Blizzard RM. Growth hormone: metabolic clearance rates, integrated concentrations, and production rates in normal adults and the effect of prednisone. J Clin Invest 1972; 51:3193.

35. Genazzani AR, Lemarchand-Beraud T, Aubert ML, Felber JP. Pattern of plasma ACTH, hGH, and cortisol during menstrual cycle. J Clin Endocrinol Metab 1975; 41:431.

36. Dawson-Hughes B, Stern D, Goldman J, Reichlin S. Regulation of growth hormone and somatomedin-C secretion in postmenopausal women: effect of physiological estrogen replacement. J Clin Endocrinol Metab 1986; 63:424.

37. Plotsky PM, Vale W. Patterns of growth hormone-releasing factor and somatostatin secretion into the hypophysial-portal circulation of the rat. Science 1985; 230:461.

38. Parker MW, Johanson AJ, Rogol AD, Kaiser DL, Blizzard RM. Effect of testosterone on somatomedin-C concentrations in prepubertal boys. J Clin Endocrinol Metab 1984; 58:87.

39. Ho KY, Evans WS, Blizzard RM, Veldhuis JD, et al. Effects of sex and age on the 24-hour profile of growth hormone secretion in man: importance of endogenous estradiol concentrations. J Clin Endocrinol Metab 1987; 64:51.

40. Veldhuis JD, Rogol AD, Johnson ML. Minimizing false positive errors in hormonal pulse detection. Am J Physiol 1985; 248:E475.

41. Crowley WF Jr, Filicori M, Spratt DI, Santoro NF. The physiology of gonadotropin-releasing hormone (GnRH) secretion in men and women. In: Greep RO, ed. Recent progress in hormone research. New York: Academic Press, 1985:473.

42. Ross JL, Barnes KM, Brody S, Merriam GR, Loriaux DL, Cutler GB Jr. A comparison of two methods for detecting hormone peaks: the effect of sampling interval on gonadotropin peak frequency. J Clin Endocrinol Metab 1984; 59:1159.

43. Veldhuis JD, Evans WS, Rogol AD, et al. Intensified rates of venous sampling unmask the presence of spontaneous, high-frequency pulsations of luteinizing hormone in man. J Clin Endocrinol Metab 1984; 59:96

44. Veldhuis JD, Evans WS, Rogol AD, et al. Performance of LH pulse-

detection algorithms at rapid rates of venous sampling in humans. Am J Physiol 1984; 247:E554.

45. Veldhuis JD, Johnson ML. Cluster analysis: a simple, versatile, and robust algorithm for endocrine pulse detection. Am J Physiol 1986; 250:E486.

46. Evans WS, Faria ACS, Ho KY, et al. Impact of intensive venous sampling on the characterization of pulsatile growth hormone release. Am J Physiol 1987; 252:E549.

47. Evans WS, Christiansen E, Faria ACS, Asplin CM. Pulsatile growth hormone secretion in insulin dependent diabetes mellitus. 69th Annual Meeting of the Endocrine Society, Indianapolis, IN, 1987.

48. Thorner MO, Vance ML, Evans WS, et al. Physiological and clinical studies of GRF and GH. In: Greep RO, ed. Recent progress in hormone research. New York: Academic Press, 1985:589.

49. Smals AEM, Pieters GFFM, Smals AGH, Benraad TJ, Van Laarhoven J, Kloppenborg PWC. Sex difference in human growth hormone (GH) response to intravenous human pancreatic GH-releasing hormone administration in young adults. J Clin Endocrinol Metab 1986; 62:336.

50. Gelato MC, Pescovitz OH, Cassorla F, Loriaux DL, Merriam GR. Dose-response relationships for the effects of growth hormone-releasing factor-$(1-44)$-NH$_2$ in young adult men and women. J Clin Endocrinol Metab 1984; 59:197.

51. Gelato MC, Malozowski S, Caruso-nicoletti M, et al. Growth hormone (GH) responses to GH-releasing hormone during pubertal development in normal boys and girls: comparison to idiopathic short stature and GH deficiency. J Clin Endocrinol Metab 1986; 63:174.

52. Vance ML, Borges JLC, Kaiser DL, et al. Human pancreatic tumor growth hormone releasing factor (hpGRF-40): dose response relationships in normal man. J Clin Endocrinol Metab 1984; 58:838.

53. Evans WS, Borges JLC, Vance ML, et al. Effects of human pancreatic growth hormone releasing factor-40 on serum growth hormone, prolactin, luteinizing hormone, follicle-stimulating hormone and somatomedin C concentrations in normal women throughout the menstrual cycle. J Clin Endocrinol Metab 1984; 59:1006.

54. Shibasaki T, Shizume K, Nakahara M, et al. Age-related changes in plasma growth hormone response to growth hormone-releasing factor in man. J Clin Endocrinol Metab 1984; 58:212.

55. Pavlov EP, Harman SM, Merriam GR, Gelato MC, Blackman MR. Responses of growth hormone (GH) and somatomedin-C to GH-releasing hormone in healthy aging men. J Clin Endocrinol Metab 1986; 62:595.

56. Evans WS, Boykin BJ, Kaiser DL, Borges JLC, Thorner MO. Biphasic LH secretion in response to GnRH during continuous perifusion of dispersed rat anterior pituitary cells: changes in total release and the phasic components during the estrous cycle. Endocrinology 1983; 112:535.

57. Evans WS, Krieg RJ, Limber ER, Kaiser DL, Thorner MO. Effects of the in vivo gonadal hormone environment on in vitro hGRF-40-stimulated GH release. Am J Physiol 1985; 249:E276.

58. Ho KY, Leong DA, Sinha YN, Johnson ML, Evans WS, Thorner MO. Sex-related differences in GH secretion in rat using reverse hemolytic plaque assay. Am J Physiol 1986; 250:E650.

59. Sinha YN, Wickes MA, Salocks CB, Vanderlaan WP. Gonadal regulation of prolactin and growth hormone secretion in the mouse. Biol Reprod 1979; 21:473.

60. Wehrenberg WB, Baird A, Ying SY, Ling N. The effects of testosterone and estrogen on the pituitary growth hormone response to growth hormone-releasing factor. Biol Reprod 1985; 32:369.

61. Hoeffler JP, Frawley LS. Capacity of individual somatotropes to release growth hormone varies according to sex: analysis by reverse hemolytic plaque assay. Endocrinology 1986; 119:1037.

62. Frawley LS, Boockfor FR, Hoeffler JP. Identification by plaque assays of a pituitary cell type that secretes both growth hormone and prolactin. Endocrinology 1985; 116:734.

63. Leong DA, Lau SK, Sinha YN, Kaiser DL, Thorner MO. Enumeration of lactotropes and somatotropes among male and female pituitary cells in culture: evidence in favor of mammosomatotrope subpopulation in the rat. Endocrinology 1985; 116:1371.

64. Goluboff LG, Ezrin C. Effect of pregnancy on the somatotroph and prolactin cell of the human adenohypophysis. J Clin Endocrinol Metab 1969; 29:1533.

65. Stratmann IE, Ezrin C, Sellers EA. Estrogen-induced transformation of somatotropes into mammotrophs in the rat. Cell Tissue Res 1974; 152:229.

15

CHRONOBIOLOGY OF GROWTH HORMONE SECRETION

Hans-Jurgen Quabbe, M.D.

Section of Endocrinology, Department of Internal
Medicine, Klinikum Steglitz, Freie Universitat Berlin,
West Germany

INTRODUCTION

The secretion of growth hormone (GH) in man occurs in episodic bursts during day and night (1). During trough periods, concentrations are below the sensitivity of the usual radioimmunoassay (approximately 0.5-1.0 ng/ml). Peak concentrations are often around 20 ng/ml, but may attain 50 ng/ml (or even more), especially in younger subjects. In man, the secretory episodes occur approximately every 4 h. Although some of these GH peaks are often missing in 24-h profiles, the rhythmicity probably persists with low-amplitude peaks occurring below the sensitivity of most current assay systems (2).

The basic pattern is subject to modulation by a multitude of influences. These include the sleep/wake and the sleep-stage cycle, the basic-rest-activity cycle (BRAC), a circadian pacemaker as well as "limbic system" influences (stress, emotions, etc.).

SLEEP, SLEEP-STAGES, BRAC

During nocturnal sleep the GH secretory episodes are related temporally to periods of deep sleep, as was first reported in 1966 and later confirmed with the use of nocturnal EEG recordings (1,3). The major secretory episode of the 24-h day usually occurs soon after sleep-onset during the first slow-wave-sleep (SWS) episode (Fig. 1).

A well-developed episode of SWS, which is characterized by high-amplitude, low-frequency synchronized waves in the cortical EEG of a sleeping person, usually occurs shortly after sleep-onset. After a transitional episode of light (stage 1/2) sleep, SWS is followed by an episode of rapid-eye-movement (REM) sleep. As sleep progresses during the night, SWS stages become less and REM stages more consolidated, such that SWS predominates during the first half and REM during the second half of the night.

During the day, periods of activity alternate with periods of inactivity (rest periods, naps). The cortical EEG during daytime naps contains more stage REM in the first part of the day and more stage SWS in the second part. Despite the similarities between the daytime naps and

nocturnal sleep stages, it is still a matter of dispute whether the
sleep-stage cycle is part of a more general 24-h BRAC or whether daytime
and nighttime rhythms are driven by different oscillators.

During undisturbed sleep, the first stage SWS is usually associated
with a large GH secretory burst. Although the delay between SWS-onset and
the beginning of the GH secretory pulse varies considerably, sleep-onset
per se (i.e., stage 2 sleep) does not seem to trigger GH secretion. It
must be recognized, however, that the EEG sleep pattern is monitored
continuously, while GH concentrations are usually determined at 15-min
intervals or even less often. Hence, it is difficult to define the onset
of a GH secretory pulse as exactly as that of sleep stage changes.

Sleep-delay, sleep-advance and sleep-reversal studies have been used
to differentiate between sleep/sleep-stage-triggered GH secretion and a
mere temporal coincidence. They have all shown an immediate entrainment
of GH secretion to the altered sleep pattern and have thus supported the
hypothesis of a link between sleep/SWS and GH secretion (4).

During daytime, GH secretion occurs primarily during nap periods (5).
When naps are not allowed, less GH is secreted. More GH is secreted
during afternoon naps which comprise more SWS than morning naps. Thus,
CNS structures/mechanisms which are involved in the generation of SWS (and
probably also of daytime naps) have a major influence on the timing and
the amount of GH secreted during the entire 24-h day.

However, the dependence of nocturnal GH secretion on SWS is not
absolute. The first SWS episode of undisturbed sleep is unique in being
almost invariably associated with a major GH secretory pulse. With
progression of nocturnal sleep, subsequent SWS stages are then less likely
to trigger a secretory episode (6). Moreover, a GH pulse sometimes begins
before the clear-cut presence of SWS. On the other hand, even sleep-onset
SWS is sometimes not accompanied by GH secretion.

Nocturnal GH secretion diminishes in the course of the night parallel
to the decrease of SWS, while the amount of stage REM sleep increases.
Does this indicate a suppressive effect of stage REM on GH secretion? The
effect of SWS deprivation clearly points to a stimulatory role for SWS

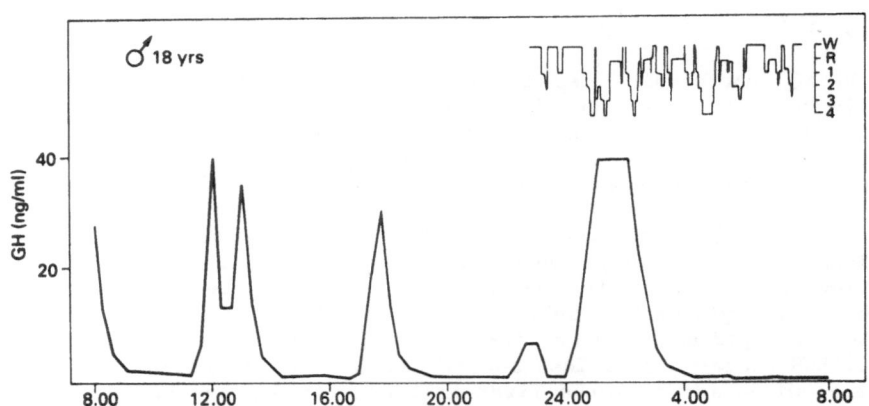

Fig. 1. Twenty-four-hour pattern of GH secretion in a
healthy male subject. Sleep histogram indicates sleep
stages wake (W), REM (R) and non-REM 1, 2, 3, 4. The major
secretory episode is associated with the sleep-onset/SWS
episode. Reprinted with permission (4).

rather than a suppressive role of REM in the control of nocturnal GH secretion. A recent analysis of the relationship between GH and the different sleep stages confirmed that GH secretion was associated primarily with SWS. However, the total amount of GH secreted during sleep was negatively correlated with the duration of REM sleep and the best overall correlation was found when both REM preceding stage SWS and SWS per se were included in the calculations (7). These and some other observations suggest a more complex relationship between the sleep-stage cycle and the GH-releasing mechanisms than was hitherto thought.

CIRCADIAN PACEMAKER

Circadian pacemakers have an important influence on the secretory pattern of many hormones, ACTH/cortisol secretion probably being the best-known example. Circadian rhythms are thought to serve the purpose of coordinating interdependent processes and separating incompatible ones. On the other hand, one function of ultradian hormonal rhythms is probably the regulation of a dependent physiological process by modulation of the frequency (rather than amplitude) of hormonal stimulation. This has been documented for the regulation of the menstrual cycle, which depends on the appropriate GnRH/LH pulse frequency. Amenorrhea can be produced by changes in the LH pulse frequency alone.

A circadian component is probably also involved in the determination of the overall 24-h pattern of GH secretion, although it is more weakly expressed than in the case of ACTH/cortisol. In one investigation, GH (and cortisol) were measured during a prolonged (10 days) artificial 3-h sleep-wake cycle (1-h sleep/2-h wake) (8). A major GH peak was absent at the clock time where the sleep-onset SWS stage would have been expected under normal conditions. Thus, the importance of SWS for sleep-linked GH secretion was confirmed. However, inspection of the data shows that an approximate 4-h cycle of GH secretion persisted with some entrainment of the secretory episodes to the 1-h sleep periods despite the disruption of the normal sleep-wake cycle. These results suggest a role for a sleep-independent ultradian cyclicity of GH secretion (9). In these studies, the total amount of GH secreted within 24 h was unchanged during the disturbed sleep pattern as compared with basal conditions. This would indicate that sleep disturbances have an influence on the pattern rather than on the amount of GH secreted.

In contrast, a set of "jet lag" studies (7) (transmeridian flights between Brussels and Chicago) showed that the amount of GH secreted was increased during the time of disturbed sleep. The increase was due to a larger amplitude and not to more frequent GH pulses. The largest secretory pulse still occurred during early sleep. An exception was the first night following eastward return to Europe, when the major GH secretory episode was shifted to late in sleep. These results again underline the importance of sleep and SWS for the regulation of GH secretion. However, the dissociation of sleep-onset SWS and the major GH secretory episode immediately after the eastward flight is best explained by the influence of a circadian pacemaker superimposed on the sleep-related mechanisms. A similar result was obtained in a laboratory sleep shift study by the same investigators.

Thus, present knowledge suggests that the nocturnal GH secretory pattern is mainly determined by the sleep-stage-generating mechanisms of the brain. SWS apparently is a powerful initiator for a GH secretory episode, but the amount of GH secreted may then depend on a more complex influence of both the REM- and the SWS-regulating mechanisms. A circadian component is also present, and its influence can be unmasked by studies in which circadian and sleep-related influences are dissociated. A link of GH secretory episodes to nap periods points to the persistence of CNS influences on the temporal pattern of GH secretion during daytime as well. It remains unclear at present whether this is a daytime extension of the mechanisms that are active during nighttime sleep or represents a link to a more general basic rest-activity cycle.

ATTEMPTS AT AN ANIMAL MODEL

In order to elucidate the neuroanatomy of the sleep-GH link and to determine its neurohumoral and electrophysiological basis, attempts have been made to establish an animal model. Some of the areas that would be candidates for such studies are shown in Figure 2.

Studies in the Rat

Studies in the rat have yielded controversial results. This is not surprising, since these animals have a much less consolidated sleep pattern than human beings, with sleep cycles often shorter than 15 min. Their GH secretory pattern, on the other hand, is dominated by a relatively regular 3-h periodicity (at least in male animals). Hence, an influence of sleep or sleep stages on GH secretion will be more difficult to detect than in man. A distinction between different sleep stages has generally not been attempted in such studies.

Willoughby et al. (11) have not found a correlation between GH secretory episodes and sleep cycles or sleep stage duration in the rat. On the other hand, a positive correlation has been reported between GH and the preceding amount of sleep as well as a fixed phase relation of the ultradian GH rhythm and the sleep cycle (12). GH secretion occurred in the early stage of each second sleep cycle at 3-h intervals. However, a relation between GH and the amount of sleep in each cycle was not found. Since the 3-h periodicity of GH secretory pulses persisted during prolonged thiopental anesthesia, the relationship between GH secretory pulses and the sleep cycle probably represents only a temporal coincidence and not a causal relationship.

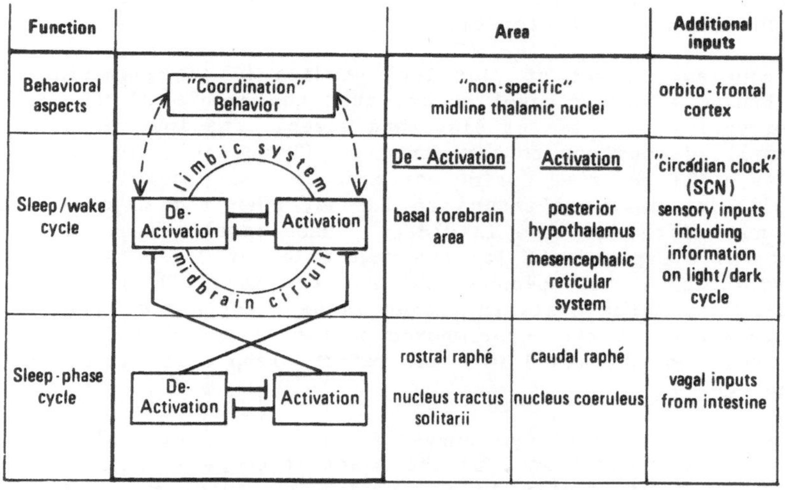

Function	Area			Additional inputs
Behavioral aspects	"Coordination" Behavior	"non-specific" midline thalamic nuclei		orbito-frontal cortex
Sleep/wake cycle	De-Activation ⊣ Activation (limbic system, midbrain circuit)	De-Activation basal forebrain area	Activation posterior hypothalamus mesencephalic reticular system	"circadian clock" (SCN) sensory inputs including information on light/dark cycle
Sleep-phase cycle	De-Activation ⊣ Activation	rostral raphé nucleus tractus solitarii	caudal raphé nucleus coeruleus	vagal inputs from intestine

Fig. 2. Highly simplified schematic presentation of the sleep/wake regulating system. Reprinted with permission (10).

It is interesting, nevertheless, that one of the sleep-substances, delta-sleep-inducing peptide (DSIP), has recently been reported to exert a stimulatory influence on GH release in the rat (13).

Studies in the Dog

The domestic dog has a sleep pattern in which short sleep periods occur intermittently throughout the 24-h day. In order to investigate a possible GH-sleep link in this species, Takahashi et al. (14) performed sleep deprivation studies in an attempt to produce consolidated sleep following forced wakefulness. Sleep deprivation was obtained by an electroshock avoidance procedure. Spontaneous GH secretion under basal conditions was not characterized by the pattern of episodic secretory bursts seen in man, monkeys and the rat. The small GH elevations which occurred bore no relationship to sleep or sleep stages. During recovery sleep, SWS was obtained and GH secretory peaks were observed in most animals. Although the authors claimed to have established an animal model for the study of sleep-related GH secretion, the influence of factors unrelated to sleep (but possibly related to the sleep deprivation procedure) remains to be determined. The value of this model for the elucidation of the mechanisms of sleep-related GH secretion still awaits confirmation.

Studies in Non-Human Primates

In non-human primates, no sleep-GH link has been detected, although a "pilot study" had suggested such a link in one of two baboons. The sleep and sleep-stage pattern of the rhesus monkey closely resembles that of man. In a series of 24-h profiles under basal conditions, we have established that the GH secretory pattern of these animals likewise resembles that of man. GH secretory episodes occur approximately every 4.5 h and are similar in shape and amplitude to those found in man (5-20 ng/ml in a typical case). However, our extensive sleep and sleep-deprivation studies have failed to produce any evidence for a link between GH secretory episodes on the one hand and the sleep-wake cycle, the sleep-stage cycle or the daytime rest-activity cycle on the other hand ([15], Fig. 3). The absence of a GH-sleep link in non-human primates has been confirmed for the cynomolgus monkey (16). However, in our series, there was a highly significant relationship of GH secretory episodes during the night to episodes of awakening, possibly indicating that changes of state may be a trigger for GH secretion in this species. This would be in accordance with the observation in another series of our studies; synchronization of the matutinal (morning) GH secretory pulses between individuals, which occurs in the colony-held animals, is related to awakening (and not the to dark-light transition, as had been expected) (17).

PHYSIOLOGICAL SIGNIFICANCE OF THE TEMPORAL PATTERN OF GH SECRETION AND OF ITS LINK TO SLEEP

The physiological significance of the temporal pattern of GH secretion, both ultradian/circadian and sleep-related, has remained unclear. However, some speculations can be formulated.

The Sleep-GH Link

Sleep is often thought to be a prerequisite for the restoration of certain body functions, especially those of the brain, following heightened activity and stressful/catabolic influences during the waking state. GH, on the other hand, is viewed to be a promotor of tissue growth and anabolic metabolism. Hence, it has been proposed that triggering of a

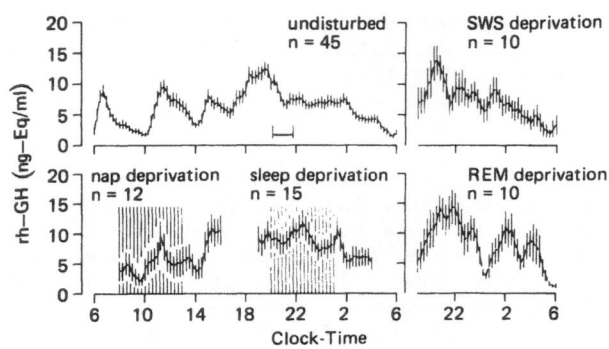

Fig. 3. 24-h and nighttime pattern respectively of GH secretion in a group of rhesus monkeys. Blood was obtained every 15 min from unanesthetized animals via remote sampling from the adjacent room. There is no indication of increased GH secretion at the time of sleep-onset during undisturbed sleep. Neither nap- nor total-sleep- nor selective-sleep-stage (SWS or REM) deprivation is accompanied by any significant reduction of GH secretion. n = number of observations. Range of sleep-onset times during undisturbed conditions is denoted by the horizontal bar. Shaded area denotes time period of nap- and total-sleep-deprivation respectively. Selective-sleep-stage deprivation (SWS and REM respectively) was done during the entire sleep time from 20.00 to 06.00 h. Data for undisturbed sleep are taken from reference 15 with permission. For details of techniques used, see reference 15.

major GH secretory episode at the time of sleep-onset/SWS helps the body to switch to restorative and anabolic conditions.

However, GH exerts its anabolic actions mainly in synergism with insulin, but insulin concentrations are low during sleep and show no link to sleep or a particular sleep stage. Another anabolic hormone, somatomedin-C, likewise decreases rather than increases during sleep.

Whether sleep is indeed a state of anabolism, growth and tissue repair is also controversial. For instance, protein synthesis proceeds predominantly when substrates are available, i.e., following food intake during daytime, especially when GH can act together with insulin. During sleep, protein catabolism provides substrates for gluconeogenesis when glucose is in short supply.

Thus, the evidence for relating sleep-onset/SWS-triggered GH secretion to anabolic/restorative demands of the body during sleep is not well-founded at the present time. However, the brain could well be an exception to this rule. There is evidence that the brain "needs" sleep and especially SWS to maintain normal function. Following prolonged total sleep deprivation in man, only part of the lost sleep-time is reclaimed in recovery sleep but SWS loss is almost totally recompensated. It is unknown, however, whether this dependence of CNS function on sleep/SWS is related to necessities of protein anabolism and "tissue repair" and what role, if any, SWS-related GH secretion might play. These conditions have recently been reviewed by Horne (18).

To date, GH has not been shown to have an influence on sleep or sleep-stage distribution. Whether it has any direct influence on brain metabolism, questions of permeability of the blood-brain-barrier notwithstanding, is unknown. There are sporadic reports in the literature, however, that GH has an effect on the maturing brain, its weight increase as well as on neuronal content and functional capacity (19). It remains possible that these effects are related to placental growth rather than being due to a direct GH effect on the developing brain. These reports still await confirmation.

Sleep-Related GH Secretion and Glucose Metabolism

GH has an early insulin-like and a late insulin-antagonistic effect on glucose metabolism. This could possibly promote early hypoglycemia and late hyperglycemia respectively following a large GH secretory episode. Nocturnal hypoglycemia is a problem in some patients with insulin-dependent diabetes mellitus (IDDM). It is due, at least in part, to a combination of the nighttime fasting state and a circadian increase in insulin sensitivity of the peripheral tissues. On the other hand, blood glucose sometimes begins to rise to unacceptably high concentrations in the early morning hours, the so-called "dawn phenomenon." Could the insulin-like and the insulin-antagonistic effects of GH participate in these dysregulations? If so, pharmacological manipulation of nocturnal, sleep-related GH secretion could possibly improve the treatment of patients with IDDM (20).

Schnure et al. (21) tested glucose tolerance during nights with normal sleep, delayed sleep-onset and total SWS-deprivation, respectively. When GH secretion occurred early in the night, glucose tolerance was normal on the following morning (i.e., 7-8 h after the physiological sleep-onset GH peak). On the other hand, when sleep-delay had moved the endogenous SWS-related GH pulse to the early morning hours, glucose tolerance was decreased to the diabetic range.

However, a comparison of the temporal spacing of these events makes it difficult to explain nighttime hypoglycemia and early-morning hyperglycemia in IDDM by an influence of sleep-related GH secretion. Nevertheless, therapeutic trials have been undertaken in IDDM patients in an attempt to improve metabolic control using somatostatin analogs for suppression of nocturnal GH secretion. The results are controversial at the present time (22). Improvement and no change in metabolic control have both been reported. Moreover, an effect need not be due to suppression of sleep-related GH secretion alone. Somatostatin analogs also have additional actions, such as suppressing glucagon secretion and delaying glucose absorption from the gut. Moreover, somatostatin treatment could also be counterproductive by augmenting the risk of nocturnal hypoglycemia. Hence, the value of suppression of sleep-related GH secretion for the treatment of IDDM remains to be established.

Physiological Significance of the Ultradian GH Periodicity

The physiological significance of the ultradian rhythmicity of GH secretory pulses during daytime (or during the entire 24-h period for that matter) is also still unknown. However, there are some indications that the temporal pattern of secretion may play a role in the metabolic as well as the growth-promoting actions of GH. An example is the GH effect in adipose tissue. In vitro GH has an acute insulin-like action in adipose tissue. It then induces a resistance to further additions of GH which lasts approximately as long as the interval between GH secretory bursts in the animal in vivo (23). Thus, in vivo the frequency of GH pulses may modulate its metabolic effects in this tissue and in others as well, possibly at the receptor or postreceptor level.

179

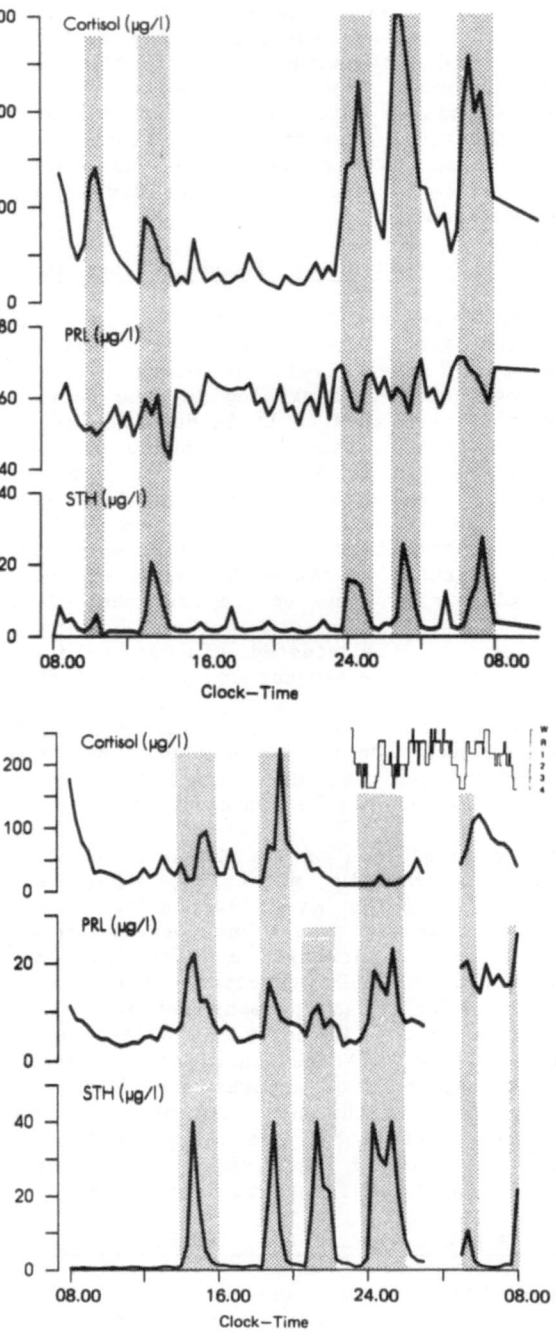

Fig. 4. Synchronization of pulsatile secretion of pituitary hormones in a 17-year-old male patient with apallic syndrome (top) and in a 16-year-old male patient with hypersomnia syndrome (bottom). Blood sampling was done every 20 min. In the hypersomnia patient (bottom), extensive clinical studies failed to reveal the cause of the syndrome. In this patient, the major GH secretory episode does occur during the sleep-onset SWS episode.

In hypophysectomized adolescent rats, GH administration results in an acceleration of the growth rate. Clark et al. (24) have shown that the magnitude of the GH effect depends on the frequency at which GH pulses are applied. A frequency which imitates the physiological pattern results in the highest growth rate. On the other hand, it has recently been shown that, during human puberty, augmented GH secretion is due to an increase in pulse amplitude rather than pulse frequency (25). Thus, whether the growth-promoting effect of GH in man is physiologically modulated by changes in the GH pulse frequency remains to be determined.

HUMAN PATHOPHYSIOLOGY

The pathophysiology of sleep-related and pulsatile GH secretion has recently been reviewed (4,10). Disturbances have, for example, been found in the psychosocial deprivation syndrome (which can cause reduced growth), in narcolepsy and possibly in myotonic dystrophy. The sleep-related GH increase is also absent in patients with the apallic syndrome (26). Patients with endogenous depression secrete less GH during sleep than normal subjects, and their major GH secretory episode precedes sleep-onset rather than being linked to the first stage SWS. This has been proposed to be part of a phase advance of a circadian pacemaker in this disease (27).

Under physiological conditions the overall 24-h patterns of the different pituitary hormones have a characteristic temporal relationship to each other. Disruption of these phase relationships occurs during flights across several time zones and is thought to be responsible for the "jet lag syndrome" (7), as has already been discussed.

The ultradian pattern of pulsatile secretion of the different pituitary hormones is not usually linked in a close phase relationship. However, under certain conditions (stress, insulin-induced hypoglycemia), the secretion of two or more pituitary hormones is stimulated simultaneously. There is some evidence that spontaneous synchronization of the ultradian rhythms of two or more pituitary hormones can also occur for more extended periods of time in the rhesus monkey (28). Similar synchronization has also been observed in certain disease states in man (Fig. 4, [29]).

The pathophysiological significance and neurophysiological basis of this synchronization of ultradian rhythm of several pituitary hormones are at present unknown. Its occurrence in the apallic syndrome would seem to suggest that removal of regulatory influences rather than active synchronization may be the cause. However, this remains to be investigated. Careful studies in selected patients may help in the future to improve our understanding of the temporal pattern of pituitary hormone secretion, its regulatory mechanisms and its physiological and pathophysiological significance.

ACKNOWLEDGMENT

Original research of the author was supported by Deutsche Forschungsgemeinschaft.

REFERENCES

1. Quabbe H-J, Schilling E, Helge H. Pattern of growth hormone secretion during a 24-hour fast in normal adults. J Clin Endocrinol Metab 1966; 26:173-7.

181

2. Drobny EC, Amburn K, Baumann G. Circadian variation of basal growth hormone in man. J Clin Endocrinol Metab 1983; 57:524-8.
3. Takahashi Y, Kipnis DM, Daughaday WH. Growth hormone secretion during sleep. J Clin Invest 1968; 47:2079-90.
4. Quabbe H-J. Growth hormone. In: Lightman SL, Everitt BJ, eds. Neuroendocrinology. Oxford: Blackwell Scientific Publications, 1986:409-49.
5. Karacan I, Rosenbloom AL, Londono JH, Williams RL, Salis PJ. Growth hormone levels during morning and afternoon naps. Behav Neuropsychiatry 1975; 6:67-70.
6. Quabbe H-J, Helge H, Kubicki S. Nocturnal growth hormone secretion: correlation with sleeping EEG in adults and pattern in children and adolescents with non-pituitary dwarfism, overgrowth and with obesity. Acta Endocrinol (Copenh) 1971; 67:767-83.
7. Golstein J, van Cauter E, Desir D, et al. Effects of "jet lag" on hormonal patterns. IV. Time shifts increase growth hormone release. J Clin Endocrinol Metab 1983; 56:433-40.
8. Weitzman ED, Nogeire C, Perlow M, et al. Effects of a prolonged 3-hour sleep-wake cycle on sleep stages, plasma cortisol, growth hormone and body temperature in man. J Clin Endocrinol Metab 1974; 38:1018-30.
9. Aschoff A. Circadiane rhythmen im endokrinen system. Klin Wschr 1978; 56:425-35.
10. Quabbe H-J. Hypothalamic control of GH secretion: pathophysiology and clinical implications. Acta Neurochirurgica 1985; 75:60-71.
11. Willoughby JO, Martin JB, Renaud LP. Pulsatile growth hormone release in the rat: failure to demonstrate a correlation with sleep phases. Endocrinology 1976; 98:991-6.
12. Mitsugi N, Kimura F. Simultaneous determination of blood levels of corticosterone and growth hormone in the male rat: relation to sleep-wakefulness cycle. Neuroendocrinology 1985; 41:125-30.
13. Iyer KS, McCann SM. Delta sleep-inducing peptide (DSIP) stimulates growth hormone (GH) release in the rat by hypothalamic and pituitary actions. Peptides 1987; 8:45-8.
14. Takahashi Y, Ebihara S, Nakamura Y, Takahashi K. A model of human sleep-related growth hormone secretion in dogs: effects of 3, 6 and 12 hours of forced wakefulness on plasma growth hormone, cortisol, and sleep stages. Endocrinology 1981; 109:262-72.
15. Quabbe H-J, Gregor M, Bumke-Vogt C, Eckhof A, Witt I. Twenty-four-hour pattern of growth hormone secretion in the rhesus monkey: studies including alterations of the sleep/wake and sleep stage cycles. Endocrinology 1981; 109:513-22.
16. Bunner DL, McNamee A Jr, Dinterman RE, Wannemacher RW Jr. Lack of enhanced nocturnal growth hormone release in tethered cynomolgus monkeys. Am J Physiol 1982; 243:R213-7.
17. Quabbe H-J, Kroll M, Thomsen P. Dissociation of light onset and wake onset: effect on rhesus monkey growth hormone secretion. Endocrinology 1983; 112:1828-31.
18. Horne JA. Human sleep and tissue restoration: some qualifications and doubts. Clin Sci 1983; 65:569-78.
19. Sara VR, Lazarus L, Stuart MC, King T. Fetal brain growth: selective action by growth hormone. Science 1974; 1986:446-7.
20. Campbell PJ, Bolli GB, Cryer PE, Gerich JE. Pathogenesis of the dawn phenomenon in patients with insulin-dependent diabetes mellitus. N Engl J Med 1985; 312:1473-9.
21. Schnure JJ, Raskin P, Lipman RL. Growth hormone secretion during sleep: impairment in glucose tolerance and nonsuppressibility by hyperglycemia. J Clin Endocrinol Metab 1971; 33:234-41.
22. Skor DA, White NH, Thomas L, Santiago JV. Influence of growth hormone on overnight insulin requirements in insulin-dependent diabetes. Diabetes 1985; 34:135-9.

23. Goodman HM, Coiro V. Induction of sensitivity to the insulin-like action of growth hormone in normal rat adipose tissue. Endocrinology 1981; 108:113–9.

24. Clark RG, Jansson J-O, Isaksson O, Robinson ICAF. Intravenous growth hormone: growth responses to patterned infusions in hypophysectomized rats. J Endocrinol 1985; 104:53–61.

25. Mauras N, Blizzard RM, Link K, Johnson ML, Rogol AD, Veldhuis JD. Augmentation of growth hormone secretion during puberty: evidence for a pulse amplitude-modulated phenomenon. J Clin Endocrinol Metab 1987; 64:596–601.

26. Fritschka E, Kroll MH, Vogel H-P, Kroll M, Quabbe H-J. Diurnal variations of growth hormone, prolactin, and cortisol secretion in patients with apallic syndrome [Abstract]. Acta Endocrinol (Copenh) 1981; 96(suppl 240):72–3.

27. Mendlewicz J, Linkowski P, Kerkhofs M, et al. Diurnal hypersecretion of growth hormone in depression. J Clin Endocrinol Metab 1985; 60:505–12.

28. Quabbe H-J. Endocrine rhythms in a nonhuman primate, the rhesus monkey. In: Mendlewicz J, van Praag HM, eds. Adv Biol Psychiatry 1983; 11:48–59.

29. Vogel H-P, Quabbe H-J. 24-hour profiles of growth hormone, prolactin and cortisol with frequent sampling in CNS-diseases (a pilot study) [Abstract]. 7th European Sleep Congress, Munich, Sept 3–7.

16

SUMMARY OF SESSION III

ASSESSMENT OF GROWTH HORMONE SECRETION IN CHILDREN

Milo Zachmann, M.D.

Department of Pediatrics
University of Zurich
CH-8032 Zurich, Switzerland

Only two or three years ago, assessment of growth hormone secretion seemed to be simple and straightforward: in most centers, two provocation tests (e.g., an insulin tolerance test and an arginine infusion) were carried out in an individual patient, and the growth hormone results were compared with established normal values from the respective laboratory. At present, even though much has been recently learned concerning the dynamics of growth hormone secretion, it is much less clear when growth hormone secretion is considered normal in a child with short stature.

The speakers of this session expertly pointed out different newly recognized aspects and better studied known factors influencing growth hormone secretion. Their observations are particularly useful at this time because recombinant human growth hormones are now available in unlimited quantities. Clinicians need guidelines to better determine which patients with short stature could benefit from treatment, and which studies should be carried out to get the most valuable information.

Dr. Albertsson-Wikland presented her interesting data on integrated growth hormone determinations from many samples obtained over a 24-h period in a large number of normal children. She showed that while there is no correlation of these integrated levels with age and sex during prepuberty, the values increased later with height and pubertal stages. It also seems to be true that taller normal children secrete somewhat more growth hormone than shorter normal children.

Dr. Bercu presented results of his studies in patients with intermediate growth hormone responses, whom he described as having "growth hormone neurosecretory dysfunction." In part, these seem to be similar patients to those described by others as having "partial growth hormone deficiency" and/or "constitutional delay of growth and adolescence." Regardless of how these patients are called, Dr. Bercu's studies show in a more clear fashion that between normal subjects and patients with classic growth hormone deficiency, there is a wide spectrum of partially insufficient growth hormone secretion due to various reasons. Such patients will probably benefit in the future from treatment with human growth hormone, even though part of the conventional testing may give normal or almost normal results.

Dr. Rappaport presented convincing data from a large series of children who had been irradiated for various reasons, and who showed reduced growth hormone secretion as a consequence. Unfortunately, the results of human growth hormone treatment in these patients are often not satisfactory, and catch-up growth generally does not seem to occur in the same manner as in other patients with growth hormone deficiency. A particular problem in these children is apparently the markedly reduced growth potential of the spine, which may lead to trunk-limb disproportion.

Dr. Evans studied the relationships between sex hormones and growth hormone secretion with advanced techniques. His in vivo results in humans, as well as in vitro studies in rat pituitary cells, partly confirm older reports concerning interactions between growth hormone and sex hormones. Partly, however, they also resolve some previous contradictions. Among others, one conclusion of his studies is that estradiol, but not testosterone, correlates with integrated growth hormone concentrations in vivo in men and women. On the other hand, GHRH-stimulated growth hormone secretion in cells from intact male rats was higher than in cells from castrated animals. Such studies are of particular importance to clinicians because they create the basis for accurate and well-timed additional treatment with sex hormones, pulsatile gonadotropin releasing hormone, or gonadotropins in patients with combined pituitary defects.

Dr. Quabbe described the chronobiological aspects of growth hormone secretion in detail, and analyzed its ultradian 3- to 5-h cycle in man and primates. Smaller peaks which may be undetectable by insensitive methods appear to prevail during daytime, while much higher peaks appear during the night. Light does not, however, seem to be as important in this regulation as was previously thought. Other factors, such as increasing frequency of the secretory peaks during puberty, further modulated the pattern.

As a general conclusion from this session, it may be stated that the factors regulating and influencing growth hormone secretory patterns are multiple involving various neurotransmitters, the balance between GHRH and somatostatin, chronobiological laws, and sex hormones, that the classic pharmacological provocative tests are clearly insufficient for evaluation in an individual patient.

IV. GROWTH HORMONE ACTION

17

GROWTH HORMONE RECEPTORS IN RAT ADIPOCYTES

H. Maurice Goodman, Erela Gorin, Genevieve Grichting,
Thomas W. Honeyman, Jaroslaw Szecowka, Lih-Ruey Tai, and
Leonard R. Waice

Department of Physiology
University of Massachusetts Medical School
Worcester, MA 01605

Like other peptide and protein hormones, GH is thought to produce its biological effects by interacting with specific receptors on the surface of target cells. Understanding of GH receptors lags behind that of other hormone receptors, in part because GH receptors are scarce, and in part because there has been little agreement on what constitutes a good in vitro model to study GH action. Furthermore, because at least some of the in vivo actions of GH are mediated by insulin-like growth factors, attention has been diverted to study of these receptors. GH, however, does produce direct metabolic effects, particularly on adipose tissue, and although we do not know how these effects are related to growth, metabolic actions may be important even after growth has terminated.

The effects of GH on rat epididymal fat can be divided into three major categories (Table 1). Insulin-like effects are seen immediately after addition of GH to adipose tissue obtained from GH deficient (1), weanling (2), or stressed (3) rats. GH virtually duplicates the entire spectrum of insulin actions (4), but only for a brief period. After about 2 h, the insulin-like response wanes, and cannot be reinitiated even with very high doses of hormone. Refractoriness is confined to insulin-like stimulation by GH, lasts many hours, and is characteristic of tissues freshly isolated from normal rats (5). Refractoriness of normal tissues gradually disappears, and when tissues are maintained in a GH-free medium in vitro for 3 or more h, sensitivity to insulin-like stimulation by GH is fully evident (5). Refractoriness can be produced with amounts of GH that are too low to produce an insulin-like response. Conversely, an insulin-like response is not followed by refractoriness when tissues are exposed to GH for less than about 60 min (6). Refractoriness, thus, is not a consequence of insulin-like stimulation per se. In the presence of either glucocorticoid or theophylline, GH also increases lipolysis after a delay of about 2 h. This response persists for many hours and is not subject to the refractory phenomenon (7). We do not yet understand whether these diverse responses all stem from interaction of GH with a single class of receptors, or result from more than one hormone-receptor interaction. In one series of experiments with chemically modified GH, insulin-like responses were severely reduced, but lipolytic responses were enhanced, suggesting that different hormone receptor interactions mediated these responses (8).

Table 1. Responses of adipose tissue to growth hormone.

Action	Minutes after GH	Concentration range
Insulin-like		
↑ glucose metabolism	15 - 120	30 - 300 ng/ml
↑ leucine or pyruvate oxidation		
↓ lipolysis		
Delayed		
↑ lipolysis	90 - 360+	1 - 30 ng/ml
↓ glucose metabolism		
Refractoriness	120 - 480+	1 - 30 ng/ml

Our studies of the nature of GH receptors have focused on adipocytes since this preparation offers the greatest opportunity for relating receptor phenomenology to biological responses (9). To study GH binding, we used isolated adipocytes that had preincubated in vitro for 3 h to allow the appearance of insulin-like responsiveness. Even when labeled with as many as 5 atoms of ^{125}I per molecule, hGH is fully active in producing both initial insulin-like and delayed lipolytic responses (10). Adipocytes bind [^{125}I]hGH in a manner that is highly specific and saturable (Fig. 1). Bound hGH was completely displaced by human, rat and ovine GH, but not by other pituitary hormones including prolactin or by insulin. Failure of unlabeled insulin to compete with [^{125}I]hGH and of unlabeled GH to compete with [^{125}I]insulin for binding to adipocytes indicates that insulin-like responses to GH are not mediated by insulin receptors.

Scatchard plots of binding data are straight lines and suggest that each fat cell has a single class of about 20,000 binding sites that appeared to be half-saturated at a GH concentration of about 1 nM (Fig. 2). More recent studies suggest somewhat fewer receptors per cell and a

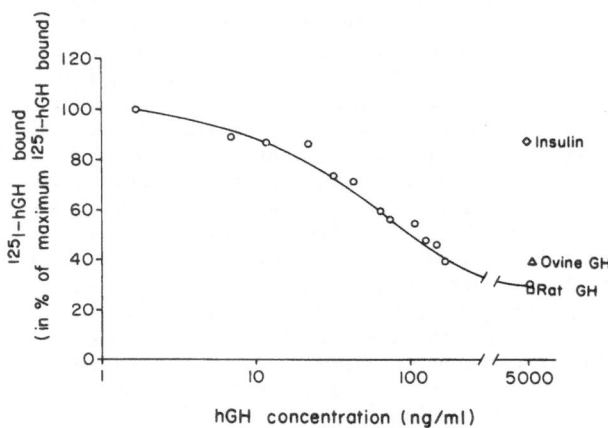

Fig. 1. Displacement of [^{125}I]hGH from binding sites on adipocytes by unlabeled insulin or human, ovine, or rat GH. Reprinted with permission (9).

higher affinity, but estimates of these constants are only approximations, since GH binding to fat cells is virtually irreversible and may not follow equilibrium kinetics. Measurement of initial rates of binding also failed to reveal any consequences of refractoriness on GH binding (4). The data indicate that refractoriness to insulin-like stimulation is not due to any change in hGH binding, and suggest that sensitivity or refractoriness is determined at a post-receptor locus.

When the concentrations of hGH needed to produce the various biological responses are compared to binding data (Fig. 3), it is evident that adipocytes contain no "spare receptors." Half maximum insulin-like responses are produced when about 65-70% of the receptors are occupied. If, indeed, there is a single class of GH receptors, considerably fewer need to be activated to produce lipolysis or refractoriness than to produce insulin-like responses.

To characterize GH receptors further, [^{125}I]hGH was cross-linked to surface proteins using the bifunctional reagent, disuccinimidyl suberate (11). Proteins were then dissolved in SDS, separated by polyacrylamide gel electrophoresis, and visualized by autoradiography (Fig. 4). The principal binding component migrated on 5% polyacrylamide gel with a mobility corresponding to a molecular weight of about 130 kDa. Assuming a single binding site for GH, the mass of this binding protein must be about 110 kDa. Autoradiography also revealed larger components corresponding to 240 and 310 kDa. Upon treatment with the sulfhydryl reducing reagent, dithiothreitol (DTT), these bands disappeared, and the cross-linked radioactivity was quantitatively recovered in the 130 kDa band. These

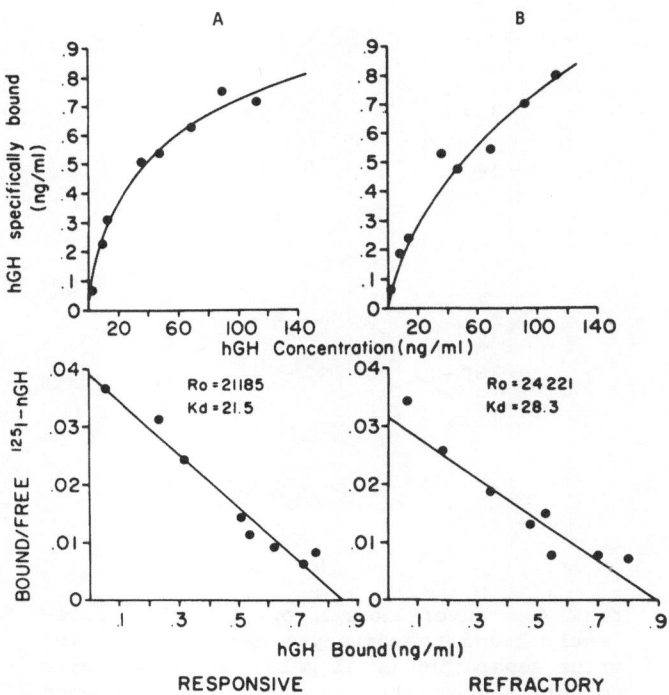

Fig. 2. Specific binding of [^{125}I]hGH to adipocytes that are responsive (A) or refractory (B) to the insulin-like action of GH. Reprinted with permission (9).

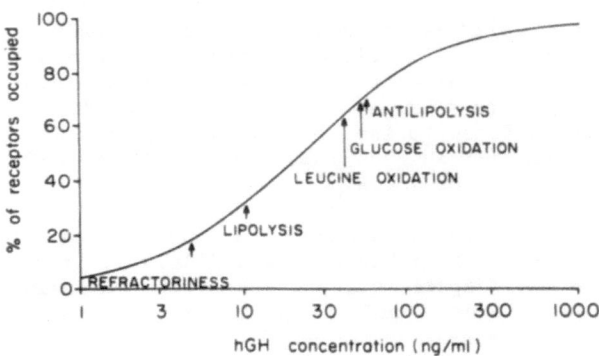

Fig. 3. Relationship between receptor occupancy and biological responses. The arrows indicate the points on the curve that correspond to half maximal responses. Reprinted with permission (9).

observations suggest that the GH receptor contains a binding unit of about 110 kDa, some of which is present in larger forms. The larger forms may represent dimers or trimers of the binding unit connected to each other or other membrane proteins by disulfide bonds.

To determine whether the GH binding protein, like other hormone receptors, contains carbohydrate, we examined the effects of lectins on

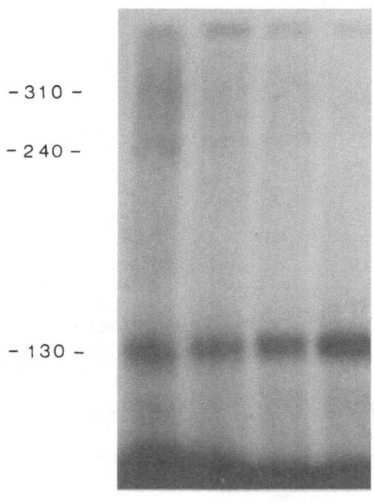

Fig. 4. Autoradiogram of [^{125}I]hGH covalently bound to adipocyte membrane proteins after separation on 5% gels. Membranes were solubilized in the absence (A) or presence of dithiothreitol at 2.5 mM (B), 10 mM (C), or 100 mM (D). No labeled bands were seen after cross-linking in the presence of excess unlabeled hGH. Reprinted with permission (11).

the binding of [^{125}I]hGH to fat cells. Wheat germ lectin (10^{-6} M) reduced GH binding by about 90%; concanavalin A had a considerably smaller effect. Since interference with binding might reflect steric hindrance produced by binding of lectin to the glucosamine or sialic acid of adjacent glycoprotein molecules rather than the receptor itself, a more direct approach was adopted. Membranes prepared from adipocytes cross-linked to [^{125}I]hGH were incubated with glycosidases prior to electrophoresis and autoradiography. After treatment with neuraminidase, which removes terminal sialic acid residues, the principal band migrated with a mobility corresponding to 120 kDa. Treatment with endoglycosidase F, which cleaves the carbohydrate-protein linkage, reduced the apparent molecular weight to about 110 kDa, suggesting that nearly 20% of the binding protein is carbohydrate.

We next examined the physiological behavior of the receptor. At 4°C, [^{125}I]hGH dissociates exceedingly slowly from binding sites on the adipocyte surface with a half-time of more than 16 h. When fat cells which had bound [^{125}IhGH] in an earlier incubation were transferred to hormone-free medium and incubated at 37°C (12), ^{125}I was released into the incubation medium with a half-time of about 30 min (Fig. 5). About 90% of the radioactivity released was soluble in trichloroacetate, and was in the form of iodotyrosines. These observations suggest that the principal route by which receptor-bound hormone is cleared from fat cells is internalization and degradation. Dissociation of ^{125}I is sensitive to temperature and to treatment of adipocytes with agents that interfere with lysosomal activity such as chloroquine, leupeptin, or ammonium chloride. Chloroquine decreased the dissociation of [^{125}I]hGH, and also caused labeled hormone to accumulate in the adipocytes (Fig. 6).

Typically, receptor-mediated endocytosis is followed by dissociation of the ligand from the receptor in the acidic environment of the endosome. The ligand is then transferred to lysosomes for degradation, and the receptor recycles back to the membrane (13). While hormones, such as insulin, dissociate from their receptors when the pH falls below 7, GH binding increased at mildly acidic pH (Fig. 7). Adipocytes bound approximately as much [^{125}I]hGH at the pH of 4.5 found in lysosomes, as at pH

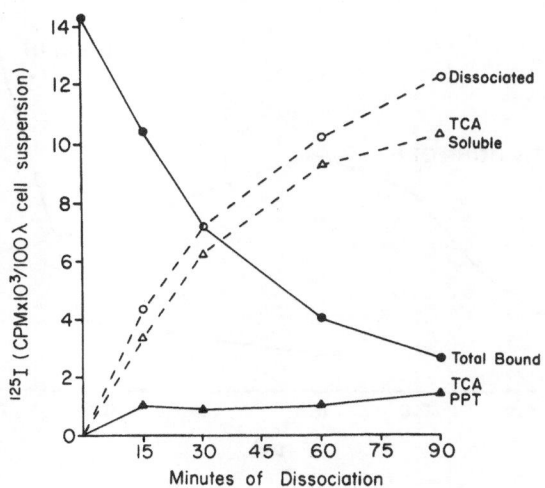

Fig. 5. Fate of ^{125}I bound to adipocytes in the form of [^{125}I] hGH during incubation at 37°C in hormone-free medium. Reprinted with permission (12).

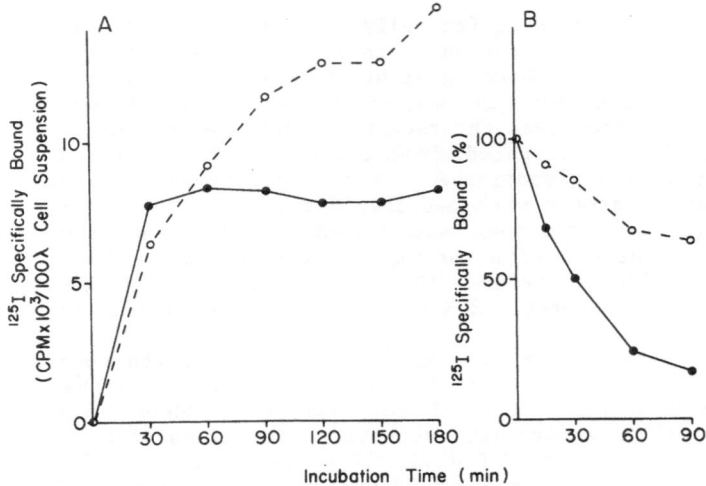

Fig. 6. Effects of chloroquine (0.1 µM) on binding of [^{125}I]hGH (A) and subsequent dissociation (B) from adipocytes. Reprinted with permission (12).

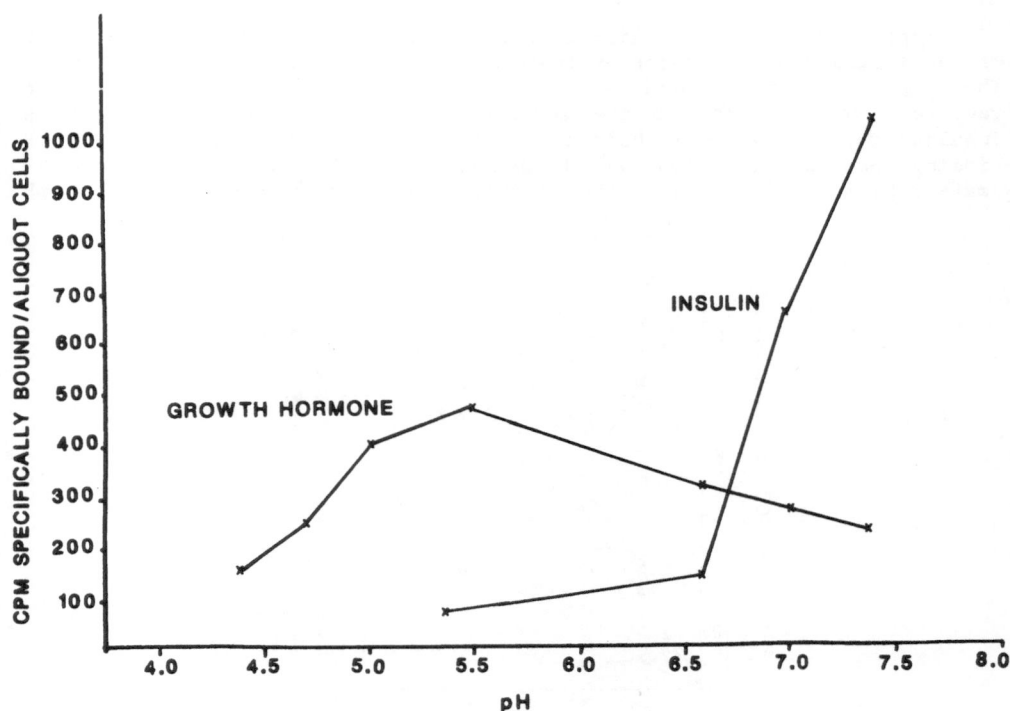

Fig. 7. Effects of pH on binding of [^{125}I]insulin or [^{125}I]hGH to adipocytes.

7.4. The failure of acidification to dissociate GH from its receptor suggests that the entire hormone-receptor complex may be degraded in lysosomes.

Insight into turnover of receptors was obtained by measuring specific binding of [^{125}I]hGH by adipocytes that were pretreated for various times with cycloheximide to inhibit protein synthesis (14). Cells were incubated with [^{125}I]hGH for the 10 min immediately following a 2.5 h incubation period in which cycloheximide was added to different flasks at 30-min intervals. Specific binding decreased as the length of exposure to the inhibitor of protein synthesis increased. Loss of binding followed first order kinetics with a half time of 45-50 min (Fig. 8). Binding declined at the same rate when labeled hormone was added along with cycloheximide, indicating that loss of binding is independent of receptor occupancy. Replacing cycloheximide with puromycin, another inhibitor of protein synthesis, produced identical effects, but actinomycin, an inhibitor of RNA synthesis, had no effect on GH binding. These results suggest that ongoing protein synthesis is necessary to sustain GH binding sites on the surface of adipocytes. Failure of actinomycin to modify GH binding, suggests that the short-lived protein required must be synthesized from a stable RNA template. The short-lived protein may be the receptor itself or some other protein that is needed to sustain affinity of receptors or the insertion of recycling receptors into the plasma membrane.

To distinguish between these possibilities, we treated cells with agents that affect the carbohydrate rather than the protein component of cellular glycoproteins. Swainsonine is an alkaloid inhibitor of a Golgi mannosidase II (15), and hence interferes with normal processing of mannose branches of the carbohydrate moiety of glycoproteins. Tunicamycin blocks the N-linked glycosylation of asparagine residues (16). Swainsonine produced no significant diminution in specific binding of [^{125}I]hGH to adipocytes even after 8 h, and after 8 h tunicamycin decreased binding by only about 50%. Since only newly synthesized glycoproteins would be affected by these agents, determination of the molecular size of GH-receptor complexes formed in swainsonine or tunicamycin-treated cells should

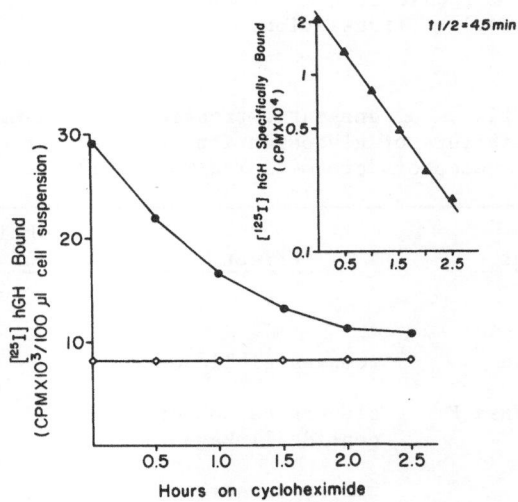

Fig. 8. Effects of preincubation with 20 µg/ml cycloheximide on subsequent binding of [^{125}I]hGH to adipocytes. Reprinted with permission (14).

provide information on receptor turnover rate. [^{125}I]hGH was covalently linked to adipocytes that had preincubated for various times with either tunicamycin or swainsonine, and the molecular sizes of the labeled membrane proteins were estimated from their mobility on polyacrylamide gels. Two h after swainsonine treatment, all of the cross-linked GH-receptor complex migrated with a mobility corresponding to 120 kDa, instead of the 130 kDa of untreated cells. In cells treated with tunicamycin, a new labeled band corresponding to a molecular weight of about 110 kDa was evident by about 4 h and was the major component by 8 h. These values correspond well with the molecular weights of crosslinked complexes isolated from membranes after treatment with neuraminidase or endoglycosidase F (Table 2).

The finding of cross-linked GH-receptor complexes of lower molecular weight soon after inhibition of glycosylation indicates that membrane receptors are replaced frequently with newly synthesized receptors, and provides strong corroboration of the idea that GH receptors turn over with a half-life of less than 1 h. The longer time needed for replacement of receptors after tunicamycin treatment reflects both incomplete inhibition of glycosylation and lowered affinity for the ligand, and also suggests that disruption of glycosylation may interfere with turnover. Since GH binds to receptors of smaller size, it is evident that the carbohydrate component is not essential either for insertion into the membrane or proper orientation.

Physiologically, the behavior of the GH receptor is also consistent with rapid turnover. Within 8 h after hypophysectomy, binding of [^{125}I]hGH to adipocytes is reduced by about 50% (17) and can be restored nearly to normal by administration of a single injection of GH 4 h before sacrifice (Fig. 9). Sixteen h after a single injection of GH to hypophysectomized rats, binding of labeled hormone was no greater than seen in adipocytes obtained from untreated hypophysectomized rats. The stress of surgery, which, in rats, inhibits GH secretion (18), also temporarily decreased GH binding. In addition, fasting inhibits GH secretion in rats (19) and decreases GH binding by adipocytes (17). These observations suggest that the GH receptor is "up regulated" rather than "down regulated" by GH, and that receptor abundance on the cell surface may be regulated at the level of translation.

Table 2. Effects of enzymatic treatment of plasma membranes or inhibitors of glycosidation on molecular size of receptors cross-linked to [^{125}I]hGH.

Treatment	Effect	Molecular weight of complex (kDa)
Control		130
Neuraminidase	removes sialic acid	120
Endoglycosidase F	cleaves carbohydrate-peptide linkage	110
Swainsonine	blocks mannose processing	120
Tunicamycin	blocks N linked glycosylation	110

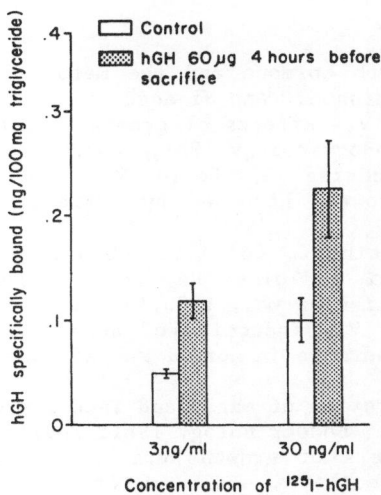

Fig. 9. Effects of treatment of hypophysectomized rats with GH in vivo on the subsequent binding of [^{125}I]hGH to adipocytes.

Some regulation of GH-receptor binding may also be accomplished by phosphorylation. Incubation of adipocytes with agents known to increase cellular concentrations of cyclic AMP or with dibutyryl cyclic AMP promptly decreased GH binding. Scatchard analysis of binding data obtained with cells treated with forskolin or dibutyryl cyclic AMP indicated a threefold decrease in receptor number, with no change in affinity (Table 3). Since these effects are also seen when isolated membranes are incubated with cyclic AMP-dependent protein kinase prior to assessment of binding, it is likely that phosphorylation of the receptor itself accounts for decreased binding.

After reviewing the state of our knowledge of the GH receptor in adipocytes, it is clear that much remains to be learned. We know little of its chemistry, of its subunit structure, of how it signals metabolic changes, or whether it shares signals with like-acting hormones. While it appears that GH binds to a single glycoprotein of about 110 kDa, the binding unit itself may be present in larger complexes. Whether these different forms of the receptor each mediate a different effect of GH in adipocytes remains to be determined.

Table 3. Effects of forskolin (10 μM) and dibutyryl cyclic
AMP (2 mM) on binding of [^{125}I]hGH to adipocytes.

Treatment	Binding sites/cell	nM producing half-saturation
Control	9120	2.4
Forskolin	3730	2.6
Dibutyryl cAMP	3026	2.4

REFERENCES

1. Goodman HM. Growth hormone and the metabolism of carbohydrate and lipid in adipose tissue. Ann NY Acad Sci 1968; 148:419-40.
2. Goodman HM, Coiro V. Effects of growth hormone on adipose tissue of weanling rats. Endocrinology 1981; 109:2046-53.
3. Goodman HM, Grichting G, Coiro V. Induction of insulin-like responses to growth hormone by stress. Endocrinology 1981; 109:2213-9.
4. Goodman HM, Grichting G, Coiro V. Growth hormone action on adipocytes. In: Raiti S, Tolman RA, eds. Human growth hormone. New York: Plenum Publishing Co., 1980:499-512.
5. Goodman HM, Coiro V. Induction of sensitivity to the insulin-like action of growth hormone in normal rat adipose tissue. Endocrinology 1981; 108:113-9.
6. Goodman HM. Separation of early and late responses of adipose tissue to growth hormone. Endocrinology 1981; 109:120-9.
7. Goodman HM. Effects of growth hormone on isolated adipose tissue. In: Muller EE, Pecile A, eds. Amsterdam: Excerpta Medica Foundation, 1968:153-71.
8. Goodman HM, Kostyo JL. Altered profiles of biological activity of growth hormone fragments on adipocyte metabolism. Endocrinology 1981; 108:553-8.
9. Grichting G, Levy L, Goodman HM. Relationship between binding and biological effects of human growth hormone in rat adipocytes. Endocrinology 1983; 113:1111-20.
10. Goodman HM, Levy LK. Preparation and biological reactivity of polyiodinated human growth hormone. Endocrinology 1983; 113:2017-23.
11. Gorin E, Goodman HM. Covalent binding of growth hormone to surface receptors on rat adipocytes. Endocrinology 1984; 114:1279-86.
12. Gorin E, Grichting G, Goodman HM. Binding and degradation of [^{125}I]-human growth hormone in rat adipocytes. Endocrinology 1984; 115:467-75.
13. Brown MS, Anderson RGW, Goldstein JL. Recycling receptors: the round-trip itinerary of migrant membrane proteins. Cell 1983; 32:663-7.
14. Gorin E, Goodman HM. Turnover of growth hormone receptors in rat adipocytes. Endocrinology 1985; 116:1796-805.
15. Tulsiani DRT, Harris TM, Touster O. Swainsonine inhibits the biosynthesis of complex glycoproteins by inhibition of Golgi mannosidase II. J Biol Chem 1982; 257:7936-9.
16. Lehle L, Tanner W. The specific site of tunicamycin inhibition in the formation of dolichol-bound N-acetylglucosamine derivatives. FEBS Lett 1976; 71:167-70.
17. Grichting G, Goodman HM. Growth hormone maintains its own receptors in rat adipocytes. Endocrinology 1986; 119:847-54.
18. Reichlin S. Regulation of somatotrophic hormone secretion. In: Knobil E, Sawyer W, eds. Handbook of physiology (section 7, vol 4, part II). Washington: American Physiological Society, 1977:405-47.
19. Tannenbaum GS, Rostad O, Brazeau P. Effects of prolonged food deprivation on the ultradian growth hormone rhythm and immunoreactive somatostatin tissue levels in the rat. Endocrinology 1979; 104:1733-8.

18

DIRECT ACTION OF GH

O. G. P. Isaksson, J. Isgaard, A. Nilsson, and A. Lindahl

Department of Physiology
University of Goteborg, P.O. Box 33031
S-400 33 Goteborg, Sweden

INTRODUCTION

Growth hormone (GH) has long been known to have a pivotal role in the regulation of somatic growth. Thus, GH deficiency results in proportionate dwarfism that is responsive to replacement therapy with GH. The physiological mechanism(s) by which GH exerts its stimulatory effect on somatic growth has not yet been elucidated. It has been demonstrated convincingly that administration of GH stimulates the growth of cartilage and other tissues by increasing the number of cells, showing that the effect of GH in vivo ultimately results in a stimulation of DNA synthesis and cell proliferation (1-3). However, efforts to demonstrate stimulatory effects of GH in vitro in explants of cartilage and other skeletal tissues have been unsuccessful in most cases.

Approximately 30 years ago, Salmon and Daughaday (4) made the important observation that rat plasma contains GH-dependent peptide growth factors that stimulate a number of cellular functions that are associated with cell multiplication and growth. The growth factors that originally were designated as sulphation factors and later as somatomedin(s), have been characterized and are presently recognized as insulin-like growth factor I (IGF-I) and II (IGF-II). The fact that somatomedin stimulates different growth-associated functions in several in vitro preparations and cell cultures, whereas GH is ineffective in most cases, led to the formulation of the somatomedin hypothesis of GH action (5). The central thesis of this theory is that the action of GH on skeletal growth is mediated by IGF-I, that is synthesized in noncartilage tissues like the liver and other nonskeletal tissues.

It is certain that GH in several species postnatally, is a main determinant of the plasma level of IGF-I and plasma levels of IGF-I are typically high in patients with an enhanced endogenous production of GH and low in GH-deficient individuals (6). Infusion of large doses of highly purified human IGF-I to hypophysectomized rats have been shown to stimulate tibial width, body weight and thymidine incorporation into costal cartilage, giving direct experimental support for a biological role of IGF-I on somatic growth in vivo (7). However, local administration of GH at the site of the epiphyseal growth plate increases longitudinal bone growth of the treated but not the untreated contralateral leg, suggesting that GH interacts directly with cells in the epiphyseal growth plate

(8–10). Recently it was shown that chondrocytes in the proliferative layer of the epiphyseal growth plate of normal rats contain IGF-I-like immunoreactivity; local administration of small doses of GH at the site of the growth plate increased the number of cells expressing IGF-I-like immunoreactivity on the injected side without a concomitant rise in the plasma level of IGF-I (11). Subsequent studies have shown that the IGF-I immunoreactivity is preferentially localized in the endoplasmatic reticulum and the Golgi apparatus of the proliferative chondrocytes, suggesting that IGF-I is synthesized and released by the chondrocytes themselves (12). IGF-I is synthesized in multiple nonhepatic tissues (13), and recent studies suggest that GH regulates the concentration of IGF-I in several tissues by stimulating the gene encoding for IGF-I (14–16).

Green and co-workers made the important discovery that GH specifically promotes the differentiation of cloned preadipose 3T3 cells into adipocytes (17,18). Subsequent studies have shown that pretreatment of 3T3 preadipose cells with GH but not IGF-I increases the responsiveness to IGF-I (19). These observations indicate that GH and IGF-I act on cells in a specific order that is dependent upon the stage of cell maturation. GH is the prime and IGF-I the second effector in this orderly sequence of events (19).

Chondrocytes in the growth plate of postnatal animals exhibit a specific spatial location depending upon their stage of differentiation/maturation. Close to the bony epiphysis there is a narrow cell layer consisting of germinal or stem cell chondrocytes (20,21). During the process of longitudinal bone growth, cells in the stem cell layer differentiate and enter the proliferative layer where the cells undergo limited clonal expansion. Concomitantly new progenitor cells start their program of differentiation and limited clonal expansion, making the epiphyseal growth plate a constantly renewing tissue until the time of epiphyseal closure.

To evaluate the effects of GH and IGF-I on colony formation of epiphyseal chondrocytes at different stages of maturation, chondrocytes have been isolated from different layers of normal rabbit tibia growth plates and cultured in suspension stabilized with agarose. The effect of in vivo pretreatment of hypophysectomized rats with GH or IGF-I on colony formation of epiphyseal chondrocytes in vitro and the subsequent responsiveness to IGF-I have also been studied.

MATERIAL AND METHODS

Eight-week-old normal male prepubertal New Zealand white rabbits were used for isolation of chondrocytes of different maturation. Male Sprague-Dawley rats were hypophysectomized at 26 days of age and used for in vivo pretreatment with GH or IGF-I 10 days later. The animals were killed and tibial bones were dissected out and trimmed free of soft tissue. The epiphyseal cartilage was dissected avoiding any loss of cartilage bordering the bony epiphysis. Intact rat tibia growth plates or segments of rabbit growth plates (see Results) were digested in a spinner bottle for 4 h at 37°C in 0.12% (wt/vol) Clostridium collagenase and 0.02% (wt/vol) deoxyribonuclease I in Ham's F-12 medium. After isolation, the cells were washed 3 times in serum-free medium and cell counts were made in a hemocytometer. Viability of cells was determined by trypan blue exclusion technique. The cell viability was over 90% in all experiments. After isolation and washings, the cells were suspended and cultured in soft agar according to Benya and Shaffer (22). Cultures with rabbit chondrocytes were supplemented with 10% newborn calf serum (NCS, Gibco) and cultures with rat epiphyseal chondrocytes with 2.5% NCS, 2.5% serum from hypophysectomized rats and 1% of the serum substitute Ultroser G (LKB, Sweden). The culture medium was further supplemented with HEPES (10 mM), gentamicin sulphate (100 ng/ml, Sigma), Fungizone (2 µg/ml, Gibco) and L-ascorbic acid (50 µg/ml). The cultures were maintained at 37C in air containing 5% CO_2 for 14 days. Cultures were terminated by fixation in buffered formaldehyde (4%), and staining with alcian blue (0.5% in 0.04 M hydrochloric acid) was utilized to identify colonies producing glyco-saminoglycans. Colonies were counted in 100 squares (2 mm grid) for each culture dish, the counts being made separately by two investigators. A cell colony was defined as a cluster of cells with the matrix stained by alcian blue and with a diameter of more than 56 µm. In some experiments the diameter of each colony was measured in a microscope with a calibrated eyepiece and the colonies were arranged in class intervals of 16 µm. Bacteriologically produced cloned methionine human growth hormone (Somatonorm®, 2 IU/mg) and yeast derived cloned human insulin-like growth factor I (IGF-I, approximately 4100 U/mg, as determined by radioreceptor-assay) were generous gifts from KabiVitrum AB, Stockholm, Sweden).

RESULTS

The epiphyseal growth plate of the proximal tibia of prepubertal male rabbits was divided in 3 different zones and the cells were subsequently isolated by collagenase digestion. The approximate extension of the 3 different zones (proximal, intermediate and distal) is indicated in Figure 1. Chondrocytes isolated from the proximal and intermediate zones formed small colonies in suspension culture after 5-8 days and colonies could easily be detected and counted under the microscope after 14 days. No colonies were seen in cultures of chondrocytes isolated from the distal zone as shown in Figure 2. Colonies consisted of varying numbers of cells and matrix containing proteoglycans as identified with alcian blue staining.

The effect of various concentrations of hGH and IGF-I on colony formation of chondrocytes isolated from the proximal and the intermediate zones is shown in Figure 3. IGF-I caused a dose-related increase in colony formation, with an apparent maximal effect at 100 ng/ml, in cells

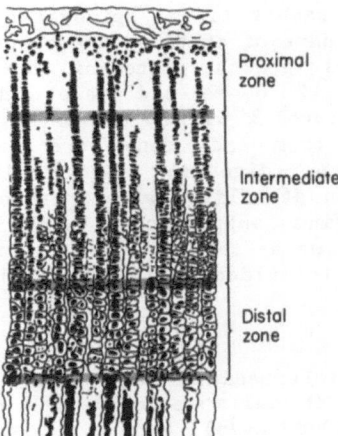

Fig. 1. Schematic drawing of rabbit epiphyseal plate cartilage. The approximate extent of the dissected zones is indicated by the brackets.

201

PROXIMAL ZONE

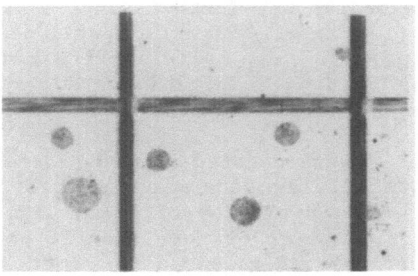

INTERMEDIATE ZONE

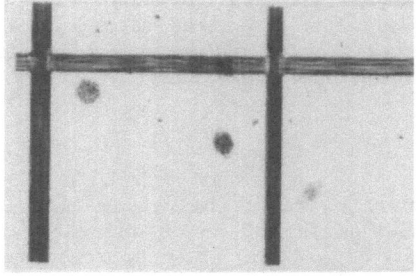

DISTAL ZONE

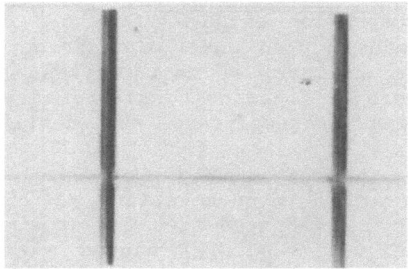

Fig. 2. Colonies of chondrocytes isolated from the proximal, intermediate and distal zones of rabbit tibial epiphyseal cartilage after 14 days of culture in suspension. The epiphyseal growth plate of the proximal tibia of 2 8-week-old male rabbits was divided into 3 different zones and chondrocytes from each zone were isolated by collagenase digestion and cultured in suspension stabilized with agarose in Ham's F-12 medium supplemented with 10% NCS. Cultures were terminated by fixation in buffered formaldehyde (4%). (Magnification x 50.)

isolated both from the intermediate and proximal zones. Human GH potentiated colony formation in cells isolated from the proximal zone at the concentration range of 10-80 ng/ml, but no potentiation was apparent at a concentration of 160 ng/ml. No stimulatory effect of GH was apparent in cells isolated from the intermediate zone. Rather, at high concentrations of hGH (40-160 ng/ml) a significant reduction in colony numbers was seen.

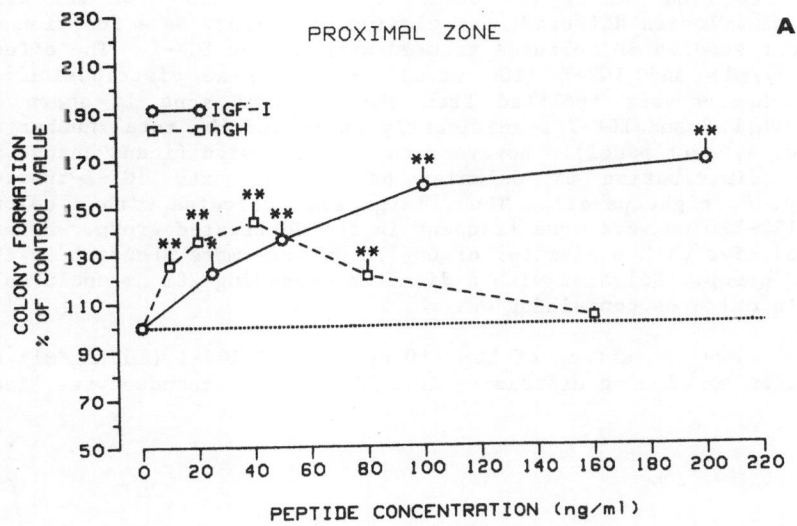

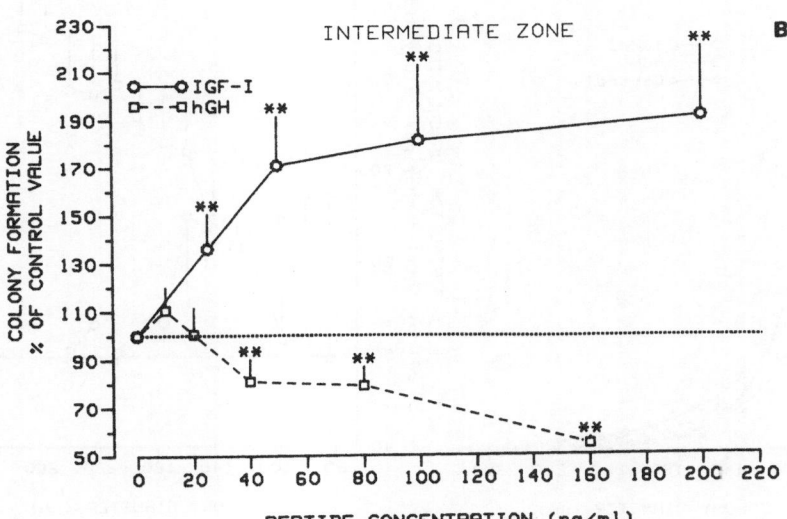

Fig. 3. Dose-response effects of hGH and IGF-I on colony formation of chondrocytes isolated from (A) the proximal zone or (B) the intermediate zone of rabbit tibia epiphyseal growth plate. Total cloning efficiency (number of colonies with a diameter exceeding 56 μm per 10^3 seeded cells) for control cultures was 9.7 ± 0.9. The stimulatory effect of GH and IGF-I is expressed as percent stimulation of control value (control value = 100%). Values are mean ± SEM of 8 different experiments using two rabbits for each cell isolation. Significances between control and treated cultures were calculated with Student's t test.

In order to find out if the effect of hGH and IGF-I on the size distribution of colonies differed, the cloning efficiency as a function of colony size was studied in cultures treated with hGH or IGF-I. The effect of hGH (40 ng/ml) and IGF-I (100 ng/ml) on the size distribution of colonies of chondrocytes isolated from the proximal zone is shown in Figure 4. Both hGH and IGF-I significantly increased the total number of colonies (Fig. 4, left panel). However, there was a significant change in the relative distribution of colonies between GH- and IGF-I-treated cultures (Fig. 4, right panel). Thus, large size colonies with a colony diameter of 112–320 μm were more frequent in the GH-treated group, whereas small size colonies with a diameter of 64–176 μm were more abundant in the IGF-I-treated group. Colonies with a diameter exceeding 288 μm could only be detected in cultures containing GH.

Figure 5 shows the effect of hGH (40 ng/ml) and IGF-I (100 ng/ml) on the distribution of cloning efficiency in cultures of chondrocytes iso-

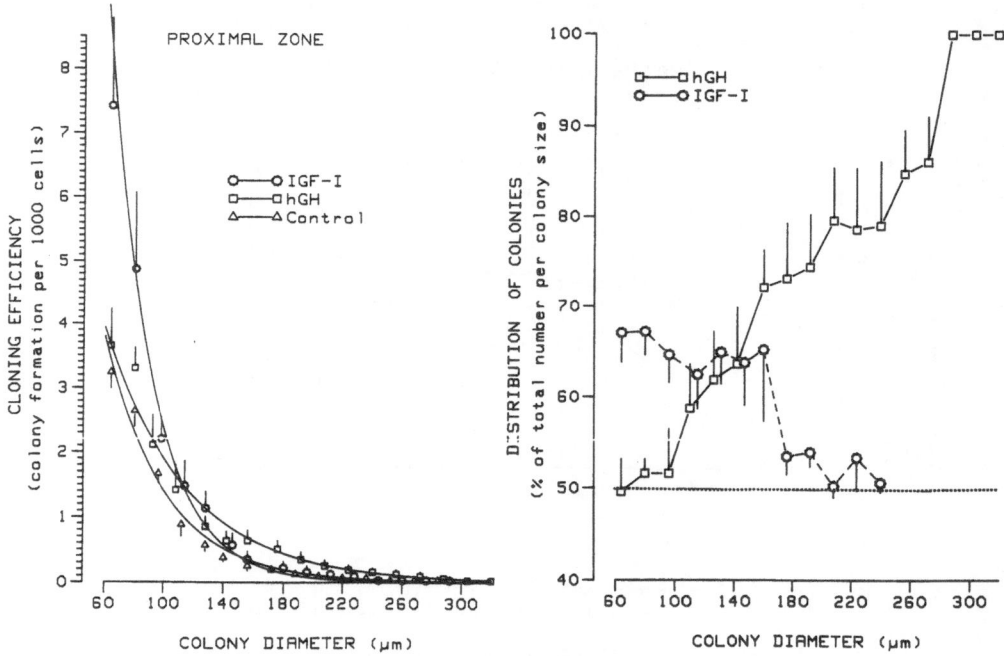

Fig. 4. Effect of hGH and IGF-I on distribution of cloning efficiency of chondrocytes isolated from the proximal zone of rabbit tibia epiphyseal growth plate. The distribution of cloning efficiency as a function of colony diameter in control, hGH- (40 ng/ml) and IGF-I- (100 ng/ml) treated cultures is shown in left panel. Values are mean ± SEM of 7 different experiments using two rabbits for each cell isolation. Total cloning efficiency (number of colonies with a diameter exceeding 56 μm per 1000 seeded cells) was 10.1 ± 0.7 (control), 14.6 ± 1.4 (hGH), and 19.0 ± 2.9 (IGF-I) respectively. Both hGH- and IGF-I-treated cultures differed in distribution compared to control cultures as calculated by X^2-analyses (P<0.001 and P<0.05 respectively). The relative distribution of colonies between control-, IGF-I- and hGH-treated cultures is shown in right panel. All distribution values differed significantly from control (P<0.001) except for the following groups: IGF-I (208 μm, 224 μm) and hGH (64 μm, 80 μm, 96 μm).

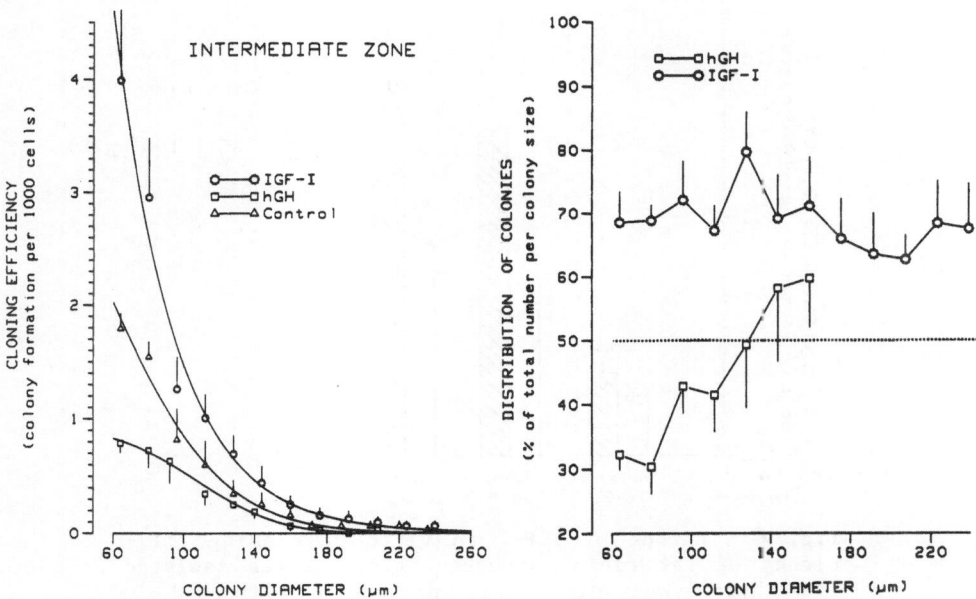

Fig. 5. Effect of hGH and IGF-I on the distribution of cloning efficiency of chondrocytes isolated from the intermediate zone of rabbit tibia epiphyseal growth plate. The distribution of cloning efficiency as a function of colony diameter in control, hGH- (40 ng/ml) and IGF-I- (100 ng/ml) treated cultures is shown in left panel. Values are mean ± SEM of 7 different experiments using 2 rabbits for each cell isolation. Total cloning efficiency (number of colonies with a diameter exceeding 56 µm per 1000 seeded cells) was 6.0 ± 0.9 (control), 3.0 ± 0.4 (hGH), and 11.4 ± 1.6 (IGF-I). The relative distribution of colonies between control, IGF-I- and hGH-treated cultures is shown in right panel. All distribution values differed significantly from control (P<0.001) except for hGH-treated cultures with colony diameters of 128 µm, 144 µm, and 160 µm.

lated from the intermediate zone of the growth plate. As shown in the left panel of Figure 5, IGF-I caused a significant increase in the total number of colonies whereas the total number of colonies was decreased in hGH-treated cultures. The right panel of Figure 5 shows that IGF-I potentiated the formation of all colonies, independent of size, whereas hGH significantly decreased the number of small size colonies.

In the next series of experiments, the effect of pretreatment with GH or IGF-I in vivo on colony formation of epiphyseal chondrocytes from hypophysectomized rats and the subsequent responsiveness to IGF-I in vitro was studied. Pretreatment of hypophysectomized rats with 10 or 100 µg of hGH 24, 12, and 2 h before cell isolation resulted in an increased cloning efficiency as shown in Figure 6. Addition of IGF-I (100 ng/ml) to cultures of chondrocytes isolated from GH-pretreated rats caused a substantial increase in cloning efficiency compared to the small effect of IGF-I in cultures of chondrocytes isolated from saline-treated control rats (Fig. 6).

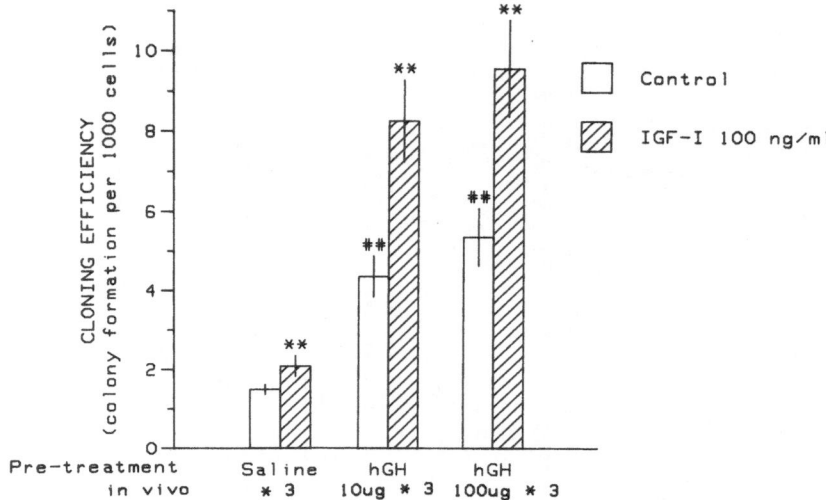

Fig. 6. Effect of IGF-I in vitro on cloning efficiency of rat tibia epiphyseal chondrocytes isolated from hypophysectomized rats pretreated with hGH in vivo. Hypophysectomized rats received 3 subcutaneous injections of 2 different doses of hGH (10 μg x 3 or 100 μg x 3) or saline 24, 12 and 2 h before decapitation. Epiphyseal growth plate chondrocytes were isolated and cultured in absence or presence of IGF-I (100 ng/ml). The total cloning efficiency for each culture was estimated after 14 days of culture. Values are mean ± SEM of 3 different experiments with 4-8 animals in each group. (## = P<0.01 vs. the control culture in saline-injected control group; ** = P<0.01 IGF-I vs. the control culture in the same group.)

To study the time course of the stimulatory effect of GH pretreatment and the subsequent responsiveness to IGF-I in vitro on colony formation, epiphyseal chondrocytes were isolated at different time periods after injection of a single dose of hGH (300 μg) and cultured in the absence or presence with IGF-I (100 ng/ml) as shown in Figure 7. The cloning efficiency as well as the responsiveness to IGF-I was significantly increased in animals that received GH replacement 12 or 24 h before the start of cell isolation, but chondrocytes isolated 4 h after administration of GH did not show an increased colony formation. This observation suggests that GH has to interact with its target cells for 4-12 h in vivo to stimulate subsequent colony formation in vitro and to increase the responsiveness to IGF-I.

To find out whether the "priming" effect of GH in vivo on the increased responsiveness to IGF-I in vitro perhaps was due to an increased plasma level of IGF-I caused by the GH-treatment, hypophysectomized rats were treated with 2 different doses of IGF-I (5 μg x 3 or 50 μg x 3) 24, 12 and 2 h before cell isolation. Figure 8 shows that pretreatment with IGF-I in vivo caused a slight stimulation of colony formation in vitro but no potentiation of the response to IGF-I in vitro could be detected. In the same experiment, hGH potentiated the effect of IGF-I in vitro. The plasma level of IGF-I in the GH-treated group was measured at the time of autopsy and found to be approximately the same as in the group of rats receiving 50 μg x 3 of IGF-I (data not shown). The results of these

series of experiments show that pretreatment of hypophysectomized rats
with GH, but not with IGF-I, promotes the formation of chondrocyte colonies and increases the responsiveness of the chondrocytes to IGF-I in
vitro. The results suggest that GH induces colony formation by IGF-I-
independent mechanisms probably due to a direct interaction between GH and
precursor cells in the growth plate.

DISCUSSION

Earlier studies showed that isolated rat epiphyseal chondrocytes,
cultured in suspension, show an enhanced colony formation in response to
both GH and IGF-I in vitro, providing evidence for a direct interaction
between chondrocytes and these two peptides (23,24). By studying the size
distribution of chondrocyte colonies isolated from whole rat tibia growth
plates, it was revealed that the effect of GH and IGF-I was different
qualitatively. It was found that GH preferentially stimulated the formation of large size colonies whereas IGF-I potentiated the formation of
middle size and small colonies (24). These results suggested that GH
interacted directly with progenitor cells with a high inherent capacity to
multiply, e.g., with prechondrocytes or "early" proliferative chondrocytes.

The present study was designed to take advantage of the fact that the
chondrocytes in the growth plate show a specific spatial orientation that
correlates to the stage of cell maturation. The topmost cells bordering

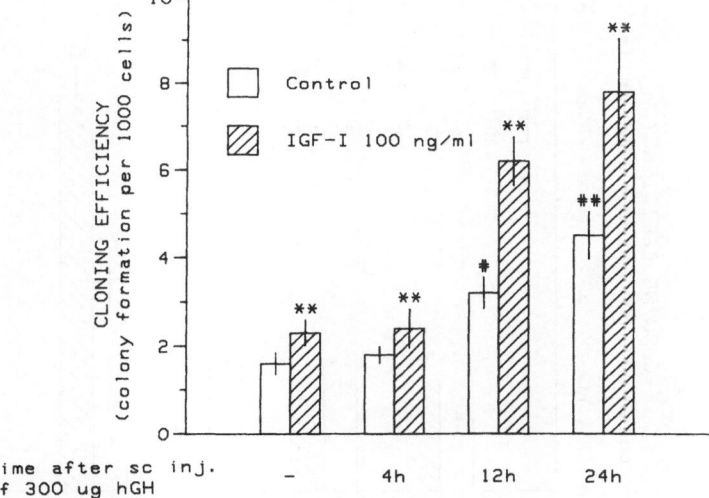

Fig. 7. Time course effect of GH pretreatment in vivo
on subsequent effect of IGF-I in vitro on cloning
efficiency of tibia epiphyseal chondrocytes of
hypophysectomized rats. Chondrocytes were isolated
from hypophysectomized rats that were treated with one
sc injection of hGH (300 µg) 4, 12 or 24 h before cell
isolation. The chondrocytes were cultured in suspension in absence or presence of IGF-I (100 ng/ml).
Values are mean ± SEM of 3 different experiments with
4-8 animals in each group. (## = P<0.01 vs. control
cultures in saline-injected control group; ** = P<0.01
IGF-I vs. control cultures.)

the bony epiphysis constitute stem cell chondrocytes or prechondrocytes. The chondrocytes become progressively more mature in the columns oriented in the direction of longitudinal bone growth towards the calcification zone (20,21). Although the division of the growth plate into 3 different zones, as performed in the present study, does not correlate to any well-defined stages of chondrocyte maturation, it is clear that the progenitor cells isolated from the different zones show different ability to form colonies when subsequently cultured in suspension. The finding that GH only stimulated the formation of large size colonies in cells isolated from the proximal part of the growth plate indicates that GH stimulated a few cells with a high inherent proliferative capacity. The observation that high concentrations of hGH reduced colony formation of chondrocytes isolated from the intermediate zone is unexplained but indicate that GH might directly influence proliferative chondrocytes as well. The notion that IGF-I potentiates the formation of middle size and small colonies in cells isolated from both the proximal and intermediate zones is compatible with the hypothesis that IGF-I stimulates clonal growth of differentiating chondrocytes. In summary, the present results indicate that the cloning efficiency of epiphyseal chondrocytes in suspension culture is dependent upon the previous spatial location of the cells in the growth plate.

The finding that pretreatment of hypophysectomized rats with GH but not IGF-I potentiated the subsequent response to IGF-I in vitro suggests that GH induced the formation of IGF-I responsive cells. This finding is analogous to the earlier demonstration that in vitro GH generates IGF-I sensitive 3T3 preadipose cells (19). The present results give additional

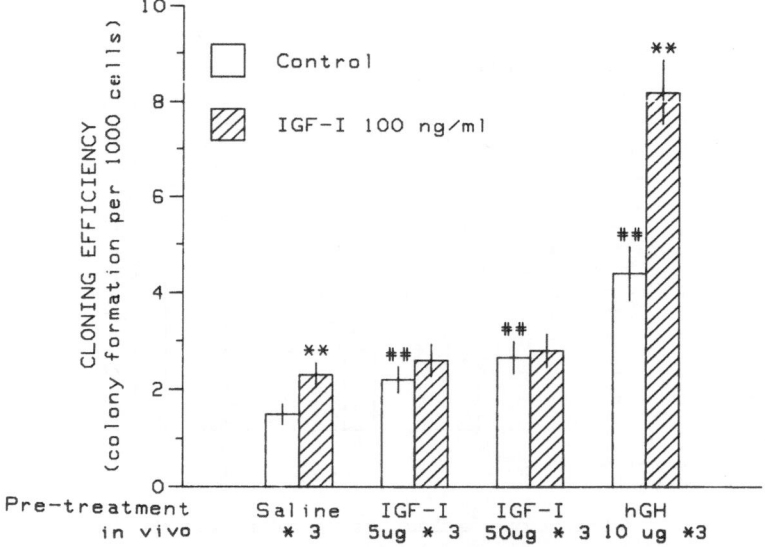

Fig. 8. Effect of IGF-I in vitro on the colony formation of tibia epiphyseal chondrocytes isolated from hypophysectomized rats pretreated with IGF-I or hGH in vivo. Hypophysectomized rats were treated with two different doses of IGF-I (5 μg x 3 or 50 μg x 3) or with hGH (10 μg x 3). Values are mean ± SEM of 3 different experiments with 4-8 animals in each group. (## = P<0.01 vs. control cultures in saline-injected control group; ** = P<0.01 IGF-I vs. control cultures.)

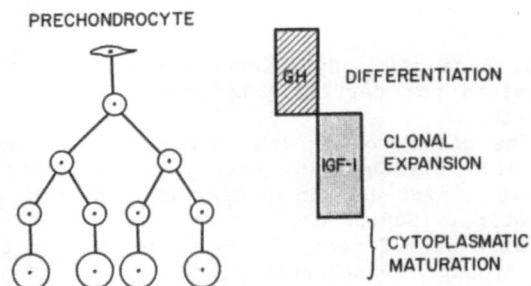

Fig. 9. A proposed model for GH and IGF-I interaction in chondrocytes of epiphyseal growth plate.

evidence for the hypothesis that GH is the prime and IGF-I the second effector in the sequence of events resulting in increased tissue mass as earlier suggested (19).

The earlier demonstration of IGF-I-like immunoreactivity in proliferating epiphyseal chondrocytes and the regulatory role of GH on the number of cells expressing IGF-I-like immunoreactivity suggests that IGF-I is produced by the proliferating cells themselves under the influence of GH (11). The possibility that locally produced IGF-I has a physiological role as an autocrine or paracrine growth factor has been suggested earlier (25,26). Recently, Schlechter et al. (27) showed that local infusion of neutralizing antibodies to IGF-I completely blocked the stimulatory effect on longitudinal bone growth of concomitantly infused GH, providing evidence for an important functional role of locally produced IGF-I. The possibility exists that circulating IGF-I could play a role for the support of clonal growth of differentiating chondrocytes. However, infusion of IGF-I to hypophysectomized rats produce small stimulatory effects on longitudinal bone growth in comparison to GH (7,28), suggesting that locally produced rather than circulating IGF-I support clonal growth of differentiating chondrocytes in intact animals.

The cellular mechanisms by which GH and IGF-I increase longitudinal bone growth are not yet completely known. We suggest that GH directly stimulates the differentiation of prechondrocytes or young differentiating chondrocytes (Fig. 9). During the process of cell differentiation, the cells become responsive to IGF-I and concomitantly the gene encoding for IGF-I is expressed which results in an increased local production of IGF-I in the differentiating cells themselves. Locally produced IGF-I subsequently support the clonal growth of IGF-I-responsive proliferating chondrocytes by autocrine or paracrine mechanism(s). This hypothesis shows great similarities to the "dual effector theory" of GH action as earlier proposed by Green and co-workers (18). In summary, GH stimulates longitudinal bone growth directly by stimulating the differentiation of precursors cells and indirectly by stimulating the local production of IGF-I and by increasing the responsiveness of differentiating cells to locally produced IGF-I.

ACKNOWLEDGMENTS

This work was supported by grants from the Swedish Medical Research Council (14X-04250), KabiVitrum, Stockholm, the Goteborg Medical Society and the Faculty of Medicine, University of Goteborg.

REFERENCES

1. Daughaday WH, Reeder C. Synchronous activation of DNA synthesis in hypophysectomized rat cartilage by growth hormone. J Lab Clin Med 1966; 68:357-68.
2. Cheek DB. The effect of growth hormone on cell multiplication and cell size. In: Blizzard RM, ed. Human pituitary growth hormone: the 54th Ross conference on pediatric research. Columbus, Ohio: Ross Laboratories, 1966:58-63.
3. Beach RK, Kostyo JL. Effect of growth hormone on the DNA content of muscles of young hypophysectomized rats. Endocrinology 1968; 92:882-4.
4. Salmon WD Jr, Daughaday WH. A hormonally controlled serum factor which stimulates sulfate incorporation by cartilage in vitro. J Lab Clin Med 1957; 49:825-36.
5. Daughaday WH, Hall K, Raben MS, Salmon WD Jr, Van Den Brande JL, Van Wyk JJ. Somatomedin: proposed designation for sulphation factor. Nature 1972; 235:107.
6. Hall K, Sara VR. Somatomedin levels in childhood, adolescence and adult life. Clin Endocrinol Metab 1984; 13:91-112.
7. Schoenle E, Zapf J, Humbel RE, Froesch ER. Insulin-like growth factor I stimulates growth in hypophysectomized rats. Nature 1982; 296:252-3.
8. Isaksson O, Jansson J-O, Gause IAM. Growth hormone stimulates longitudinal bone growth directly. Science 1982; 216:1237-9.
9. Russell SM, Spencer EM. Local injections of human or rat growth hormone or of purified human somatomedin-C stimulate unilateral tibial epiphyseal growth in hypophysectomized rats. Endocrinology 1985; 116:2563-7.
10. Isgaard J, Nilsson A, Lindahl A, Jansson J-O, Isaksson OGP. Effects of local administration of GH and IGF-I on longitudinal bone growth in rats. Am J Physiol 1986; 250(Endocrinol Metab 13):E367-72.
11. Nilsson A, Isgaard J, Lindahl A, Dahlstrom A, Skottner A, Isaksson O. Regulation by growth hormone of number of chondrocytes containing IGF-I in rat growth plate. Science 1986; 233:571-4.
12. Wroblewski J, Engstrom M, Skottner A, Madsen K, Friberg U. Subcellular location of IGF-I in chondrocytes from rat rib growth plate. Acta Endocrinol (Copenh) 1987; 115:37-43.
13. D'Ercole AJ, Stiles AD, Underwood LE. Tissue concentrations of somatomedin C: further evidence for multiple sites of synthesis and paracrine or autocrine mechanisms of action. Proc Natl Acad Sci USA 1984; 81:935-9.
14. Lund PK, Moats-Staats BM, Hynes MA, et al. Somatomedin-C/insulin-like growth factor-I and insulin-like growth factor-II mRNAs in rat fetal and adult tissues. J Biol Chem 1986; 261:14539-44.
15. Roberts CT Jr, Laky SR, Lowe WL, Seaman WT, LeRoith D. Molecular cloning of rat IGF-I cDNSs: differential mRNA processing and regulation by growth hormone in extrahepatic tissues. Mol Cell Endocrinol 1987 (in press).
16. Isgaard J, Nilsson A, Isaksson O, Moller C, Norsted G. Regulation of IGF-I mRNA in rat growth plate by growth hormone [Abstract]. Endocrine Society, 1987.
17. Morikawa M, Nixon T, Green H. Growth hormone and the adipose conversion of 3T3 cells. Cell 1982; 29:783-9.
18. Green H, Morikawa M, Nixon T. A dual effector theory of growth hormone action. Differentiation 1985; 29:195-8.
19. Zezulak KM, Green H. The generation of insulin-like growth factor-I sensitive cells by growth hormone action. Science 1986; 233:551-3.
20. Kember NF, Sissons HA. A quantitative histology of the human growth plate. J Bone Joint Surg 1976; 58B:426-35.

21. Kember NF. Cell kinetics and the control of growth in long bones. Cell Tissue Kinet 1978; 11:477-85.
22. Benya PD, Shaffer JD. Dedifferentiated chondrocytes reexpress the differentiated collagen phenotype when cultured in agarose gels. Cell 1982; 30:215-24.
23. Lindahl A, Isgaard J, Nilsson A, Isaksson OGP. Growth hormone potentiates colony formation of epiphyseal chondrocytes in suspension culture. Endocrinology 1986; 118:1843-8.
24. Lindahl A, Isgaard J, Carlsson L, Isaksson OGP. Differential effects of growth hormone and insulin like growth factor I (IGF-I) on colony formation of epiphyseal chondrocytes in suspension culture in rats of different ages. Endocrinology 1987 (in press).
25. D'Ercole AJ, Applewhite GT, Underwood LE. Evidence that somatomedin is synthesized by multiple tissues in the fetus. Dev Biol 1980; 75:315-28.
26. Clemmons DR, Van Wyk JJ. Evidence for a functional role of endogenously produced somatomedin like peptides in the regulation of DNA synthesis in cultured human fibroblasts and porcine smooth muscle cells. J Clin Invest 1985; 75:1914-8.
27. Schlechter NL, Russell SM, Spencer EM, Nicoll CS. Evidence suggesting that the direct growth-promoting effect of growth hormone on cartilage in vivo is mediated by local production of somatomedin. Proc Natl Acad Sci USA 1986; 83:7932-4.
28. Skottner A, Clark RG, Robinson ICAF, Fryklund L. Recombinant human insulin-like growth factor: testing the somatomedin hypothesis in hypophysectomized rats. J Endocrinol 1987; 112:123-33.

19

COMPARISON OF GROWTH EFFECTS OF rhIGF-I IN DIABETIC AND HYPOX RATS WITH THOSE OF INSULIN AND GROWTH HORMONE

E. R. Froesch, H. P. Guler, M. Ernst, C. Schmid,
E. Scheiwiller, and J. Zapf

Metabolic Unit, Department of Medicine
University of Zurich
Zurich, Switzerland

INTRODUCTION

Insulin-like growth factor I (IGF-I) stimulates replication of cultured cells in vitro (1-3). In contrast to other growth factors, IGF-I does not lead to dedifferentiation of differentiated cells in culture, but rather maintains or even enhances the degree of differentiation of cultured cells (2,4,5). In view of (1) these in vitro findings, (2) the similarity of action between insulin and IGF-I on differentiation (2-5), and (3) several reports on growth stimulation by IGF-I in hypox and other animals (6-8), we decided to investigate the action of recombinant human IGF-I (rhIGF-I) on diabetic and hypophysectomized rats. In addition, acute effects of IGF were studied in man (9,10).

IGF-I IS HYPOGLYCEMIC IN MAN

These studies were performed with rhIGF-I obtained from Drs. W. H. Rutter and J. Nuesch, San Francisco and Basel. RhIGF-I was injected intravenously as a bolus at a dose of 100 µg/kg b.w. in 8 healthy medical doctors engaged in IGF research. The results were compared with those of a conventional insulin tolerance test using 0.15 IU/kg b.w. Figure 1A shows the results of the blood glucose response to insulin and to rhIGF-I. The hypoglycemic curves as a whole, the nadir of hypoglycemia and the time course of recovery from hypoglycemia were identical. From these data one can compute the hypoglycemic potency of IGF-I to be approximately 7% of that of insulin under these conditions of an acute intravenous injection. The response of counterregulatory hormones such as epinephrine, norepinephrine, glucagon, cortisol and growth hormone were indistinguishable in the two tests. The only significant difference was found in the behavior of the free fatty acid levels shown in Figure 1B. Free fatty acid levels fell to a nadir 30 min after injection of either hormone. However, after rhIGF-I free fatty acid levels rose to fasting levels significantly faster than after insulin. These results indicate that insulin is a far better antilipolytic agent than IGF-I as suggested by results of in vivo experiments in rats (11). There, glycogen synthesis of muscle is preferentially stimulated by IGF-I whereas insulin is comparatively significantly more active on adipose tissue (11-13). This difference points to a potential for the use of IGF-I in the treatment of diabetes where the aim is to achieve an anabolic response in tissues other than adipose tissue. IGF-I appears to be the most potent naturally occurring hypoglycemic hormone, second only to insulin, and proinsulin ranks third. The major difference between IGF-I and proinsulin is that proinsulin acts on the same tissues as insulin whereas IGF-I has a preferential affinity for cartilage, bone and muscle (3,4,11).

GROWTH-PROMOTING EFFECTS OF IGF-I IN THE DIABETIC RAT (7)

One-hundred twenty to 140 g male rats were rendered diabetic by the IV injection of 120 mg of streptozotocin/kg b.w. Body weight of the diabetic rats was monitored closely and the only rats which were included in these experiments were those animals which gained less than 2 g of weight in 7 days during week 2 and 3 after the injection of streptozoto-cin. The rats were severely diabetic, had lost a considerable amount of lean body weight and had a much greater bowel content than normal rats. Three weeks after the injection of streptozotocin, rats which remained constant in weight were sc implanted with osmotic mini-Alza pumps which contained either saline, growth hormone (hGH), rhIGF-I or insulin. The hormone doses were: insulin, 0.5 IU or 2.5 IU/day; rhIGF-I, 150 or 300 µg/day; hGH, 200 mU/day. The rats were bled by aortic puncture 6 days after starting the infusion. Glucosuria was identical in untreated diabetic rats and in growing IGF-I (300 µg/day) treated diabetic rats and averaged in both groups 30 g/24 hours x 100 g b.w. In the normoglycemic, insulin-treated (2.5 U/day) rats, glucosuria was reduced to 3 g/day. Growth hormone had no effect on glucosuria. The severity of diabetes is also reflected by the food consumption which averaged (g/day): 21 in

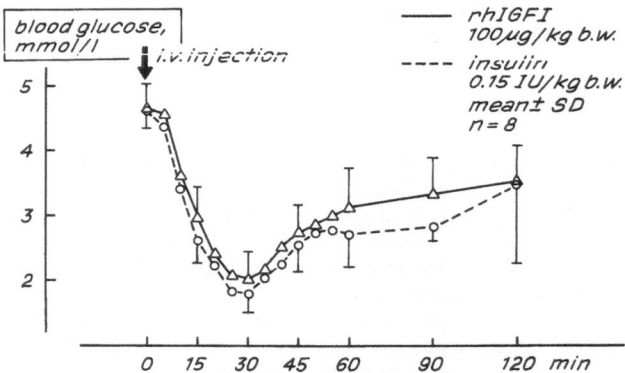

Fig. 1A. Comparison of blood glucose after IV rhIGF-I and insulin. Eight healthy normal subjects received either 0.15 IU of insulin or 100 µg/kg b.w. of rhIGF-I (Professors W. J. Rutter and J. Nuesch, San Francisco and Basel) IV as a bolus after an overnight fast. Venous blood was obtained from an indwelling catheter and blood glucose determined on a YSI-analyzer. The classical symptoms of hypo-glycemia occurred during both tests and none of the subjects felt any difference between insulin- and rhIGF-I-hypoglycemia. From Guler et al. (10).

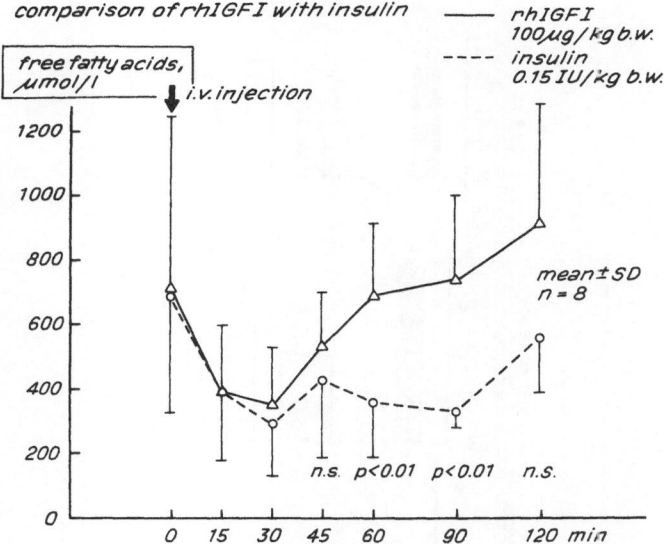

Fig. 1B. Free fatty acid levels during acute hypoglycemia caused by an IV injection of insulin or rhIGF-I. The free fatty acid levels were determined in the same plasma samples of the 8 subjects receiving insulin or rhIGF-I (see Fig. 1A). RhIGF-I lowers the free fatty acid levels to the same extent as insulin but the duration of the antilipolytic action is much shorter. From Guler et al. (10).

untreated diabetic rats; 7 in control rats; 24 in diabetic rats treated with 300 μg of IGF-I/day; 13 in diabetic, insulin-treated normoglycemic rats (15). Further data on the degree of diabetes are also shown in Figure 2A. Whereas insulin normalized the blood sugar, rhIGF-I had a significant, but small blood sugar-lowering effect and growth hormone had no effect at all on blood sugar. Figure 2B shows that body weight increased most in the normoglycemic insulin-treated rats and that IGF-I also had a clear-cut dose-dependent effect on body weight in contrast to growth hormone. Tibial epiphyseal width increased most with insulin therapy and both doses of rhIGF-I also had marked effects. These data demonstrate that rhIGF-I has anabolic growth-stimulating effects on cartilage and bone in diabetic rats. Body weight gain, tibial epiphyseal width and thymidine incorporation in insulin-treated diabetic rats correlate with the endogenous IGF-I levels suggesting that insulin stimulates growth of diabetic rats mainly by inducing endogenous IGF-I synthesis.

IGF-I MIMICS ALL EFFECTS OF HUMAN GROWTH HORMONE IN THE HYPOX RAT (16,17)

Hypophysectomized rats were obtained from Ciba-Geigy AG and used 3-6 weeks after operation for these experiments only if they gained less than 2 g of body weight per week. At that time, mini-osmotic Alzet pumps were implanted subcutaneously into the abdomen. These pumps delivered 300 μg of rhIGF-I or 200 mU of human growth hormone per day. After 14 days, they were replaced by another pump delivering the same amount of hormone. Hypox control rats received saline and were treated in the same way as the rats receiving the hormones. Figure 3 shows the response of the body

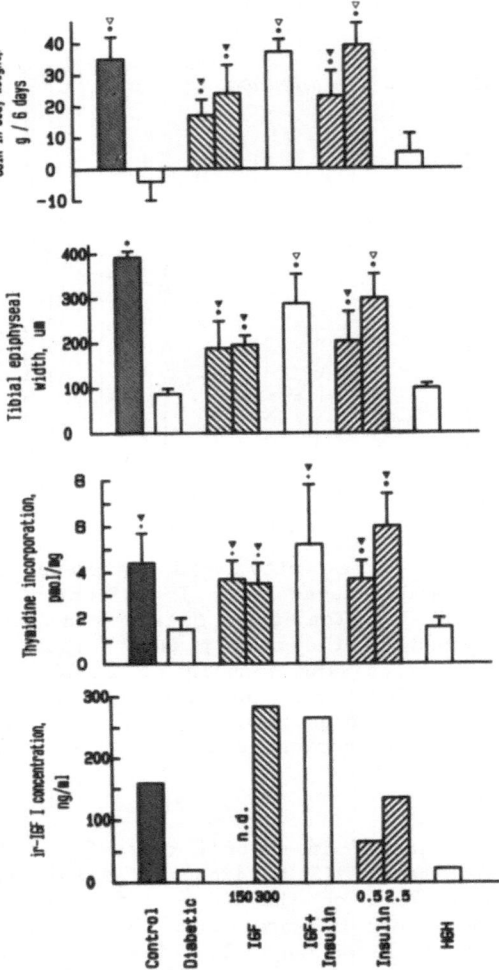

Fig. 2A. Stimulation of growth indices in diabetic rats by insulin, IGF-I and hGH. From top to bottom panels: Gain in body weight, tibial epiphyseal width, thymidine (TdR) incorporation, immunoreactive IGF-I concentration. Hormones were administered over 6 days by osmotic minipumps in the following daily amounts: insulin, 0.5 IU (n=5) and 2.5 IU (n=6); hGH, 400 mU (n=5); rhIGF-I, 150 µg (n=4) and 300 µg (n=11); a combination of 300 µg rhIGF-I and 0.5 IU insulin (n=6). Controls and non-diabetic rats are of the same age. Bars represent means; brackets, standard deviations. Student's t test was used for statistical analysis. All values in each panel were tested against the value of the untreated diabetic rats: •, P<0.001; +, P<0.01. All values of each treatment group were also tested against each other: ▼, no significant difference against values designated by ▼; ▽, no significant differences against values designated by ▽; ▽ versus ▼, P<0.05-0.001. In the radio-immunoassay for IGF-I, human ^{125}I-IGF-I served as a tracer and human IGF-I for standard dilutions. Rat IGF-I levels are, therefore, equivalents of human IGF-I and should not be considered as absolute values. It is impossible to distinguish between endogenous rat IGF-I and infused rhIGF-I. ND, not determined. From Scheiwiller et al. (7).

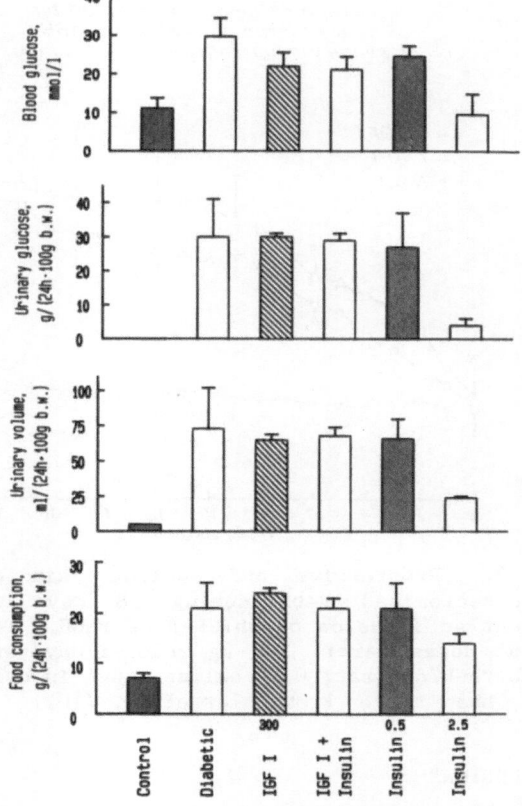

Fig. 2B. Metabolic indices in diabetic rats treated with IGF-I, 2 doses of insulin or IGF-I + insulin. The data are from the same rats of which growth parameters are shown in Figure 1. Glucosuria, urine volume and food consumption of diabetic rats are barely influenced by 300 μg of rhIGF-I ± 0.5 IU of insulin per day, although both hormones alone or together stimulate all growth parameters (see Fig. 1); 2.5 IU of insulin per day bring all metabolic indices towards normal. From Scheiwiller et al. (7) and Froesch and Zapf (15).

weight to 200 mU of growth hormone/day or 300 μg of rhIGF-I/day. The two curves are superimposable. Both IGF-I and growth hormone have a more pronounced effect on body weight early on in the experiment and the gain of body weight tends to diminish towards the end of the third week. Longitudinal bone growth was determined by the injection of tetracycline at the beginning of the experiment and by measuring the distance between the tetracycline band in the trabecular bone and the epiphysis (Fig. 4). This distance was 73 ± 12 μm in the control hypox rats receiving saline, 666 ± 36 μm in the hypox rats treated with rhIGF-I and 945 ± 194 μm in those receiving human growth hormone. The difference between the growth hormone-treated and IGF-I-treated rats is not statistically significant. Thymidine incorporation into costal cartilage in vitro was the same in IGF-I- and growth hormone-treated rats; both were stimulated about twofold above baseline. The weight of the kidneys, spleen and thymus was increased by both hormones but significantly more by rhIGF-I than by growth hormone.

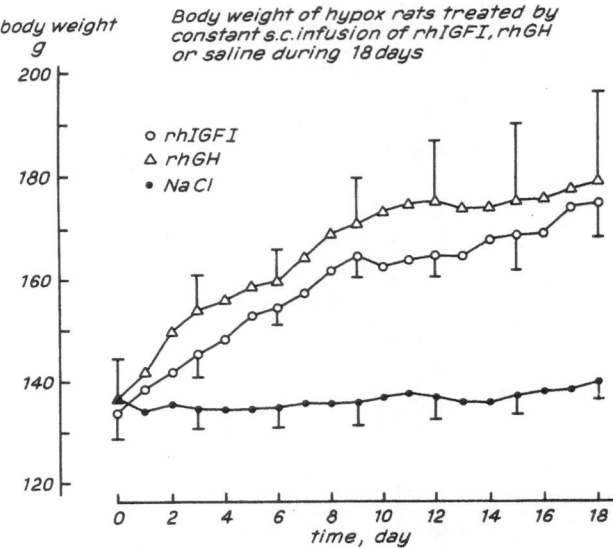

Fig. 3. Progressive body weight gain of hypophysectomized rats during 18 days of constant sc infusion of rhIGF-I or rhGH. The hormone doses were: 300 μg rhIGF-I/day/rat; 200 mU rhGH/day/rat; 0.9% saline. n=4 in each group, mean ± SD. From Guler et al. (10).

DISCUSSION AND CONCLUSIONS

RhIGF-I is a potent growth-stimulating hormone in vitro which enhances the degree of differentiation of many different cells (2-4,18,19). Insulin has similar effects but only in pharmacological concentrations usually above 1000 μU/ml which are rarely reached in vivo (2-4). In contrast, IGF-I exerts these effects well within the physiological range, and the dose response curves usually begin between 3 and 10 ng/ml, i.e., far below physiological serum levels which are around 100-200 ng/ml (20). IGF-I also stimulates metabolic processes of several tissues in vitro and in vivo; cartilage, bone and muscle are particularly sensitive and adipose tissue the least sensitive (3,4,11,14,23). Whether IGF-I has any effect on glucose homeostasis by the liver is not known although metabolic effects on chick liver cells in culture have been demonstrated (24). IGF-I appears to cause hypoglycemia only when it occurs in the blood as the free molecule, i.e., when the binding proteins are saturated (20). We have observed hypoglycemic effects of IGF-I only after acute intravenous bolus injections and in one situation, where more than 30 μg of rhIGF-I per kg and h were infused in a healthy normal subject (10). The daily dose of rhIGF-I required for an anabolic response over 24 h is about 3-4 times the dose which causes acute hypoglycemia after an IV bolus (rat, dog, mini-pig, man) (9-11).

As suggested earlier (14), IGF-I may yet become a useful compound in the therapy of diabetes since its spectrum of activity is so different from that of insulin and, particularly, because it has very little activity on adipose tissue.

Our data validate the somatomedin hypothesis originally formulated by Salmon and Daughaday (25). We show that the administration of IGF-I in vivo over a prolonged period of time causes hypophysectomized animals to

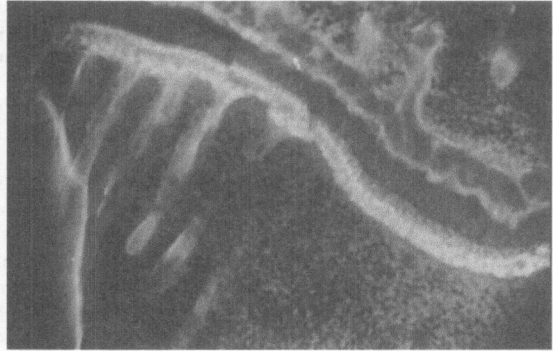

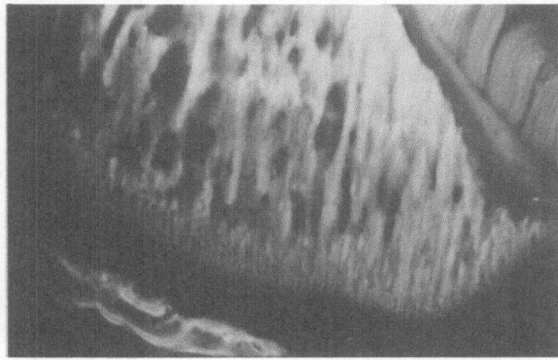

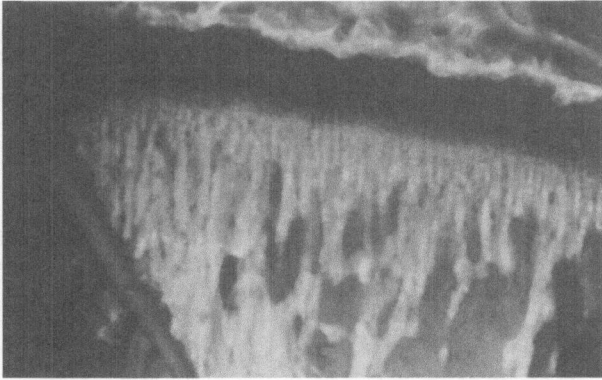

Fig. 4. Tetracycline staining of the tibia as a measure of longitudinal bone growth in hypophysectomized rats infused with saline, rhGH or rhIGF-I. Hypophysectomized rats whose growth curves are shown in Figure 3 were injected with tetracycline. At the time of sacrifice, i.e., 3 weeks later, the tibiae were prepared for microscopic examination under a mercury lamp. A = saline controls; B = rhGH (200 mU/day and rat); C = rhIGF-I (300 µg/day and rat). From Guler et al. (10).

grow just as well as with growth hormone. Our results also reopen the discussion about the dual role of growth hormone and IGF-I in sequentially stimulating differentiation and replication of cells. According to Nixon and Green (28) and Isaksson et al. (27), growth hormone is needed to favor a differentiation step of preadipocytes and of prechondrocytes at an early stage followed by the action of IGF-I stimulating mostly the replication of competent cells. In several culture systems, IGF-I alone stimulates replication and differentiation of cells (erythroid precursor cells [18], chondrocytes [23], osteoblasts [3,4], Leydig and granulosa cells [19,26] and thymocytes [Froesch P, to be published]).

Hypophysectomized rats grew just as well with IGF-I alone as with growth hormone. What may be more important in this respect was the finding that longitudinal bone growth was the same, and that by histologic examination of the growth plate and adjacent trabecular bone, it was impossible to distinguish between IGF-I and GH treatment (17).

Our data speak in favor of the endocrine mode of action of IGF-I which, of course, does not exclude a physiological role as a paracrine or autocrine hormone. Thus, IGF-I was shown to be fully active on growth when it reached tissues by the classical endocrine route. Growth hormone may still have a dual mode of action by stimulating the synthesis of IGF-I in the liver and at the sites of growth.

For the first time, rhIGF-I has been shown to act in vivo on tissues other than cartilage and bone. Hypox rats treated during 18 days with rhIGF-I had larger kidneys and spleens than the rats treated with growth hormone (17). Here again we found nothing specific about growth hormone since rhIGF-I was more potent. Nevertheless, these results are of interest since they point to the importance of the vectors presenting IGF-I to cells. Growth hormone administration leads to an increase of the 150 kD binding protein to which most of the IGF-I is bound. In contrast, the administration of rhIGF-I to hypox rats does not induce the 150 kD carrier protein so that large amounts of IGF-I are circulating either free and/or bound to the 50 kD carrier protein. In the latter forms, IGF-I appears to have particularly pronounced effects on the kidneys, spleen and thymus. In the future, the binding proteins will certainly be recognized as important factors which determine the relative tissue distribution and bioavailability of circulating IGF-I.

ACKNOWLEDGMENTS

This work was supported by a grant (No. 3.051-0.84) from the Swiss National Science Foundation and by a grant from Ciba Geigy, Basel. The expert secretarial help of Mrs. M. Salman and the excellent technical assistance of Mrs. L. Marxer, C. Hauri, I. Einschenk, E. Futo and K. Froesch is gratefully acknowledged.

REFERENCES

1. Morell B, Froesch ER. Fibroblasts as an experimental tool in metabolic and hormone studies. II. Effects of insulin and non-suppressible insulin-like activity (NSILA-s) on fibroblasts in culture. Eur J Clin Invest 1973; 3:119.
2. Schmid C, Steiner T, Froesch ER. Preferential enhancement of myoblast differentiation by insulin-like growth factors (IGF-I and IGF-II) in primary cultures of chicken embryonic cells. FEBS Lett 1983; 161:117.
3. Schmid C, Steiner T, Froesch ER. Insulin-like growth factor I

supports differentiation of cultured osteoblast-like cells. FEBS Lett 1984; 173:48.

4. Ernst M, Froesch ER. Osteoblastlike cells in a serum-free methylcellulose medium form colonies: effects of insulin and insulinlike growth factor I. Calcif Tissue Int 1987; 40:27.

5. Froesch ER, Schmid C, Zangger I, Schoenle E, Eigenmann E, Zapf J. Effects of IGF/somatomedins on growth and differentiation of muscle and bone. J Anim Sci 1986; 63(suppl 2):57.

6. Schonle E, Zapf J, Humbel RE, Froesch ER. Insulin-like growth factor I stimulates growth in hypophysectomized rats. Nature 1982; 296:252.

7. Scheiwiller E, Guler HP, Merryweather J, et al. Growth restoration of insulin-deficient diabetic rats by recombinant human insulin-like growth factor I. Nature 1986; 323:169.

8. Van Buul-Offers S, Ueda I, Van den Brande JL. Biosynthetic somatomedin C (SM-C/IGF-I) increases the length and weight of snell dwarf mice. Pediatr Res 1986; 20:825.

9. Guler HP, Zenobi P, Zapf J, et al. IGF-I and II and recombinant human (rh) IGF-I are hypoglycemic in the rat, mini-pig and men [Abstract]. Anaheim, CA: The Endocrine Society, 1986.

10. Guler HP, Zapf J, Froesch ER. Acute metabolic effects of recombinant human insulin-like growth factor I (rhIGF-I) in healthy adult men. N Engl J Med (in press) 1987.

11. Zapf J, Hauri C, Waldvogel M, Froesch ER. Acute metabolic effects and half-lives of intravenously administered insulinlike growth factors I and II in normal and hypophysectomized rats. J Clin Invest 1986; 77:1768.

12. Oelz O, Jakob A, Froesch ER. Non-suppressible insulin-like activity (NSILA) of human serum. V. Hypoglycaemia and preferential metabolic stimulation of muscle by NSILA-S. Eur J Clin Invest 1970; 1:48.

13. Froesch ER. Nonsuppressible insulin-like activity of human serum. II. Biological properties of plasma extracts with nonsuppressible insulin-like activity. Biochim Biophys Acta 1966; 121:360.

14. Froesch ER, Zapf J. Insulin-like growth factors and insulin: comparative aspects. Diabetologia 1985; 28:485.

15. Froesch ER, Zapf J. Insulin, IGF-I and growth in diabetic rats [Reply]. Nature 1987; 326:549.

16. Guler HP, Zapf J, Froesch ER. S.c. infusion of recombinant human insulin-like growth factor I (rhIGF-I) stimulates growth of hypophysectomized rats continuously during 18 days [Abstract]. Copenhagen: First European Congress of Endocrinology, 1987.

17. Guler HP, Zapf J, Scheiwiller E, Froesch ER. Recombinant human insulin-like growth factor I stimulates growth and has specific effects on organ size in hypophysectomized rats. (Submitted.)

18. Kurtz A, Jelkmann W, Bauer C. A new candidate for the regulation of erythropoiesis. FEBS Lett 1982; 149:105.

19. Bernier M, Chatelain P, Mather JP, Saez JM. Regulation of gonadotropin receptors, gonadotropin responsiveness, and cell multiplication by somatomedin-C and insulin in cultured pig Leydig cells. J Cell Physiol 1986; 129:257.

20. Zapf J, Walter H, Froesch ER. Radioimmunological determination of insulin-like growth factors I and II in normal subjects and in patients with growth disorders and extrapancreatic tumor hypoglycemia. J Clin Invest 1981; 68:1321.

21. Poggi C, le Marchand-Brustel Y, Zapf J, Froesch ER, Freychet P. Effects and binding of insulin-like growth factor I in the isolated soleus muscle of lean and obese mice: comparison with insulin. Endocrinology 1979; 105:723.

22. Meuli C, Froesch ER. Insulin and nonsuppressible insulin-like activity (NSILA-S) stimulate the same glucose transport system via two separate receptors in rat heart. Biochem Biophys Res Commun 1977; 75:689.

23. Vetter U, Zapf J, Heit W, et al. Human fetal and adult chondrocytes. Effect of insulinlike growth factors I and II, insulin, and growth hormone on clonal growth. J Clin Invest 1986; 77:1903.
24. Widmer U, Schmid C, Zapf J, Froesch ER. Effects of insulin-like growth factors on chick embryo hepatocytes. Acta Endocrinol (Copenh) 1985; 108:237.
25. Salmon WD Jr, Daughaday WH. A hormonally controlled serum factor which stimulates sulfate incorporation into cartilage. J Lab Clin Med 1957; 49:825.
26. Veldhuis JD, Furlanetto RW. Trophic actions of human somatomedin C/insulin-like growth factor I in ovarian cells: in vitro studies with swine granulosa cells. Endocrinology 1985; 116:1235.
27. Isaksson OGP, Eden S, Jansson J-O. Mode of action of pituitary target cells. Annu Rev Physiol 1985; 47:483.
28. Nixon BT, Green H. Growth hormone promotes the differentiation of myoblasts and preadipocytes generated by azacytidine treatment of 10 T ½ cells. Proc Natl Acad Sci USA 1984; 81:3429.

20

BIOLOGICAL ACTION OF INSULIN-LIKE GROWTH FACTOR-I IN VIVO

Naomi Hizuka, Kazue Takano, Kumiko Asakawa, Izumi Sukegawa, Reiko Horikawa, Hiroyuki Kikuchi,* and Kazuo Shizume

Department of Medicine, Institute of Clinical Endocrinology Tokyo Women's Medical College, Tokyo, 162, Research Laboratory, The Foundation for Growth Science, Tokyo, 162, and *Fujisawa Pharmaceutical Co., Osaka, 532, Japan

INTRODUCTION

It has been well known that somatomedin-C/insulin-like growth factor-I (SmC/IGF-I) stimulates cell proliferation and cell differentiation and an insulin-like action in vitro (1). However, there have been only a few reports on the effects of SmC/IGF-I in vivo because of scarcity of pure extracted SmC/IGF-I (2-4). Recently, insulin-like growth factor-I (IGF-I) has been synthesized by recombinant DNA technology (5-7). With the availability of large quantities of the biosynthetic IGF-I, the biological effects of IGF-I in vivo in rats have been studied (8-12). In this paper, the results of our study for biological action of IGF-I in vivo are reported.

PREPARATION OF IGF-I AND RADIOIMMUNOASSAY OF IGF-I

IGF-I preparation used for this study was synthesized by recombinant DNA technology as described by Niwa et al. (5). The amino acid sequence of this preparation is the same as that of natural IGF-I.

Serum IGF-I levels were measured by radioimmunoassay as described earlier (13). The antiserum to IGF-I was prepared by immunizing a rabbit with an IGF-I-ovalbumin conjugate emulsified in Freund's adjuvant. The antiserum did not cross-react with multiplication stimulating activity or insulin. The rat serum was extracted with acid-ethanol (14) and the dilution curve of the rat serum extract was parallel to that for standard IGF-I. Rat serum IGF-I levels can therefore be measured by in this assay.

HALF-LIFE OF IGF-I

10 µg IGF-I was administered as IV bolus to male Wistar normal and hypophysectomized (hypox) rats, and serum IGF-I levels were measured by radioimmunoassay after the injection of IGF-I. Serum IGF-I levels in hypox rats decreased more rapidly than IGF-I concentrations in normal rats. The half-life of IGF-I in blood was calculated. In normal rats, half-lives of IGF-I for phase I and phase II disappearance curves were 3.6

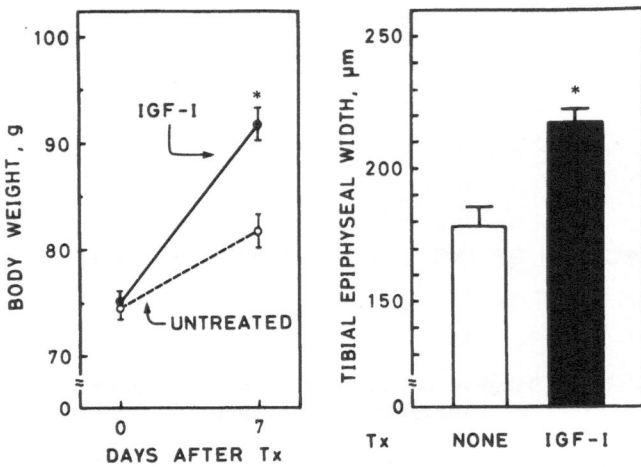

Fig. 1. Effect of IGF-I treatment (120 μg/day
for 7 days) on body weights (left) and tibial
epiphyseal widths (right) in hypox rats. The
mean values of the body weights and tibial
epiphyseal widths in IGF-I treated rats (n=6)
and untreated rats (n=6) were plotted. Vertical
lines indicate mean ± SEM. *P<0.001.

and 195 min, respectively. In hypox rats, half-lives of IGF-I for phase I
and phase II were 1.5 and 14.5 min, respectively. The half-life of IGF-I
in hypox rats was shorter than that in normal rats, and the difference in
the half-life might be due to the difference in the IGF-I binding protein.
These values are similar to those reported by Zapf et al. (9).

BIOLOGICAL EFFECTS OF IGF-I IN HYPOPHYSECTOMIZED AND
NORMAL RATS IN VIVO

Normal male Wistar rats aged 23 days, and hypophysectomized male
Wistar rats aged 33 days previously operated at 24 days of age, were used
for this study. 120 μg/day of IGF-I was administered continuously for 7
days via subcutaneous implanted osmotic minipump (model 2001, Alzet, Palo
Alto, CA) to either hypox or normal rats. In controls (untreated rats),
0.1 M acetic acid was administered for 7 days using the same method.

Serum IGF-I levels after the 7-day treatment were measured by radioimmunoassay. In the untreated hypox rats, the mean serum IGF-I value was
37.3 ± 7.3 ng/ml (mean ± SEM) and for the IGF-I treated rats it was 157.8
± 10.2 ng/ml. In the normal rats, the mean value for the untreated rats
was 239.5 ± 53.5 ng/ml and for the IGF-I treated rats it was 440.2 ± 21.9
ng/ml. The serum IGF-I levels in both hypox and normal rats treated with
IGF-I were greater than those for the untreated rats (P<0.001, P<0.001,
respectively). Therefore, the subcutaneous administration of IGF-I was
validated.

In hypox rats, the body weights and the tibial epiphyseal widths
after 7-day treatment of IGF-I were significantly greater than those in
the untreated rats (91.8 ± 1.5 vs. 81.8 ± 1.6 g, 217.2 ± 4.5 vs. 178.7 ±
6.9 μm, respectively) (Fig. 1). These data demonstrate that biosynthetic
IGF-stimulate growth in vivo in GH deficient rats and confirm the results
previously reported using extracted IGF-I (3,4).

We next studied whether IGF-I could stimulate growth in vivo in normal rats. One hundred twenty µg/day of IGF-I was administered to normal rats for 7 days. After 7 days of administration of IGF-I, the body weight increased to 107.4 ± 1.2 g, which was significantly greater than that of control rats (95.6 ± 3.2 g, P<0.01) (Fig. 2). The mean value for body lengths of rats after 7-day administration of IGF-I was 14.8 ± 0.1 cm, and that for the untreated rats was 14.2 ± 0.2 cm (Fig. 2). There was a significant difference between these two values (P<0.05). The tibial epiphyseal widths in IGF-I treated and untreated rats were 336.2 ± 6 µm, and 302.0 ± 5.9 µm, respectively (Fig. 3); these values are significantly different (P<0.01). These data indicate that IGF-I stimulates growth in vivo in normal rats as well as GH deficient rats.

After 7 days, both treated and untreated normal rats were sacrificed, and individual tissues were removed and weighed. The weights of kidneys, liver, testes in IGF-I treated rats were significantly greater than those in untreated rats (Fig. 4). Thus, in normal rats, IGF-I treatment not only caused an increase in body weights, body lengths, and tibial epiphyseal widths, but also in tissue weights.

Unexpectedly, the pituitary weights in IGF-I treated rats were greater than those in untreated rats (4.05 ± 0.07 vs. 2.81 ± 0.23 mg, P<0.01). Therefore, we measured rat growth hormone (GH) and TSH content in the pituitary. The rat pituitary extracted GH values, expressed as ng/µg extracted protein, in IGF-I treated rats were significantly greater than those in untreated rats (528.3 ± 55.8 vs. 310.3 ± 23.0 ng/µg protein, P<0.01). However, the extracted TSH values in the pituitary for IGF-I treated rats were not different from those for untreated rats. Thus, IGF-I administration to normal rats increased pituitary GH but not TSH

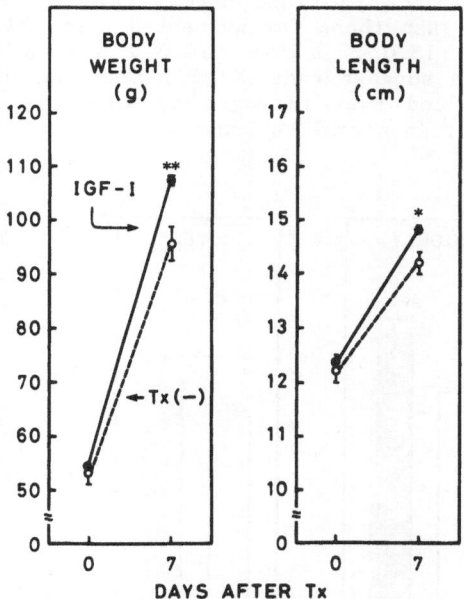

Fig. 2. Effect of IGF-I treatment (120 µg/day for 7 days) on body weights and lengths in normal rats. The mean values were plotted in IGF-I treated(●—●, n=6) and untreated rats (o---o, n=5). Vertical lines indicate the mean ± SEM. **P<0.01, *P<0.05.

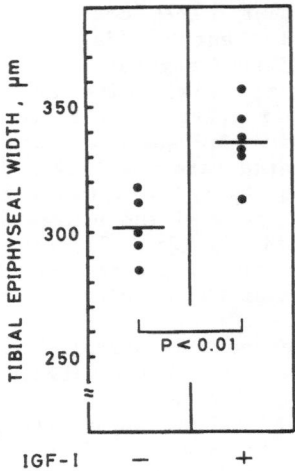

Fig. 3. Tibial epiphyseal widths in normal rats after 7-day administration of IGF-I (120 μg/day). Horizontal lines indicate the mean values.

content. Therefore, these results suggest that IGF-I might inhibit the release of GH from pituitary.

Blood urea nitrogen levels were measured in both hypox and normal rats after 7-day administration of IGF-I (Fig. 5). The blood urea nitrogen levels in both hypox and normal rats treated with IGF-I were significantly lower than those for untreated rats (21.1 ± 1.2 vs. 43.4 ± 0.3 mg/dl, P<0.001; 13.0 ± 0.5 vs. 16.0 ± 1.1 mg/dl, P<0.05, respectively). These data suggest that IGF-I has an anabolic effect in vivo. The reduction of blood urea nitrogen by IGF-I in hypox rats is more significant than that in normal control rats.

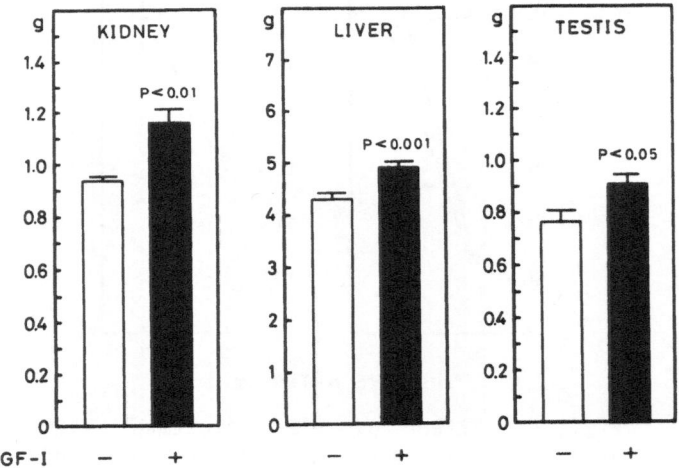

Fig. 4. Effect of IGF-I treatment on organ weights in normal rats. Vertical lines indicate mean + SEM.

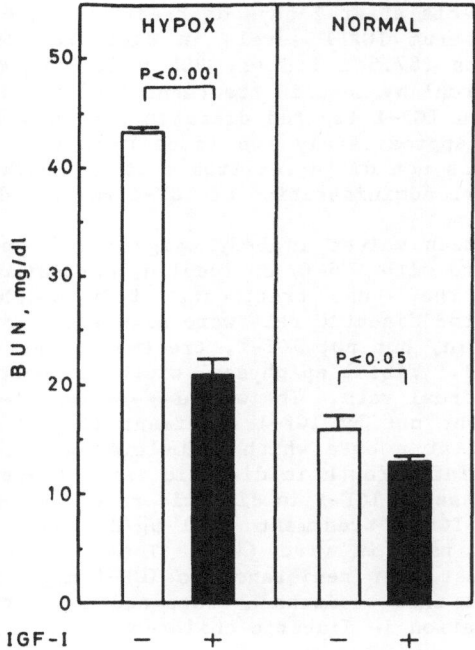

Fig. 5. Blood urea nitrogen levels in hypox
and normal rats after 7-day treatment of
IGF-I (120 µg/day). Vertical lines indicated mean + SEM.

Serum total cholesterol levels were measured in hypox rats after
7-day administration of IGF-I and/or human growth hormone. Serum total
cholesterol levels in hypox rats treated with human growth hormone were
lower than those in untreated rats (83.4 ± 5.4 vs. 120.1 ± 7.8 mg/dl,
P<0.01). However, the levels in hypox rats treated with IGF-I were not
different from those in untreated rats (121.5 ± 5.0 vs. 120.1 ± 7.8
mg/dl). As in hypox rats, the serum total cholesterol levels in normal
rats treated with IGF-I were not different from those in untreated rats.
These data suggest that the lowering effect of GH on total cholesterol is
not mediated by IGF-I.

BIOLOGICAL EFFECTS OF IGF-I IN DIABETIC RATS IN VIVO

Children with uncontrolled diabetes mellitus are retarded in growth.
Low levels of serum SmC/IGF-I might be one of the causes of the growth
retardation. Insulin-deficient diabetic rats have low SmC/IGF-I levels
(15,16). The serum SmC/IGF-I levels and body weight are restored to
normal by insulin treatment (15) but not GH treatment (16). Therefore, we
studied whether IGF-I could have an effect on stimulating growth in
diabetic rats in vivo.

Male Wistar rats, aged 23 days, were used for this study. Streptozotocin, 100 mg/kg, was administered as an IV bolus to the rats. After 3
days, the streptozotocin-treated diabetic rats were treated with 120
µg/day IGF-I, or 1 U/day insulin for 7 days by subcutaneous implanted
osmotic minipump. As controls, 0.1 M acetic acid was administered for 7
days using the same method.

Serum IGF-I levels after 7 days of treatment were measured by radio-immunoassay. The serum IGF-I levels in diabetic rats were lower than those in normal rats (87.5 ± 6.3 vs. 308 ± 10.6 ng/ml), and the levels were restored to normal by insulin treatment (243 ± 28.2 ng/ml). The mean serum IGF-I level in IGF-I treated diabetic rats was 190.8 ± 16.4 ng/ml, and the level was approximately two times more than that for untreated diabetic rats and was not different from that in insulin treated diabetic rats. Therefore, the administration of IGF-I was validated.

In Figure 6, mean values in body weights and lengths are shown for diabetic rats treated with IGF-I, or insulin, untreated diabetic rats, and normal rats after the 7-day treatment. Body weights and lengths in streptozotocin treated diabetic rats were significantly less than those in normal rats. Insulin, but not IGF-I, treatment restored the body weight and length to normal. Tibial epiphyseal widths in untreated diabetic rats were shorter than normal rats. The widths were restored towards normal by insulin treatment but not by IGF-I treatment (Fig. 7). These data demonstrate that IGF-I at a dose which stimulates growth in vivo in normal rats does not stimulate growth in diabetic rats, suggesting that there is a poor growth response to IGF-I in diabetic rats. Recently Scheiwiller et al. reported that IGF-I treatment (300 µg/day for 6 days) stimulated growth in diabetic rats in vivo (10). These data, together with our present data, suggest that resistance to IGF-I might be present in diabetic rats, and that this resistance state and low serum IGF-I levels may cause growth retardation in diabetic children.

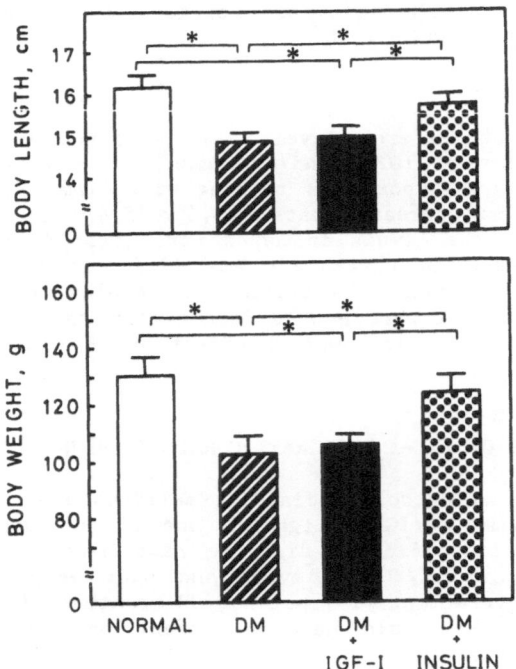

Fig. 6. Body lengths and weights in diabetic (DM) rats after 7-day administration of IGF-I (120 µg/day) or insulin (1 U/day), and in untreated diabetic rats and normal rats. Vertical lines indicate mean + SEM. *P<0.05.

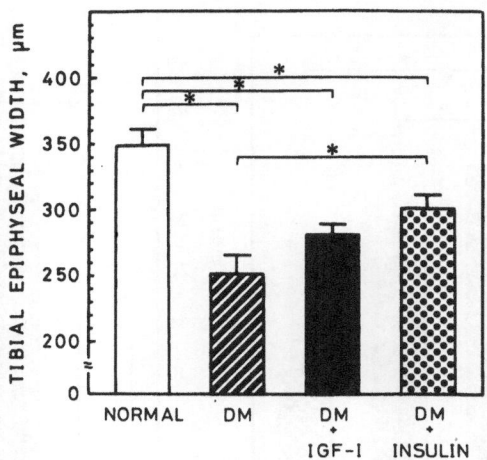

Fig. 7. Tibial epiphyseal widths in diabetic rats treated with IGF-I or insulin,
and in untreated diabetic rats, and normal
rats. Vertical lines indicate mean + SEM.
*P<0.05.

We next studied whether the low response to IGF-I could be due to
decreased binding sites of IGF-I. ^{125}I-IGF-I binding to kidney membrane
from diabetic and normal rats was measured. The ^{125}I-IGF-I binding for
normal and diabetic rats was not significantly different.

We assessed whether IGF-I treatment had an effect on lowering blood
glucose levels in diabetic rats in vivo. The mean value in IGF-I treated
diabetic rats was 425 ± 56.2 mg/dl, and in untreated diabetic rats it was
603.7 ± 37.1 mg/dl (Fig. 8). The blood glucose levels for IGF-I treated
rats were slightly but significantly lower than those for untreated
diabetic rats.

The blood urea nitrogen levels after 7 days of treatment were measured (Fig. 8). The mean value of blood urea nitrogen in IGF-I treated
diabetic rats was 24.4 ± 1.7 mg/dl, and in the untreated diabetic rats it
was 30.5 ± 0.9 mg/dl. The blood urea nitrogen levels for IGF-I treated
diabetic rats were slightly but significantly lower than those for
untreated diabetic rats, suggesting that IGF-I has anabolic effects in
diabetic rats in vivo.

INSULIN-LIKE EFFECTS IN VIVO

IGF-I (100-1000 µg/kg BW) was administered as an IV bolus to normal
and hypox rats (17). The blood glucose levels decreased after IV bolus
injection of the peptide in both normal and hypox rats. The hypoglycemic
effect of IGF-I in hypox rats was greater than that in normal rats. The
hypoglycemic effect of IGF-I was 100 times less than that of insulin.

SUMMARY AND CONCLUSION

The present study demonstrates that IGF-I has growth promoting,
anabolic and insulin-like effects in rats both in vivo and in vitro.

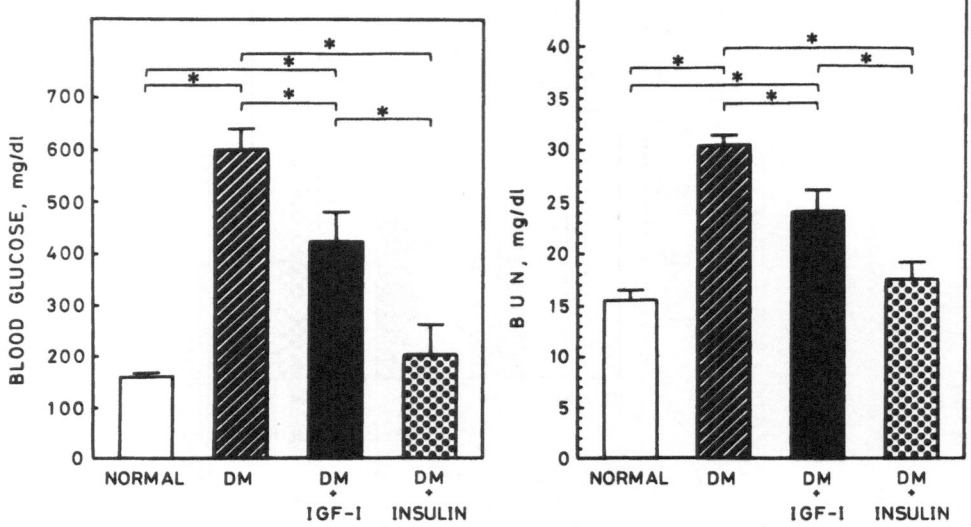

Fig. 8. Blood glucose (left) and blood urea nitrogen (right) levels in diabetic rats treated with IGF-I or insulin, and in untreated diabetic rats, and normal rats. Vertical lines indicate mean + SEM. *P<0.05.

ACKNOWLEDGMENTS

This work was partly supported by Grants in Aid for Scientific Research from the Ministry of Education, Science and Culture, Japan (No. 61770872, No. 61570566, and No. 61440052), and a Research Grant from the Intractable Diseases Division, Public Health Bureau, Ministry of Health and Welfare.

REFERENCES

1. Zapf J, Schimid CH, Froesch ER. Biological and immunological prop-
    erties of insulin-like growth factors (IGF) I and II. Clin Endo-
    crinol Metab 1984; 13:3-30.
2. Van Buul-Offers S, Van den Brande JL. Effect of growth hormone and
    peptide fractions containing somatomedin activity on growth and
    cartilage metabolism of snell dwarf mice. Acta Endocrinol (Copenh)
    1979; 92:242-57.
3. Schoenle E, Zapf J, Humbel RE, Froesch ER. Insulin-like growth
    factor I stimulates growth in hypophysectomized rats. Nature 1982;
    296:252-3.
4. Schoenle E, Zapf J, Hauri C, Steiner T, Froesch ER. Comparison of in
    vivo effects on insulin-like growth factor I and II and growth
    hormone in hypophysectomized rats. Acta Endocrinol (Copenh) 1985;
    108:167-74.
5. Niwa M, Sato S, Saito Y, et al. Chemical synthesis, cloning and
    expression of genes for human somatomedin C (insulin-like growth
    factor I) and ^{59}Val-somatomedin C. Ann NY Acad Sci 1986; 469:31-52.
6. Schalch D, Reismann D, Emler C, et al. Insulin-like growth factor
    I/somatomedin C (IGF-I/Sm C): comparison of natural, solid phase
    synthetic and recombinant DNA analog peptides in two radioligand
    assays. Endocrinology 1984; 115:2490-2.
7. Horlein D, Buell G, Schultz F, Hirschi M, Burleigh BD. Characteriza-

tion of two forms of somatomedin-C produced by recombinant bacteria [Abstract No. 250]. 67th Annual Meeting of The Endocrine Society, Baltimore, 1985.

8. Hizuka N, Takano K, Shizume K, et al. Insulin-like growth factor I stimulates growth in normal growing rats. Eur J Pharmacol 1986; 125:143-6.

9. Zapf J, Hauri C, Waldvogel M, Froesch ER. Acute metabolic effects and half lives of intravenously administered insulinlike growth factor I and II in normal and hypophysectomized rats. J Clin Invest 1986; 77:1768-75.

10. Scheiwiller E, Guler H-P, Merryweather J, et al. Growth restoration of insulin-deficient diabetic rats by recombinant human insulin-like growth factor I. Nature 1986; 323:169-71.

11. Valliant SW, Peters M, Finley S, Fagin K. Insulin-like growth factor-I[Thr59]: hypoglycemic potency and pharmacokinetics in conscious rats [Abstract No. 392]. 68th Annual Meeting of The Endocrine Society, Anaheim, 1986.

12. Asada T, Seki J, Horiai H, et al. Bioactivity of IGF-I/somatomedin C produced by recombinant DNA technology [Abstract No. 351]. Folia Endocrinol Japon 1985; 61(suppl):1030.

13. Miyakawa M, Hizuka N, Takano K, et al. Radioimmunoassay for insulin-like growth factor I (IGF-I) using biosynthetic IGF-I. Endocrinol Jpn 1986; 33:795-801.

14. Daughaday WH, Mariz IK, Blethen SL. Inhibition of access of bound somatomedin to membrane receptor and immunobinding sites: a comparison of radioreceptor and radioimmunoassay of somatomedin in native and acid-ethanol-extracted serum. J Clin Endocrinol Metab 1980; 51:781-8.

15. Takano K, Hizuka N, Shizume K, Hasumi Y, Kogawa M, Tsushima T. Effect of insulin and nutrition on serum levels of somatomedin A in the rat. Endocrinology 1980; 107:1614-9.

16. Phillips LS, Orawski AT. Nutrition and somatomedin III. Diabetic control, somatomedin, and growth in rats. Diabetes 1977; 26:864-9.

17. Seki J, Asada T, Horiai H, et al. Biological activity of IGF-I/Somatomedin C produced by recombinant DNA technology; insulin-like effect [Abstract No. 798]. Folia Endocrinol Japon 1986; 62(suppl):495.

21

INSULIN-LIKE GROWTH FACTORS IN FETAL GROWTH

Matthew M. Rechler, Yvonne W-H. Yang, Alexandra L. Brown,
Joyce A. Romanus, Sallie O. Adams, Wieland Kiess, and
S. Peter Nissley

National Institutes of Health
Bethesda, MD 20892

INTRODUCTION

The insulin-like growth factors, IGF-I and IGF-II, are single-chain polypeptides chemically related to insulin that are synthesized in multiple fetal and adult tissues, and stimulate DNA synthesis and cell differentiation (1,2). IGF-I is regulated by growth hormone and nutritional factors, and promotes bone elongation in childhood (2). Based on results initially obtained in rats, IGF-II was proposed to play a role in fetal growth and development. This paper will review some of the evidence in support of this hypothesis, and discuss its applicability to human fetal development.

IGF-II BIOSYNTHESIS IN FETAL RAT TISSUES

Developmental Regulation of Rat IGF-II

Rat IGF-II was purified from serum-free media conditioned by an established line of rat liver cells, BRL-3A (3). A 7.5 kilodalton (kDa) species of rat IGF-II is identical to human plasma IGF-II in amino acid sequence at 63 of 67 residues (4). Radioligand assays developed using rat IGF-II (rIGF-II) purified from BRL-3A cells established that short-term explants of fetal rat liver (5) and cultures of rat embryo fibroblasts (6) synthesize peptides indistinguishable in chemical, biological, and immunological properties from rIGF-II produced by BRL-3A cells. Fetal rat serum contains high levels of immunoreactive IGF-II which decrease to low adult levels by 3 weeks after birth (7). IGF-I shows an opposite developmental pattern, namely, it is present at low levels in the rat fetus and increases within the first few weeks after birth (8).

Fibroblasts cultured from rats at different ages show the same developmental pattern of IGF synthesis (9). Fibroblast cultures established from fetal rat skin or lung and studied during their third passage in culture synthesize IGF-II, whereas fibroblasts from adult tissues synthesize IGF-I (9). These results suggest that IGF is synthesized in peripheral tissues (exemplified by rat embryo fibroblast cultures) as well as in liver, and that hepatic and extrahepatic IGF synthesis exhibit the same developmental regulation.

Recent studies utilizing molecular cloning techniques have confirmed and extended these results. As shown in Figure 1, the single rat IGF-II gene contains 2 noncoding exons (-2 and -1) and 3 coding exons (1, 2, and 3) (10,11). It is transcribed from two noncontiguous promoters (upstream from exons -2 and -1) into multiple RNA transcripts: 5, 4, 2.2, 1.7, and 1.2 kilobases (kb) (13,14). The 4 kb RNA arising from the exon -1 promoter is the most abundant IGF-II RNA; the 5 kb RNA, tenfold less abundant, arises from the exon -2 promoter (10).

As seen in Figures 2 and 3, the IGF-II gene is transcribed from both promoters in multiple fetal and neonatal rat tissues: at higher levels in muscle, liver, intestine, lung, skin, and thymus; at lower levels in heart, kidney, brain stem, cerebral cortex, and hypothalamus. Similar results have been reported by other laboratories (11,16,17). In each tissue, the 5 kb RNA was less abundant than the 4 kb RNA, and the distribution of other IGF-II RNA species was similar. In nonneural tissues, IGF-II RNA abruptly decreased with developmental age, either before birth (lung, thymus, and kidney) or early in the postnatal period (muscle, liver, etc.) (Fig. 4). Each IGF-II RNA species showed the same developmental pattern. IGF-I mRNA in liver showed the opposite devel-

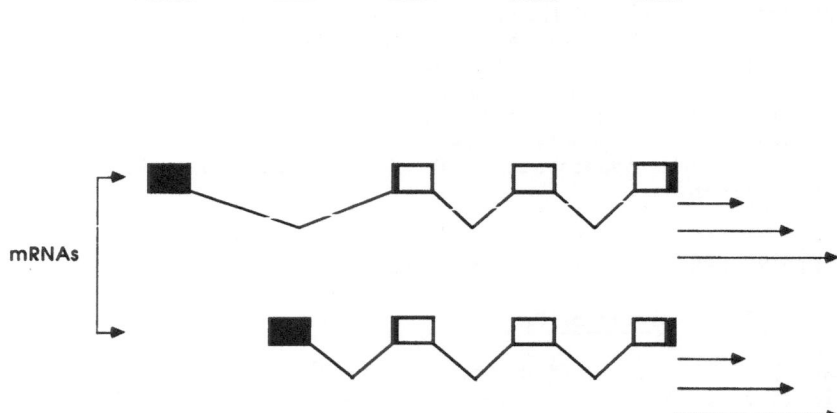

Fig. 1. Generation of multiple mRNAs from the rat IGF-II gene through the use of alternate promoters and alternate polyA addition sites. The rat IGF-II gene contains three coding exons (1, 2, and 3) and two 5'-noncoding exons (-2 and -1) (10,11). Two families of mRNAs arise by initiation of transcription at the 5'-end of exon -2 or exon -1. Untranslated regions of the mRNAs are shown as solid bars, protein-coding regions as open bars. The biosynthetic precursor for IGF-II, pre-pro-IGF-II, contains a prepeptide, the B-C-A-D domains of mature IGF-II (67-residues), and an 89-residue COOH-terminal propeptide or E-domain. Exon 1 contains the prepeptide and most of the B-domain. Exon 2 contains the C, A and D domains, and the first part of the E domain. Exon 3 contains the E domain and the 3'-untranslated region which varies in length (indicated by the arrows) depending on the polyA addition site used. Since exons -2 and -1 differ in size by only 1000 nucleotides, we believe that most of the size heterogeneity of IGF-II mRNAs results from the use of different 3'-polyA sites (12).

opmental profile: like serum IGF-I, levels were low at birth and increased in older animals (18). IGF-II RNA persists to a greater extent in adult neural tissues. Although IGF-II RNA is much less abundant in fetal rat cerebral cortex than in fetal liver, in adult rats IGF-II RNA levels are higher in cortex than liver (11,14,19,20).

Biosynthesis of IGF-II in Rat Embryo Fibroblasts

In BRL-3A cells, we have demonstrated that IGF-II is synthesized as 22 kDa pre-pro-rIGF-II in a reticulocyte lysate cell-free translation system (21). (The size of the precursor agrees with that predicted from the nucleotide sequence [15,16,22]). Addition of microsomal membranes to the translation incubation removes the signal peptide to generate 20 kDa pro-rIGF-II (23). Pro-rIGF-II also was demonstrated by biosynthetic labeling of intact BRL-3A cells (23). Mature 7.5 kDa rIGF-II is at the amino terminus of the precursor (24). The 20 kDa protein appears intracellularly after brief periods of labeling, but is not secreted. A similar conclusion recently was reached from studies using an antibody raised to a synthetic peptide corresponding to the COOH-terminal 40 amino acids of pro-rIGF-II (25). At later times, intermediate (10 and 8.7 kDa) and mature (7.5 kDa) forms appear intracellularly and in the media. The 7.5 kDa and 8.7 kDa forms have been purified and shown to possess biological activity (26).

The pathway for IGF-II biosynthesis seen in BRL-3A cells also was observed in rat embryo fibroblast cultures (27), indicating that this pathway was not limited to an established cell line of hepatic origin. As seen in Figure 5, a 20 kDa protein (pro-rIGF-II) was specifically immunoprecipitated from fibroblast lysates by 4 antibodies to BRL-3A rIGF-II; immunoprecipitation was inhibited by excess unlabeled IGF-II but not by unlabeled rat insulin. The 20 kDa protein was labeled rapidly intracellularly, but is not secreted to the culture media (Fig. 6). Intermediate (10 kDa) and mature forms are observed in the media at later times (Figure 6 and reference 9). RNA from rat embryo fibroblasts directs the synthesis of 22 kDa pre-pro-rIGF-II in cell-free translation, which is converted by microsomal membranes to 20 kDa pro-rIGF-II (Fig. 7). Thus, the biosynthesis of IGF-II in embryonic rat fibroblasts appears to be identical to that in BRL-3A cells.

IGF-II RNA in Different Tissues is Translated into pre-pro-rIGF-II

The question remained whether hybridizable IGF-II RNA in different tissues is translatable. RNAs extracted from term fetal rat liver, muscle, lung, intestine and stomach, neonatal mouse liver and lung, and rat placenta were examined in a reticulocyte lysate cell-free translation system (28). Each RNA directed the synthesis of 22 kDa pre-pro-rIGF-II, identified by specific immunoprecipitation of the translated proteins. Moreover, in rat liver, muscle, and intestine, the 22 kDa protein was not observed in translations directed by RNA from adult tissues, indicating that translatable IGF-II RNA exhibited the same developmental regulation as hybridizable IGF-II RNA.

The constancy of seeing only 22 kDa pre-pro-rIGF-II in different tissues suggests that if alternative splicing involving exons in the coding region of the rIGF-II gene occurs, it does not generate precursor proteins of appreciably different size. In the rat IGF-II gene, introns occur within sequences encoding the B-domain (exons 1 and 2) and the E-domain propeptide (exons 2 and 3). Introns occur in similar locations in the human genes for IGF-II (22,29,30) and for the related polypeptide IGF-I (31). In the human IGF-II gene, alternate splicing does occur between exons 1 and 2, generating a variant protein containing an addi-

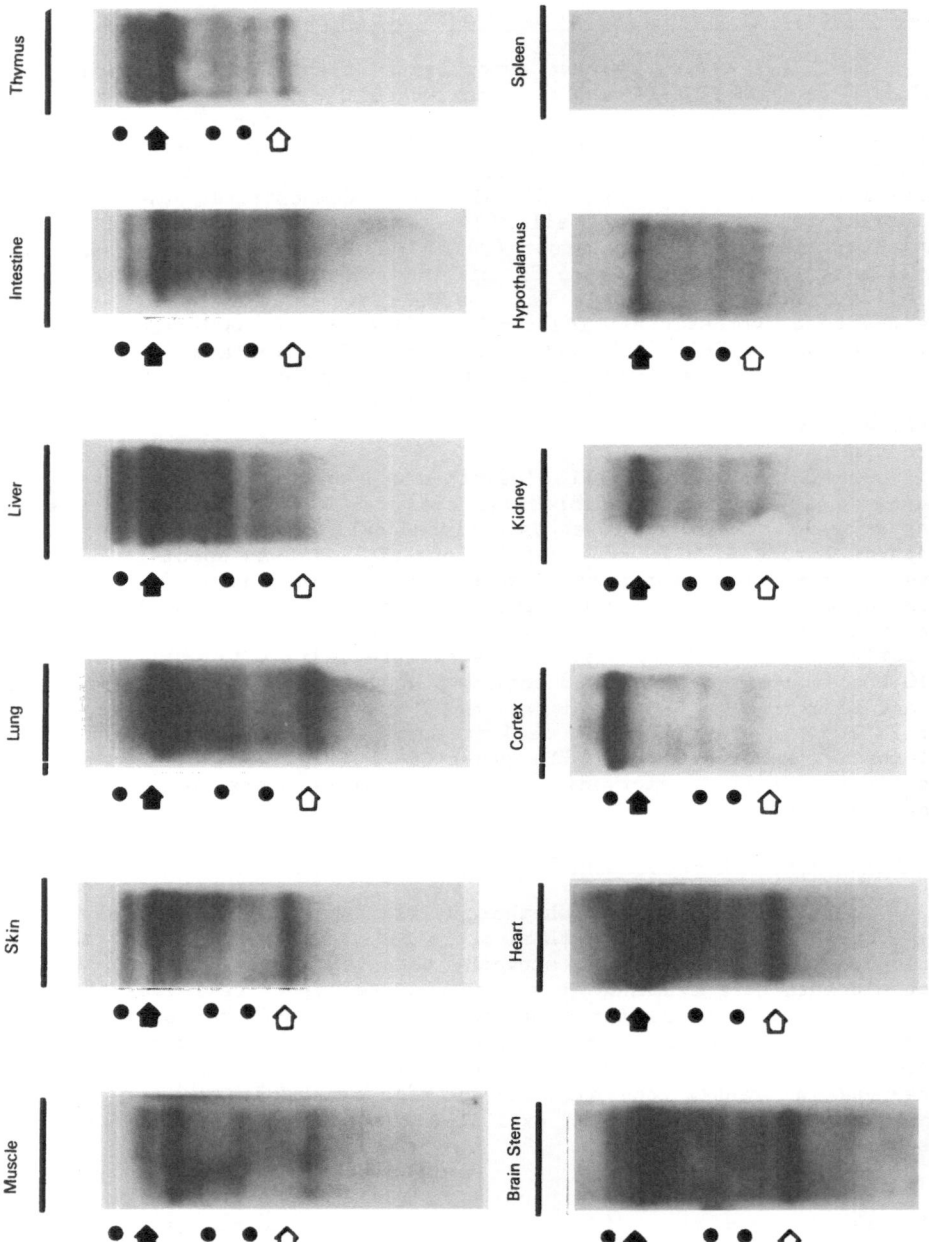

tional 3 amino acids at the end of the B-domain (30,32). Human (31,33,34) and rodent (35,36) cDNA clones for IGF-I have been isolated corresponding to mRNAs in which the proximal E-domain is spliced to different acceptor sites. This could potentially generate 2 pro-IGF-I molecules in each species with E-domain propeptides of different sequence and length (35 and 77 amino acids for human IGF-I, 35 and 41 residues for rodent IGF-I). Mills et al. (37) recently identified a 14 kDa translation product using human placental RNA and a monoclonal antibody to human IGF-I. This may correspond to the mRNA reported by Jansen et al. (33). The other putative precursors have not yet been directly demonstrated by biosynthetic studies.

Processing of IGF-II Biosynthetic Precursors in Different Tissues

We next examined whether pre-pro-rIGF-II is processed to biologically active, lower molecular weight forms in different tissues (28). In the case of mouse epidermal growth factor (EGF), the submaxillary gland is able to process the 130 kDa EGF precursor to mature 6 kDa EGF, but kidney is not (38). Tissues from 19-day gestation rats were extracted with acid-ethanol, and the extracts fractionated by gel-filtration on Sephadex G-75 at acid pH to separate low molecular weight IGF from IGF binding proteins (28). The IGF pool of each tissue contained 8.7 and 7.5 kDa IGF-II species, and was examined in a radioimmunoassay specific for rIGF-II. Each fractionated tissue extract gave a dose response curve parallel to the rat IGF-II standard. IGF-II levels of 1-2 μg/g tissue (similar to the concentration of IGF-II in rat serum at the same age [7]) were observed in liver, limb, intestine, and lung; lower levels were seen in kidney and heart. The relative abundance of immunoreactive IGF-II was similar to the abundance of IGF-II mRNA in these tissues seen by hybridization (14).

Thus, in fetal rat tissues, the rat IGF-II gene is transcribed, IGF-II mRNA translated, and pre-pro-rIGF-II processed to mature biologically active IGF-II species. Although we have not formally proven that the low molecular weight IGF in these tissue extracts is synthesized rather than sequestered in the tissues, the demonstration that IGF-II mRNA extracted from these tissues is translated into pre-pro-rIGF-II makes this

---

Fig. 2 (opposite page). Distribution of IGF-II RNA species in different fetal or postnatal rat tissues (closed arrow = 4 kb; open arrow = 1.2 kb; closed circle = 5.0, 2.2, 1.7 kb). Total RNAs extracted from different rat tissues were fractionated on agarose gels, which were blotted to nylon membranes and hybridized to a rat IGF-II cDNA probe (15) containing coding region and 3'-untranslated sequences. Tissues were obtained from fetal rats at 16-days gestation (muscle, skin, lung, intestine, brain stem) or 21-days gestation (thymus, heart, kidney), or from 2-day (spleen) or 11-day (liver, cerebral cortex) postnatal rats. Although similar amounts of RNA were examined, the times of autoradiographic exposure vary from 2 h to 4 days, so that the results do not reflect the relative abundance of IGF-II RNA in the different tissues. Solid circles designate the 5.0, 2.2 and 1.7 kb RNAs; solid arrows, the 4 kb RNA; and open arrows, the 1.2 kb RNA. IGF-II RNAs were detected in each tissue except spleen. RNAs arising from the exon -1 promoter (e.g., 4 kb and 1.2 kb) and the exon -2 promoter (5 kb) were identified in each tissue (10,12). (The 5 kb RNA was visible in hypothalamus after longer autoradiographic exposures.) (Adapted from reference 14.)

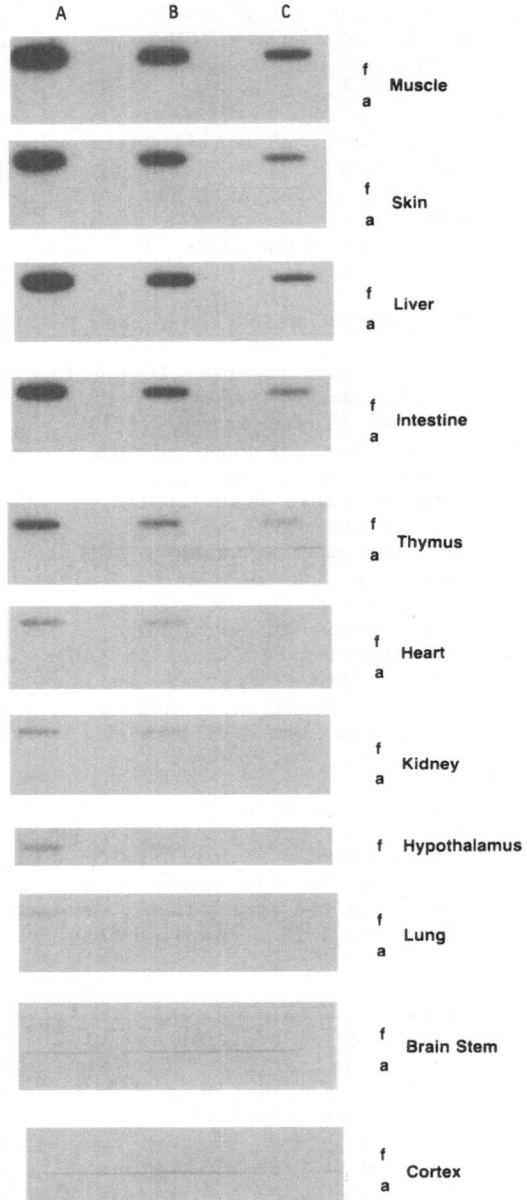

Fig. 3. Hybridization of an oligonucleotide probe specific for exon -2 to slot-blots of total RNAs from the indicated fetal (f) and adult (a) rat tissues. Serial threefold dilutions of each RNA are shown in lanes A, B, and C. The relative abundance of IGF-II RNAs transcribed from the exon -2 promoter in different tissues is the same as that observed using a cDNA probe that principally measures 4 kb IGF-II RNA transcribed from the exon -1 promoter (14). In each tissue, IGF-II RNA was detected in fetal but not adult RNA samples. (Reprinted from reference 10).

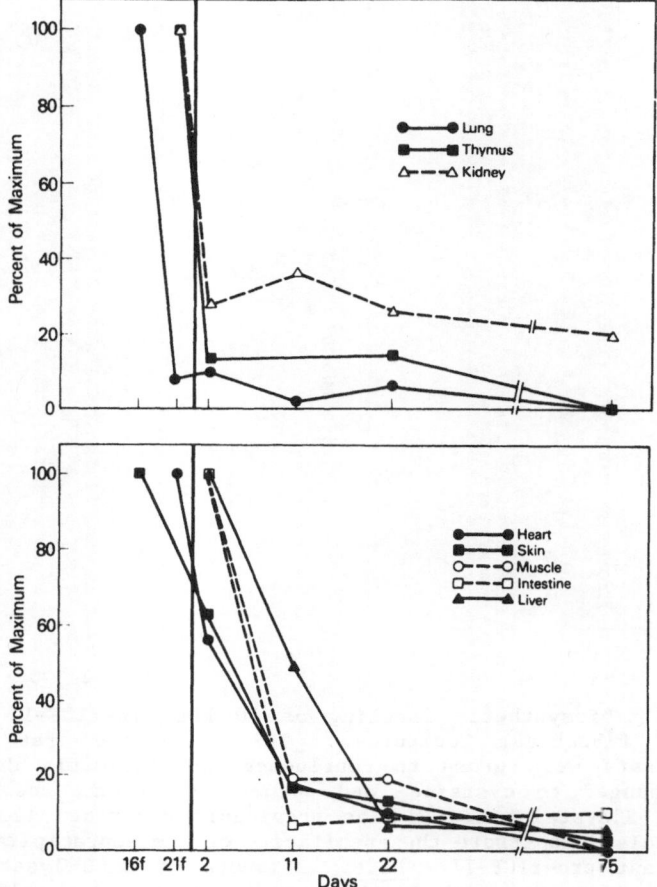

Fig. 4. Relative abundance of IGF-II RNA in
rat tissues at different ages. RNA was
extracted from rat tissues at 16 and 21 days
of gestation, and 2, 11, 22, and 75 days after
birth. Slot-blots of serial dilutions of each
RNA were hybridized to the rat IGF-II cDNA
probe (which predominantly measures the most
abundant 4·kb IGF-II RNA) and the hybridization signal quantitated by densitometry. IGF-
II RNA abruptly decreases with developmental
age in·each tissue. In lung, thymus and kid
ney shown in the upper panel, IGF-II RNA only
was elevated before birth. In liver, muscle
and other tissues, elevated IGF-II RNA levels
persisted into the early postnatal period, but
decreased to low adult levels by 11 or 22 days
after birth (lower panel). (Redrawn from reference 14.)

a more than reasonable supposition. By contrast, in other studies in
which IGF-II levels determined by hybridization and radioimmunoassay are
discordant (e.g., in pheochromocytomas and Wilms' tumors [39,40]), it
remains to be demonstrated that the RNAs are translationally competent.

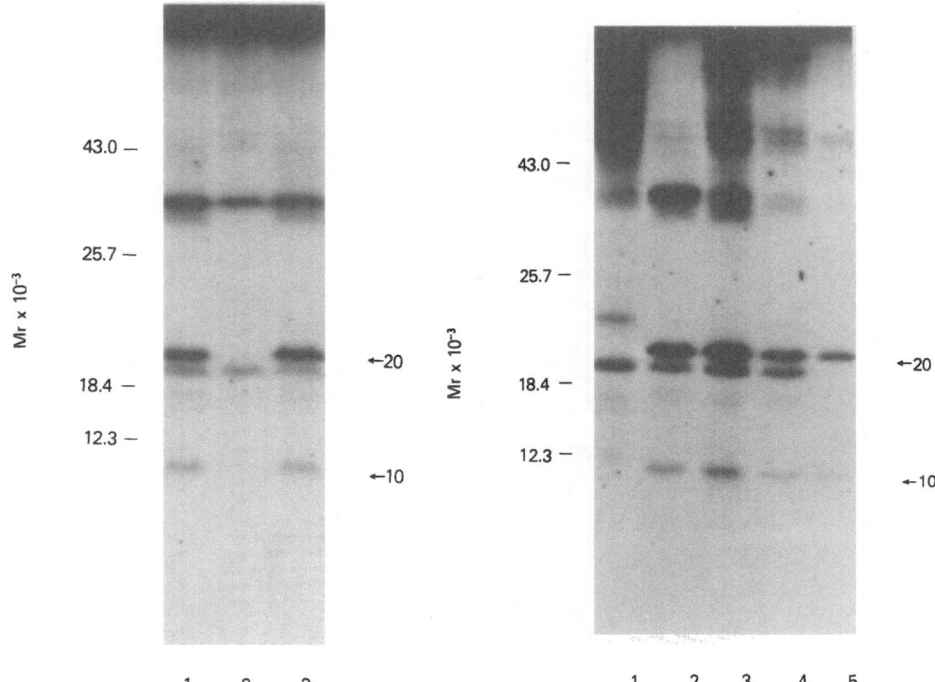

Fig. 5. Biosynthetic labeling of 20 kDa pro-rIGF-II in rat embryo fibroblast cultures. Third passage rat embryo fibroblasts were grown to confluence as previously described (6), changed to cysteine- and serum-free medium, and labeled with [^{35}S]cysteine for 2 h as previously described (23). The two panels demonstrate the specificity of immunoprecipitation of fibroblast pro-rIGF-II. Left: Aliquots of cell lysates were immunoprecipitated with 20 µl of antiserum no. 2 to rIGF-II in the absence of unlabeled peptides (lane 1), or in the presence of 20 µg of unlabeled rIGF-II (lane 2) or rat insulin (lane 3). The immunoprecipitates were examined by sodium dodecyl sulfate-polyacrylamide gel electrophoresis (15% gels) and fluorography (23). Proteins of 20 and 10 kDa (arrows) were specifically immunoprecipitated, and represent pro-rIGF-II and a partially processed intermediate, respectively. The 33 kDa IGF carrier protein also was immunoprecipitated (since this antiserum contains a second population of antibodies directed to the carrier protein). Right: The 20 kDa pro-rIGF-II was not immunoprecipitated from labeled cell lysates by nonimmune serum (lane 1), but was immunoprecipitated by 4 different antisera to rIGF-II (lane 2, antiserum no. 422; lane 3, antiserum no. 2; lane 4, antiserum no. 777; lane 5, antiserum no. 775). A closely migrating 19 kDa protein is not precipitated specifically, since it is not precipitated by antiserum no. 775 (lane 5), it is precipitated by nonimmune serum (lane 1), and its precipitation by antiserum no. 2 is not inhibited by unlabeled rIGF-II (left panel, lane 2).

IGF RECEPTORS

The preceding results strongly suggest that most fetal rat tissues are capable of synthesizing biologically active 7.5 and 8.7 kDa rIGF-II.

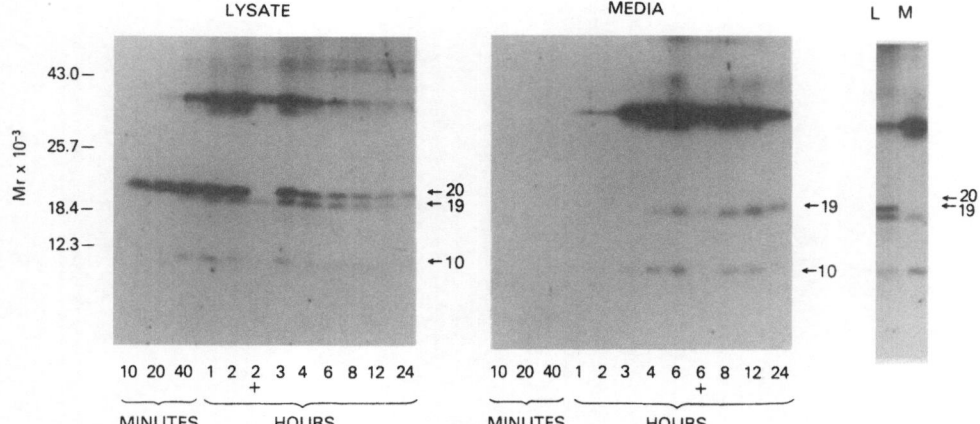

Fig. 6. Kinetics of biosynthesis and secretion of rIGF-II
in rat embryo fibroblast cultures. Fibroblast cultures were
incubated continuously with [^{35}S]cysteine for the indicated
times ranging from 10 min to 24 h. Aliquots of cell lysate
(left panel) and equivalent aliquots of cell media (center
panel) were immunoprecipitated with antiserum no. 2 to
rIGF-II (20 µl). Excess unlabeled rIGF-II (20 µg) was
included in the immunoprecipitation of one of the 2-h lysate
samples (designated 2+) and one of the 6-h media samples
(designated 6+). The right panel compares immunoprecipitates of lysate (L) and media (M) from a different experiment electrophoresed in adjacent lanes of the same gel.
This experiment demonstrates that 20 kDa pro-rIGF-II is
present in cell lysates but not secreted to the media, and
that the nonspecifically precipitated 19 kDa protein is
clearly distinct from 20 kDa pro-rIGF-II.

However, in order to conclude that locally synthesized IGF-II acts as a
local growth factor, it must be demonstrated that tissues have appropriate
receptors through which its biological actions may be mediated. Both type
I IGF receptors (heterotetramers with tyrosine kinase activity that are
homologous to the insulin receptor) and type II IGF receptors (single
chain proteins without tyrosine kinase activity) are widely distributed
(41). Although type II IGF receptors have a higher affinity for IGF-II
than IGF-I, IGF-II also binds to type I IGF receptors, in some cases with
especially high affinity (42,43), so that its biological actions might be
mediated by either receptor subtype.

Both type I and type II IGF receptors are present in rat embryo
fibroblasts, with type II receptors being more abundant (44). Exogenous
IGFs act as progression factors to stimulate DNA synthesis in serum-
starved rat embryo fibroblasts. Preliminary experiments (W. Kiess,
unpublished results) indicate that a polyclonal antiserum that blocks
IGF-II binding to the type II IGF receptor does not block this stimulation, suggesting that these effects are not mediated by the type II
receptor. Similarly, blockade of type II IGF receptors in L6 rat
myoblasts by these antibodies did not inhibit IGF stimulation of amino
acid or glucose transport, or protein synthesis (45). By contrast, in
human fibroblasts, experiments using antibodies to the type I IGF receptor
establish that IGF-I stimulates DNA synthesis and amino acid transport via
the type I IGF receptor (46,47).

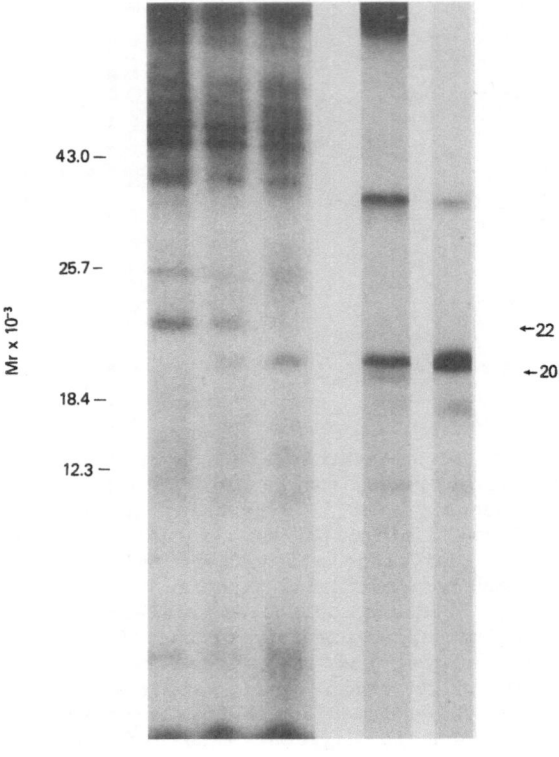

Fig. 7. Rat embryo fibroblast RNA directs the cell-free synthesis of pre-pro-rIGF-II. Lanes 1-3: PolyA RNA (2 μg/lane) was translated in a rabbit reticulocyte lysate system containing [^{35}S]cysteine and [^{35}S]methionine as previously described (21,23). Different concentrations of microsomal membranes were added to the translation incubation: 0, 0.2, and 1 μl in lanes 1, 2, and 3, respectively. The translation mixture then was immunoprecipitated with antiserum no. 2 (20 μl), and the immunoprecipitates examined by sodium dodecyl sulfate-polyacrylamide gel electrophoresis and fluorography as described above. Lanes 4 and 5: Rat embryo fibroblast cultures (lane 4) or BRL-3A cells (lane 5) were biosynthetically labeled with [^{35}S]cysteine (2 h and 40 min, respectively) as previously described (23). Lysates (0.5 ml and 0.1 ml, respectively) were immunoprecipitated with antiserum no. 2, and the immunoprecipitates resuspended and examined by electrophoresis and fluorography. Increasing concentrations of microsomal membranes providing signal peptidase convert 22 kDa pre-pro-rIGF-II to 20 kDa pro-rIGF-II. The 20 kDa pro-rIGF-II synthesized in cell-free translation migrates identically to 20 kDa pro-rIGF-II synthesized by intact rat embryo fibroblasts and BRL-3A cells.

A recent intriguing observation suggests that the type II IGF receptor may have a special role in the rat fetus. A circulating form of the type II IGF receptor was detected in fetal rat serum. It is present at high levels for 20 days after birth, and then markedly decreases in abundance (48). This time course is similar to the time of disappearance of IGF-II from the circulation (7). The circulating receptor is 240 kDa under reducing conditions, 10 kDa smaller than the type II receptor purified from rat placental membranes. The role and significance of the circulating type II IGF receptor remain to be determined.

IGF BINDING PROTEINS

In plasma and other extracellular fluids, the IGFs are complexed to specific carrier proteins (reviewed in [49]). The predominant carrier protein in the fetus has a molecular weight of ~40 kDa, and in adult serum, ~150 kDa. (The transition from 40 to 150 kDa forms occurs early in the third trimester in the human fetus [50], and approximately 3 weeks after birth in the rat [51].) The fetal and adult carrier proteins are antigenically distinct (52-55).

Recently we demonstrated in BRL-3A cells and rat embryo fibroblasts that the fetal IGF carrier protein is synthesized as a 35 kDa precursor containing a prepeptide, and is converted to a stable 33 kDa form which is secreted to the medium where it accumulates without change in size (56). RNA from fetal and neonatal liver stimulates the synthesis of the fetal carrier protein precursor in a cell-free translation system, whereas RNA from adult liver does not. This suggests that the developmental regulation of the carrier protein also may occur at the level of RNA abundance. Further study is required to elucidate the relationship between the regulation of IGF-II, the fetal carrier protein, and possibly the type II IGF receptor.

DISCUSSION

The striking developmental pattern of IGF-II levels in rat serum (7,57) initially suggested the possibility that IGF-II played a role in fetal development. Subsequently, it was demonstrated that the rat IGF-II gene is expressed in most fetal rat tissues (but at low levels in adult tissues), that this RNA is translated, and that the precursor proteins are processed to biologically active forms (7,9,11,13,14,28). These results indicated that IGF-II might act in the fetus either as a classical circulating hormone or as a local growth factor.

Most of the previous studies utilized late-gestation or early postnatal rat tissues. Other evidence suggests that the IGF-II gene is expressed at quite early stages of development. Mouse embryonal carcinoma cell lines corresponding to the sixth day postimplantation express IGF-II RNA (11) and secrete low molecular weight IGF-II into the culture medium (58). Greater expression if the IGF-II gene was observed in several more differentiated embryonal carcinoma cell lines: Dif 5, PSA-5E, and PYS (58), and PC13END (59). Heath and Shi (59) demonstrated immunoprecipitation of IGF-II precursors secreted to the culture medium following biosynthetic labeling of explants of 9-day postimplantation mouse extraembryonic tissues of mesodermal origin.

The relevance of the rodent model indicating that IGF-II is a fetal growth factor to the human fetus has been questioned (60), largely based on the low levels of immunoreactive IGF-II in human fetal blood from 15 weeks gestation to term (61,62). Recent molecular cloning studies, however, clearly indicate that IGF-II RNA is present at high levels in human fetal tissues throughout gestation (39,63-65), as well as in placenta (39). Levels of IGF-II mRNA in human fetal tissue are considerably greater than those of IGF-I mRNA (63). Immunoreactive IGF-II is present at fivefold higher levels than IGF-I in early and midterm amniotic fluid (66). IGF-II (and IGF-I) are expressed in human fetal brain (67) and placenta (68). Human tissues also developmentally regulate IGF-II gene expression, with higher expression in fetal than adult tissues (39,65). The difference between the developmental expression of IGF-II in human and rat, then, lies more in the greater persistence of IGF-II in the adult human (reflected in the high serum IGF-II [69] and detectable IGF-II mRNA [39,64,65]) than to differences during the fetal period.

Although the striking developmental regulation of IGF-II expression certainly suggests a special role in fetal development, IGF-I also is expressed during fetal life. Chick embryonic hepatocytes synthesize IGF-I but not IGF-II (70). Rat liver, lung, intestine, and brain synthesize IGF-I mRNA (detected using a highly homologous mouse IGF-I cDNA probe) (17). IGF-I mRNA is detected in human fetal tissues (albeit at significantly lower levels than IGF-II RNA [63]), and IGF-I is present in extracts of multiple fetal tissues (60) and in the media of cultured human fetal islet cells (71). IGF-I is expressed in human placenta (37,68) and human brain (67). Thus, postulating a special role for IGF-II in fetal development in no way precludes a role for IGF-I in the fetus. In the case of rat myoblast cultures (72) and human placental explants (68), both IGF molecules are synthesized.

Fetal tissues develop the capacity to respond to IGFs early in gestation. IGF receptors are present in 2-day chick embryos (73), mouse embryonal carcinomas (74), rat embryo fibroblasts (75), human brain and liver membranes <17 weeks gestation (76), and human placental membranes at >6 weeks gestation (77). The relative contributions of the two types of IGF receptors to fetal development remain to be determined. Certainly, IGF-II is capable of binding with high affinity to either type I or type II IGF receptors (41-43). It also has been suggested that fetal chondrocytes have an enhanced capacity to respond to IGF-II: (a) IGF-II stimulates DNA synthesis in human fetal, but not postnatal, chondrocytes (78); and (b) IGF-II stimulates the clonal growth of fetal chondrocytes more effectively than IGF-I, whereas IGF-I is more effective for adult chondrocytes (79).

The role of IGF carrier proteins remains elusive. It is striking that the ~40 kDa carrier protein predominates in the fetus, and the antigenically-distinct 150 kDa carrier protein predominates in the adult (49-51). Although it has generally been assumed that IGF complexed to carrier protein is a biologically inert storage form, this concept has been challenged by the provocative report of Elgin et al. (80) that a purified component of the low molecular weight carrier protein from human amniotic fluid enhances the mitogenic activity of IGF-I. Whether this is a special property of the fetal carrier protein as opposed to the 150 kDa carrier protein remains to be determined.

Although it is clear that fetal tissues synthesize IGF-II and IGF-I, and possess receptors through which these peptides might act, it remains to be elucidated what the role of the IGFs is in fetal tissues. Certainly, they may exert anabolic and mitogenic effects in responsive cells. Perhaps more intriguing is the possibility that their primary role is in inducing a differentiated phenotype in particular cells. Observations supporting such a role have been presented in muscle (81,82), erythroblasts (83), ovarian granulosa cells (84), nerve cells (85), and the lens (86).

REFERENCES

1. Humbel RE. Insulin-like growth factors, somatomedins, and multiplication-stimulating activity: chemistry. In: Li CH, ed.

Hormonal proteins and peptides; vol 12. New York: Academic Press, 1985:57-79.

2. Froesch ER, Schmid C, Schwander J, Zapf J. Actions of insulin-like growth factors. Annu Rev Physiol 1985; 47:443-67.

3. Nissley SP, Adams SO, Acquaviva AM, et al. Multiplication-stimulating activity for cells in culture. In: Spencer EM, ed. Insulin-like growth factors/somatomedins: basic chemistry, biology, and clinical importance. New York: Walter de Gruyter Co., 1983:31-48.

4. Marquardt H, Todaro GJ, Henderson LE, Oroszlan S. Purification and primary structure of a polypeptide with multiplication-stimulating activity from rat liver cell cultures. J Biol Chem 1981; 256:6859-65.

5. Rechler MM, Eisen HJ, Higa OZ, et al. Characterization of a somatomedin (insulin-like growth factor) synthesized by fetal rat liver organ cultures. J Biol Chem 1979; 254:7942-50.

6. Adams SO, Nissley SP, Greenstein LA, Yang YW-H, Rechler MM. Synthesis of multiplication-stimulating activity (rat insulin-like growth factor II) by rat embryo fibroblasts. Endocrinology 1983; 112:979-87.

7. Moses AC, Nissley SP, Short PA, et al. Increased levels of multiplication-stimulating activity, an insulin-like growth factor, in fetal rat serum. Proc Natl Acad Sci USA 1980; 77:3649-53.

8. Sara VR, Hall K, Lins P-E, Fryklund L. Serum levels of immunoreactive somatomedin A in the rat: some developmental aspects. Endocrinology 1980; 107:622-5.

9. Adams SO, Nissley SP, Handwerger S, Rechler MM. Developmental patterns of insulin-like growth factor-I and -II synthesis and regulation in rat fibroblasts. Nature 1983; 302:150-3.

10. Frunzio R, Chiariotti L, Brown AL, Graham DE, Rechler MM, Bruni CB. Structure and expression of the rat insulin-like growth factor II (rIGF-II) gene: rIGF-II RNAs are transcribed from two promoters. J Biol Chem 1986; 261:17138-49.

11. Soares MB, Turken A, Ishii D, et al. Rat insulin-like growth factor II gene: a single gene with two promoters expressing a multi-transcript family. J Mol Biol 1986; 192:737-52.

12. Brown AL, Chiariotti L, Clemmons DR, Frunzio R, Bruni CB, Rechler MM. Regulation of rat insulin-like growth factor II (rIGF-II) gene expression by polyadenylation at different sites [Abstract]. Clin Res 1987; 35:620A.

13. Graham DE, Rechler MM, Brown AL, et al. Coordinate developmental regulation of high and low molecular weight mRNAs for rat insulin-like growth factor II. Proc Natl Acad Sci USA 1985; 83:4519-23.

14. Brown AL, Graham DE, Nissley SP, Hill DJ, Strain AJ, Rechler MM. Developmental regulation of insulin-like growth factor II mRNA in different rat tissues. J Biol Chem 1986; 261:13144-50.

15. Whitfield HJ, Bruni CB, Frunzio R, Terrell JE, Nissley SP, Rechler MM. Isolation of a cDNA clone encoding rat insulin-like growth factor-II precursor. Nature 1984; 312:277-80.

16. Soares MB, Ishii DN, Efstratiadis A. Developmental and tissue-specific expression of a family of transcripts related to rat insulin-like growth factor II mRNA. Nucleic Acids Res 1985; 13:1119-34.

17. Lund PK, Moats-Staats BM, Hynes MA, et al. Somatomedin-C/insulin-like growth factor-I and insulin-like growth factor-II mRNAs in rat fetal and adult tissues. J Biol Chem 1986; 261:14539-44.

18. Roberts CT Jr, Brown AL, Graham DE, et al. Growth hormone regulates the abundance of insulin-like growth factor I RNA in adult rat liver. J Biol Chem 1986; 261:10025-8.

19. Hynes MA, Van Wyk JJ, Brooks PJ, D'Ercole AJ, Jansen M, Lund PK. Growth hormone dependence of somatomedin-C/insulin-like growth

factor-I and insulin-like growth factor II messenger ribonucleic acids. Mol Endocrinol 1987; 1:233-42.

20. Murphy LJ, Bell GI, Friesen HG. Tissue distribution of insulin-like growth factor I and II messenger ribonucleic acid in the adult rat. Endocrinology 1987; 120:1279-82.

21. Acquaviva AM, Bruni CB, Nissley SP, Rechler MM. Cell-free synthesis of rat insulin-like growth factor II. Diabetes 1982; 31:656-8.

22. Dull TJ, Gray A, Hayflick JS, Ullrich A. Insulin-like growth factor II precursor gene organization in relation to insulin gene family. Nature 1984; 310:777-81.

23. Yang YW-H, Romanus JA, Liu T-Y, Nissley SP, Rechler MM. Biosynthesis of rat insulin-like growth factor II. I. Immunochemical demonstration of a 20-kilodalton precursor of rat insulin-like growth factor II in metabolically labeled BRL-3A rat liver cells. J Biol Chem 1985; 260:2570-7.

24. Yang YW-H, Rechler MM, Nissley SP, Coligan JE. Biosynthesis of rat insulin-like growth factor II. II. Localization of mature rat insulin-like growth factor II (7484 daltons) to the amino terminus of the 20-kilodalton biosynthetic precursor by radiosequence analysis. J Biol Chem 1985; 260:2578-82.

25. Hylka VW, Kent SBH, Straus DS. E-domain peptide of rat proinsulin-like growth factor-II: validation of a radioimmunoassay and measurement in culture medium and rat serum. Endocrinology 1987; 120:2050-8.

26. Moses AC, Nissley SP, Short PA, Rechler MM, Podskalny JM. Purification and characterization of multiplication-stimulating activity. Insulin-like growth factors purified from rat-liver-cell-conditioned medium. Eur J Biochem 1980; 103:387-400.

27. Yang YW-H, Terrell JE, Nissley SP, Rechler MM. Insulin-like growth factor-II (IGF-II) biosynthesis in short-term rat embryo fibroblasts: demonstration of molecular weight 22,000 (pre-pro-) and molecular weight 20,000 (pro-) precursors [Abstract]. Program of the 7th International Congress of Endocrinology, 1984.

28. Romanus JA, Adams SO, Sofair A, Tseng L, Nissley SP, Rechler MM. Synthesis of mature insulin-like growth factor II in fetal rat tissues [Abstract]. Program, the Endocrine Society, 69th Annual Meeting. Indianapolis, IN, June 10-12:125.

29. Bell GI, Gerhard DS, Fong NM, Sanchez-Pescador R, Rall LB. Isolation of the human insulin-like growth factor genes: insulin-like growth factor II and insulin genes are contiguous. Proc Natl Acad Sci USA 1985; 6450-4.

30. De Pagter-Holthuizen P, Van Schaik FMA, Verduijn GM, et al. Organization of the human genes for insulin-like growth factors I and II. FEBS Lett 1986; 195:179-84.

31. Rotwein P, Pollock KM, Didier DK, Krivi GG. Organization and sequence of the human insulin-like growth factor I gene: alternative RNA processing produces two insulin-like growth factor I precursor peptides. J Biol Chem 1986; 261:4828-32.

32. Jansen M, Van Schaik FMA, Van Tol H, Van den Brande JL, Sussenbach JS. Nucleotide sequences of cDNAs encoding precursors of human insulin-like growth factor II (IGF-II) and an IGF-II variant. FEBS Lett 1985; 179:243-6.

33. Jansen M, Van Schaik FMA, Ricker AT, et al. Sequence of cDNA encoding human insulin-like growth factor I precursor. Nature 1983; 306:609-11.

34. Rotwein P. Two insulin-like growth factor I messenger RNAs are expressed in human liver. Proc Natl Acad Sci USA 1986; 83:77-81.

35. Bell GI, Stempien MM, Fong NM, Rall LB. Sequences of liver cDNAs encoding two different mouse insulin-like growth factor I precursors. Nucleic Acids Res 1986; 14:7873-82.

36. Roberts CT Jr, Lasky SR, Lowe WL Jr, Seaman WT, LeRoith D. Molecular

cloning of rat insulin-like growth factor I complementary deoxyribonucleic acids: differential messenger ribonucleic acid processing and regulation by growth hormone in extrahepatic tissues. Mol Endocrinol 1987; 1:243-8.

37. Mills NC, D'Ercole AJ, Underwood LE, Ilan J. Synthesis of somatomedin C/insulin-like growth factor I by human placenta. Mol Biol Rep 1986; 11:231-6.

38. Rall LB, Scott J, Bell GI, et al. Mouse prepro-epidermal growth factor synthesis by the kidney and other tissues. Nature 1985; 313:228-31.

39. Scott J, Cowell J, Robertson ME, et al. Insulin-like growth factor-II gene expression in Wilms' tumour and embryonic tissues. Nature 1985; 317:260-2.

40. Haselbacher GK, Irminger J-C, Zapf J, Ziegler W-H, Humbel RE. Insulin-like growth factor II in human adrenal pheochromocytomas and Wilms tumors: expression at the mRNA and protein level. Proc Natl Acad Sci USA 1987; 84:1104-6.

41. Rechler MM, Nissley SP. The nature and regulation of the receptors for insulin-like growth factors. Annu Rev Physiol 1985; 47:425-42.

42. Rechler MM, Zapf J, Nissley SP, et al. Interactions of insulin-like growth factors I and II and multiplication-stimulating activity with receptors and serum carrier proteins. Endocrinology 1980; 107:1451-9.

43. Casella SJ, Han VK, D'Ercole AJ, Svoboda ME, Van Wyk J. Insulin-like growth factor II binding to the type I somatomedin receptor. J Biol Chem 1986; 261:9268-73.

44. Adams SO, Nissley SP, Kasuga M, Foley TP Jr, Rechler MM. Receptors for insulin-like growth factors and growth effects of multiplication-stimulating activity (rat insulin-like growth factor II) in rat embryo fibroblasts. Endocrinology 1983; 112:971-8.

45. Kiess W, Haskell JF, Lee L, et al. An antibody that blocks insulin-like growth factor (IGF) binding to the type II IGF receptor is neither an agonist nor an inhibitor of IGF-stimulated biologic responses in L6 myoblasts. J Biol Chem 1987 (in press).

46. Van Wyk JJ, Graves DC, Casella SJ, Jacobs S. Evidence from monoclonal antibody studies that insulin stimulates deoxyribonucleic acid synthesis through the type I somatomedin receptor. J Clin Endocrinol Metab 1985; 61:639-43.

47. Flier JS, Usher P, Moses AC. Monoclonal antibody to the type I insulin-like growth factor (IGF-I) receptor blocks IGF-I receptor-mediated DNA synthesis: clarification of the mitogenic mechanisms of IGF-I and insulin in human skin fibroblasts. Proc Natl Acad Sci USA 1986; 83: 664-8.

48. Kiess W, Greenstein LA, Lee L, White RM, Nissley SP. The type II insulin-like growth factor (IGF) receptor is present in rat serum [Abstract]. In: Program, The Endocrine Society 69th Annual Meeting, Indianapolis, IN, 1987:125.

49. Nissley SP, Rechler MM. Insulin-like growth factors: biosynthesis, receptors, and carrier proteins. In: Li CH, ed. Hormonal proteins and peptides, vol 12. New York: Academic Press, 1985:127-203.

50. D'Ercole AJ, Willson DF, Underwood LE. Changes in the circulating form of serum somatomedin-C during fetal life. J Clin Endocrinol Metab 1980; 51:674-6.

51. White RM, Nissley SP, Short PA, Rechler MM, Fennoy I. The developmental pattern of a serum binding protein for multiplication-stimulating activity in the rat. J Clin Invest 1982; 69:1239-52.

52. Romanus JA, Terrell JE, Yang YW-H, Nissley SP, Rechler MM. Insulin-like growth factor carrier proteins in neonatal and adult rat serum are immunologically different: demonstration using a new radioimmunoassay for the carrier protein from BRL-3A rat liver cells. Endocrinology 1986; 118:1743-58.

53. Povoa G, Roovete A, Hall K. Cross-reaction of serum somatomedin-binding protein in a radioimmunoassay developed for somatomedin-binding protein isolated from human amniotic fluid. Acta Endocrinol (Copenh) 1984; 107:563-70.

54. Drop SLS, Kortleve DJ, Guyda HJ, Posner BI. Immunoassay of a somatomedin-binding protein from human amniotic fluid: levels in fetal, neonatal, and adult sera. J Clin Endocrinol Metab 1984; 59:908-15.

55. Baxter RC, Martin JL. Radioimmunoassay of growth hormone-dependent insulinlike growth factor binding protein in human plasma. J Clin Invest 1986; 78:1504-12.

56. Romanus JA, Yang YW-H, Nissley SP, Rechler MM. Biosynthesis of the low molecular weight carrier protein for insulin-like growth factors in rat liver and fibroblasts. Endocrinology 1987 (in press).

57. Daughaday WH, Parker KA, Borowsky S, Trivedi B, Kapadia M. Measurement of somatomedin-related peptides in fetal, neonatal and maternal rat serum by insulin-like growth factor (IGF-I) radioimmunoassay, IGF-II radioreceptor assay (RRA) and multiplication stimulating activity RRA after acid ethanol extraction. Endocrinology 1982; 110:575-81.

58. Nagarajan L, Anderson WB, Nissley SP, Rechler MM, Jetten AM. Production of insulin-like growth factor-II (MSA) by endoderm-like cells derived from embryonal carcinoma cells: possible mediator of embryonic cell growth. J Cell Physiol 1985; 124:199-206.

59. Heath JK, Shi W-K. Developmentally regulated expression of insulin-like growth factors by differentiated murine teratocarcinomas and extraembryonic mesoderm. J Embryol Exp Morphol 1986; 95:193-212.

60. D'Ercole AJ, Hill DJ, Strain AJ, Underwood LE. Tissue and plasma somatomedin-C/insulin-like growth factor I concentrations in the human fetus during the first half of gestation. Pediatr Res 1986; 20:253-5.

61. Bennett A, Wilson DM, Liu F, Nagashima R, Rosenfeld RG, Hintz RL. Levels of insulin-like growth factors I and II in human cord blood. J Clin Endocrinol Metab 1983; 57:609-12.

62. Ashton IK, Zapf J, Einschenk I, MacKenzie IZ. Insulin-like growth factors (IGF) 1 and 2 in human foetal plasma and relationship to gestational age and foetal size during midpregnancy. Acta Endocrinol (Copenh) 1985; 110:558-63.

63. Han VKM, D'Ercole AJ, Lund PK. Cellular localization of somatomedin (insulin-like growth factor) messenger RNA in the human fetus. Science 1987; 230:193-7.

64. Voutilainen R, Miller WL. Coordinate tropic hormone regulation of mRNAs for insulin-like growth factor II and the cholesterol side-chain-cleavage enzyme, P450ssc, in human steroidogenic tissues. Proc Natl Acad Sci USA 1987; 84:1590-4.

65. De Pagter-Holthuizen P, Jansen M, Van Schaik FMA, et al. The human insulin-like growth factor II gene contains two development-specific promoters. FEBS Lett 1987; 214:259-64.

66. Merimee TJ, Grant M, Tyson JE. Insulin-like growth factors in amniotic fluid. J Clin Endocrinol Metab 1984; 59:752-5.

67. Sara VR, Carlsson-Skwirut C, Andersson C, et al. Characterization of somatomedins from human fetal brain: identification of a variant form of insulin-like growth factor I. Proc Natl Acad Sci USA 1986; 83:4904-7.

68. Fant M, Munro H, Moses AC. An autocrine/paracrine role for insulin-like growth factors in the regulation of human placental growth. J Clin Endocrinol Metab 1986; 63:499-505.

69. Zapf J, Walter H, Froesch ER. Radioimmunological determination of insulin-like growth factors I and II in normal subjects and in patients with growth disorders and extrapancreatic tumor hypoglycemia. J Clin Invest 1981; 68:1321-30.

70. Haselbacher GK, Andres RY, Humbel RE. Evidence for the synthesis of

a somatomedin similar to insulin-like growth factor I by chick embryo liver cells. Eur J Biochem 1980; 111:245-50.

71. Hill DJ, Frazer A, Swenne I, Wirdnam PK, Milner RDG. Somatomedin-C in human fetal pancreas: cellular localization and release during organ culture. Diabetes 1987; 36:465-71.

72. Hill DJ, Crace CJ, Nissley SP, Morrell D, Holder AT, Milner RDG. Fetal rat myoblasts release both rat somatomedin-C (SM-C)/insulin-like growth factor I (IGF I) and multiplication-stimulating activity in vitro: partial characterization and biological activity of myoblast-derived SM-C/IGF I. Endocrinology 1985; 117:2061-72.

73. Bassas L, De Pablo F, Lesniak MA, Roth J. Ontogeny of receptors for insulin-like peptides in chick embryo tissues: early dominance of insulin-like growth factor over insulin receptors in brain. Endocrinology 1985; 117:2321-9.

74. Nagarajan L, Nissley SP, Rechler MM, Anderson WB. Multiplication-stimulating activity stimulates the multiplication of F9 embryonal carcinoma cells. Endocrinology 1982; 110:1231-7.

75. Adams SO, Nissley SP, Kasuga M, Foley TP Jr, Rechler MM. Receptors for insulin-like growth factors and growth effects of multiplication-stimulating activity (rat insulin-like growth factor II) in rat embryo fibroblasts. Endocrinology 1983; 112:971-8.

76. Sara VR, Hall K, Misaki M, Fryklund L, Christensen N, Wetterberg L. Ontogenesis of somatomedin and insulin receptors in the human fetus. J Clin Invest 1983; 71:1084-94.

77. Grizzard JD, D'Ercole AJ, Wilkins JR, Moats-Staats BM, Williams RW. Affinity-labeled somatomedin-C receptors and binding proteins from the human fetus. J Clin Endocrinol Metab 1984; 58:535-43.

78. Ashton IK, Otremski I. In vitro effect of multiplication stimulating activity (MSA) on human fetal and postnatal cartilage. Early Hum Dev 1986; 13:161-7.

79. Vetter U, Zapf J, Heit W, et al. Human fetal and adult chondrocytes. Effect of insulinlike growth factors I and II, insulin, and growth hormone on clonal growth. J Clin Invest 1986; 77:1903-8.

80. Elgin RG, Busby WH Jr, Clemmons DR. An insulin-like growth factor (IGF) binding protein enhances the biologic response to IGF-I. Proc Natl Acad Sci USA 1987; 84:3254-8.

81. Florini JR, Ewton DZ, Falen SL, Van Wyk JJ. Biphasic concentration dependency of stimulation of myoblast differentiation by somatomedins. Am Physiol Soc 1986; 250:C771-8.

82. Schmid Ch, Steiner Th, Froesch ER. Preferential enhancement of myoblast differentiation by insulin-like growth factors (IGF I and IGF II) in primary cultures of chicken embryonic cells. FEBS Lett 1983; 161:117-21.

83. Kurtz A, Jelkmann W, Bauer CH. FEBS Lett 1982; 149:105-8.

84. Adashi EY, Resnick CE, Svoboda ME, Van Wyk JJ. A novel role for somatomedin C in the cytodifferentiation of the ovarian granulosa cell. Endocrinology 1984; 115:1227-9.

85. Recio-Pinto E, Ishii DN. Effects of insulin, insulin-like growth factor-II and nerve growth factor on neurite outgrowth in cultured human neuroblastoma cells. Brain Res 1984; 302:323-34.

86. Beebe DC, Silver MH, Belcher KS, Van Wyk JJ, Svoboda ME, Zelenka PS. Lentropin, a protein that controls lens fiber formation, is related functionally and immunologically to the insulin-like growth factors. Proc Natl Acad Sci USA 1987; 84:2327-30.

22

ORGANIZATION AND EXPRESSION OF THE GENES

ENCODING THE HUMAN SOMATOMEDINS

J. S. Sussenbach, P. de Pagter-Holthuizen, M. Jansen,*
and J. L. Van den Brande*

Laboratory for Physiological Chemistry and
*Department of Pediatrics, State University of Utrecht,
Utrecht, The Netherlands

INTRODUCTION

The somatomedins or insulin-like growth factors (IGF) are small polypeptides which play an important role in fetal and postnatal growth and
development (1,2). Two major human IGFs have been fully characterized:
IGF-I is a basic peptide of 70 amino acids, which is required for postnatal growth, while IGF-II is a neutral peptide containing 67 residues
probably involved in fetal development (3,4). Recently, the nucleotide
sequences of cDNAs encoding IGF-I and IGF-II were reported (5-9). From
the cDNA sequences it can be derived that both IGFs are synthesized as
larger precursor molecules which undergo extensive processing. Employing
the IGF-specific cDNAs as probes, the chromosomal assignment and structure
of the IGF genes has been established. In this communication, our current
insight in the organization and expression of the IGF genes will be
presented.

STRUCTURE AND EXPRESSION OF THE IGF-I GENE

The gene for IGF-I has been mapped to the long arm of human chromosome 12 and consists of at least five exons (Fig. 1) (10). The entire
gene is at least 85 kilobases (kb) long (11-13). The precise length of
the stretch of chromosomal DNA encompassing these five exons is still
unknown, since the cDNAs isolated thus far are incomplete copies of IGF-I
mRNA and the cosmids containing the known IGF-I exons do not overlap.
Analysis of IGF-I cDNA suggests that initiation of translation may occur
at three different AUG codons coding for Met(-48), (-25) and (-22) relative to the first amino acid residue of mature IGF-I. Comparison of the
potential IGF-I signal peptide with signal peptide sequences of pre-
proinsulin and the IGF-II precursor favors initiation at Met(-25) or
Met(-22).

The IGF-I gene can be transcribed into two mRNA species. Jansen et
al. (5) have reported a liver cDNA, which corresponds to an mRNA (IGF-Ia)
consisting of exons 1, 2, 3 and 5, while Rotwein (9,13) has isolated from
an adult liver cDNA library a cDNA species (IGF-Ib) containing exons 1, 2,
3 and 4 (Fig. 1). The mRNAs IGF-Ia and IGF-Ib must arise by alternative
splicing of a single primary transcript and code for precursor molecules,

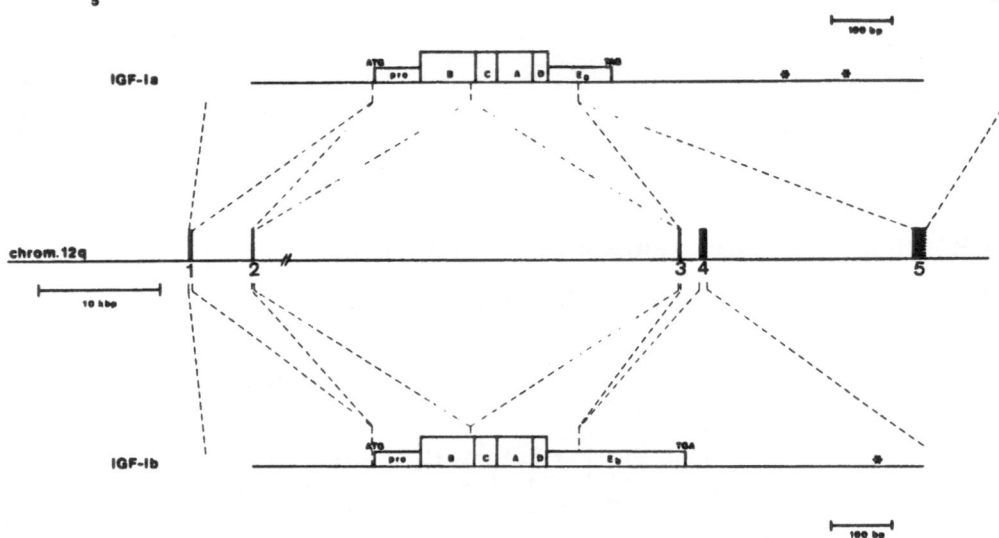

Fig. 1. Schematic representation of the human IGF-I gene and of
two different IGF-I specific cDNAs, IGF-Ia (5) and IGF-Ib
(9,13). The exons are numbered consecutively 1 to 5. Asterisks
indicate possible polyadenylation signals.

which differ only in the amino acid sequence of the carboxyl-terminal
E-domain. Whether the different E-domains lead to differential functions
of the two IGF-I precursors is still unknown.

In order to study expression of the IGF-I gene, polyA$^+$ RNA from fetal
and adult liver has been subjected to Northern blotting analysis employing
IGF-I cDNA as a probe (Fig. 2). As a comparison, rat and mouse liver
mRNAs were also analyzed. In adult human liver distinct bands of 7.6 and
1.1 kb are found, while in fetal human liver IGF-I specific mRNA is hardly
detectable. In adult rat and mouse liver IGF-I specific mRNAs have the
same length as in human liver. The results with fetal and adult human
liver are in agreement with the notion that IGF-I is predominantly
involved in postnatal growth. Further, the large size of some IGF-I mRNA
species suggests very strongly that the IGF-I gene is larger than the sum
of the IGF-I specific exons isolated thus far. Unfortunately, the number
and size of the IGF-I cDNAs currently available are insufficient to
characterize the entire IGF-I gene.

STRUCTURE AND EXPRESSION OF THE IGF-II GENE

We have mapped the gene for IGF-II to the short arm of human chromosome 11 (14). For a detailed characterization of this gene we have
isolated several IGF-II specific cDNAs from an adult human liver cDNA
library. However, none of them contained the 5'-terminus of IGF-II mRNA
(6). Localization of the cDNA sequences on cosmid clones showed that the
IGF-II gene contains at least two 5'-noncoding exons and three coding
exons (12). On further analysis of one of these cDNAs, we found that it
also contained sequences derived from a third 5'-noncoding exon (15). A
schematic presentation of this cDNA and the nucleotide sequence of its
5'-terminus are shown in Figure 3. These results imply that IGF-II mRNA

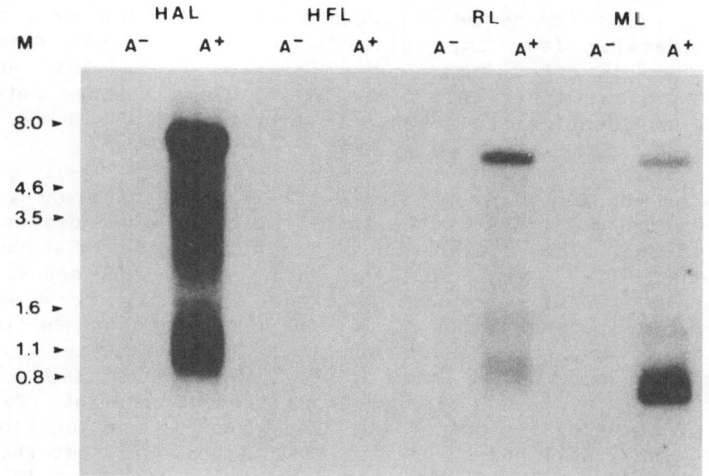

Fig. 2. Northern blot of polyA⁻ and polyA⁺ RNAs isolated from human adult liver (HAL), human fetal liver (HFL), adult rat liver (RL) and adult mouse liver (ML). Each lane contains 10 μg of RNA. Hybridization was performed with an IGF-I specific probe containing exons 1, 2, 3 and 5 (Fig. 1).

from adult liver is transcribed from three 5'-nontranslated exons and three exons coding for the IGF-II precursor.

In our search for new IGF-II cDNAs we also screened a cDNA library from the human hepatoma cell line HepG2, kindly provided by Drs. P. Berg and M. McPhaul (Stanford, USA), and isolated one IGF-II-specific clone. Nucleotide sequence analysis of this cDNA reveals that it consists of the

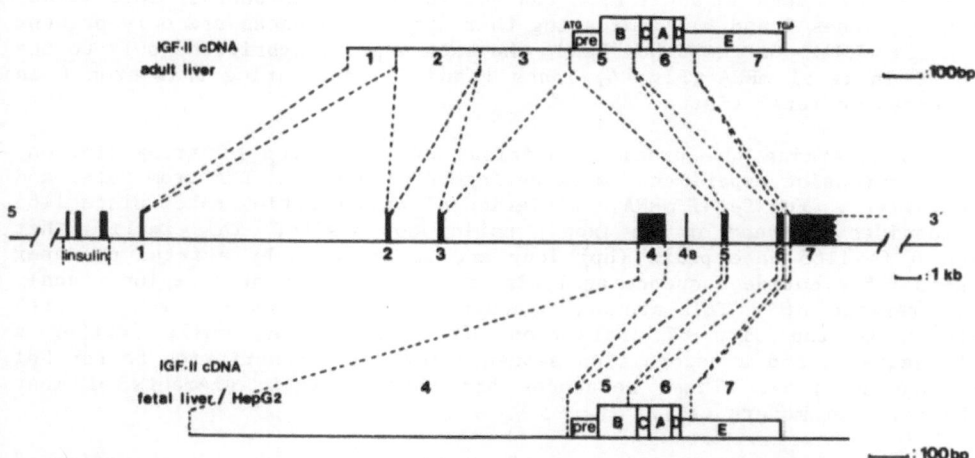

Fig. 3. Schematic representation of the human insulin and IGF-II genes and two different IGF-II specific cDNAs derived from an adult liver and a HepG2 cDNA library, respectively (12,14,15). The structure of the insulin gene was reported previously by Bell et al. (22). The exons are numbered consecutively 1 to 7.

three coding exons (exons 5-7) preceded at the 5'-end by a nucleotide sequence, diverging from the splice site onward. This has not been detected before in other human cDNAs (Fig. 3) (15). This sequence is homologous to a rat liver cell line (BRL3A) cDNA sequence determined by Dull et al. and identical to a sequence localized on the human chromosome (16).

Employing the two above-mentioned IGF-II cDNAs as probes, we determined the precise positions of the IGF-II specific sequences on chromosomal cosmid clones. The complete map of the IGF-II gene is shown in Figure 3. The human IGF-II gene contains seven exons and spans 28 kb of chromosomal DNA. Four 5'-noncoding exons (exons 1, 2, 3 and 4) are followed by three exons (exons 5, 6, and 7) coding for the IGF-II precursor. The 5'-noncoding exons are used in alternative transcripts. Adult liver mRNA consists of exons 1, 2, 3, 5, 6 and 7, while HepG2 mRNA contains exons 4, 5, 6 and 7, suggesting the presence of two different promoters. A striking feature of the IGF-II gene is its location close to the insulin gene. Bell and co-workers (11) established that the genes for insulin and IGF-II are contiguous with a maximal distance of 12.6 kb. Our data further reduce this distance to only 1.4 kb (Fig. 3). Both genes have a similar organization of the coding exons; however, the presence of the 5'-noncoding exons of IGF-II suggests a different mechanism for regulation of expression. Since the two characterized cDNAs contain different 5'-nontranslated sequences, while only a single IGF-II gene is present, we established at which stage in development the mRNAs are expressed. PolyA$^+$ RNA was isolated from fetal and adult human liver. Northern blots of polyA$^+$ RNA were hybridized with three different ^{32}P-labeled probes. Hybridization with an IGF-II probe containing exon 6 to RNA blots containing 10 μg polyA$^+$ RNA from fetal and adult human liver reveals strong expression of a 6.0 kb mRNA in fetal liver, while in adult liver mRNA a weak band of 5.3 kb is detected (Fig. 4, lanes 3 and 4). This indicates that the IGF-II gene is predominantly expressed in fetal tissue. To establish the expression of the different 5'-noncoding exons, polyA$^+$ blots were hybridized with fragments containing exon 1 and exon 4 sequences, respectively. The probe containing exon 1 sequences hybridizes to the 5.3 kb band in adult mRNA and not to the 6.0 kb band in fetal liver (Fig. 4, lanes 5 and 6), indicating that exon 1 sequences are only present in adult mRNA. On the other hand, the exon 4 probe hybridizes only to the 6.0 kb in fetal mRNA (Fig. 4, lanes 1 and 2), suggesting that exon 4 is expressed in fetal tissue.

To determine the precise positions of initiation of transcription, primer extension experiments were performed with polyA$^+$ RNA from fetal and adult liver. For fetal mRNA, initiation of transcription takes place 1165 nucleotides upstream of the exon 4 splice donor site. This implies that exon 4 is 1165 base pairs (bp) long and is preceded by a fetal promoter region. Nucleotide sequence analysis of the fetal promoter region reveals the presence of a TATA-promoter sequence at positions -25 to -19 with respect to the site of initiation of transcription, while further a CAAT-sequence and a recognition sequence for the transcription factor Sp1 are present (15). These sequences are characteristic elements of most eukaryotic promoters (17).

For the characterization of the adult promoter, we have performed similar primer extension experiments with polyA$^+$ RNA from adult liver. Initiation of transcription was localized 115 bp upstream of the exon 1 splice donor site. To characterize the adult promoter, we have determined the complete nucleotide sequence of the intergenic region between the insulin gene and exon 1 of the IGF-II gene (15). This region is 1.4 kb long and exhibits a number of remarkable features. First, the region upstream of exon 1 does not contain TATA- and CAAT-sequences, but a SP1

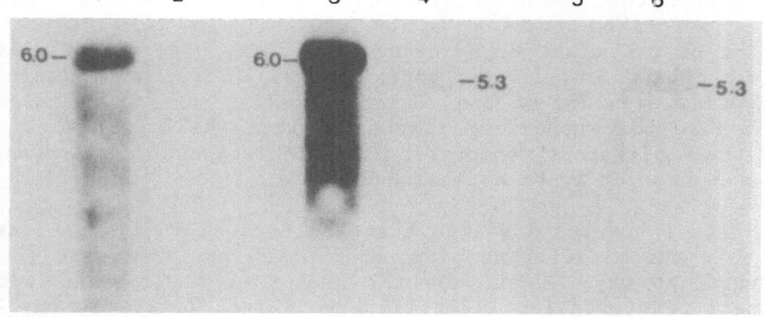

Fig. 4. Northern blot of fetal and adult human liver mRNA. PolyA$^+$ RNA was isolated from human fetal and adult liver. RNAs were size-fractionated on 0.8% agarose gels (10 µg per lane), transferred onto nylon hybridization membranes (Hybond N, Amersham England) and hybridized to different ^{32}P-labeled probes: lanes 1 and 2: an 852 bp genomic fragment of the IGF-II exon 4; lanes 3 and 4: an 825 bp genomic fragment containing IGF-II exon 6 sequences; lanes 5 and 6: a 945 bp genomic fragment containing IGF-II exon 1 sequences.

recognition site is present. Further, a GC-rich region of about 80 nucleotides precedes the site of initiation of transcription. These features have also been found for a number of so-called housekeeping genes, which are expressed at low levels in a variety of tissues (18). Finally, the intergenic region contains a number of direct and inverted repeats. Besides several small repeats, there is an almost perfect 66 bp inverted repeat. These repeats might be involved in regulation of expression by interaction with regulatory proteins.

Since the nucleotide sequences upstream of exon 1 do not contain typical eukaryotic promotor elements, we have tested whether this region exhibits promoter activity. Therefore, we constructed a eukaryotic expression plasmid in which a 266-bp long fragment of the intergenic region immediately preceding the initiation site of transcription was inserted in front of a promoter-defective neomycin-resistance gene. A mouse hepatoma cell line was transfected with this plasmid and the transfected cells were tested for expression of the neomycin-resistance gene. Preliminary results show that this fragment acts as a strong promoter (data not shown). This confirms the notion that the region upstream of exon 1 is involved in expression of the IGF-II gene in adult liver. Further analysis of the promoter regions of the IGF-II gene is in progress.

Recently, two reports have appeared describing the structure of the rat IGF-II gene (19,20). Comparison of the human IGF-II gene with the rat gene reveals striking homologies and differences between both genes. The rat IGF-II gene contains four exons which are highly homologous to the human exons 4, 5, 6 and 7. However, expression of rat analogs of the human exons 1, 2 and 3 was not detected. In contrast, a new very small 5'-noncoding exon preceded by a promoter sequence was detected in the rat genome. By comparing our nucleotide sequences of the human IGF-II gene with the rat sequence of this small 5'-noncoding exon, we can confirm that a homologous sequence is also present in the human genome (Fig. 5). We have designated this human exon, exon 4B (Fig. 3). Whether this exon is actually transcribed remains to be proven. In this respect, it is interesting to note that P. Rotwein (St. Louis, USA) recently isolated a human liver cDNA which, indeed, contains exon 4B (personal communication). The nucleotide sequence of the region preceding exon 4B contains a TATA-box and a CAAT-box supporting the notion that the human IGF-II gene has actually three different promoters. In which stage of development exon 4B is expressed has yet to be established.

The data presented indicate that the human IGF-II gene contains two and probably three different promoters, which are expressed in a development-dependent way. Until now the number of known genes with development-specific expression is still very limited (21). To our knowledge the IGF-II gene is the first human single-copy gene described with multiple promoters which are activated in a development-dependent way. It is striking that the regulation of expression of the human IGF-II gene seems to differ considerably from the corresponding rat gene. The implications of this phenomenon are still unknown.

In summary, the analysis of the somatomedin genes has revealed a number of potential levels of regulation of the somatomedin biological activity. Quantitative modulation of the activity is possible at the level of transcription by differential promoter activation and at the level of translation by using different 5'-noncoding exons (IGF-II). The nucleotide sequence of these exons might affect the efficiency of translation of the corresponding messengers. Another possibility of quantitative regulation of somatomedin expression exists at the level of mRNA stability. The different sizes of the IGF mRNAs suggest that alternative polyadenylation sites are used and preliminary results (not shown) support this notion. This might affect the lifetime of the somatomedin mRNAs. Finally, the structure of the IGF genes also suggests that quantitative regulation of the somatomedin activity is possible by alternative splicing of the primary transcript (IGF-I). This leads to synthesis of IGF precursors of different composition, which might undergo differential proteolytic processing. Alternative splicing opens also the possibility

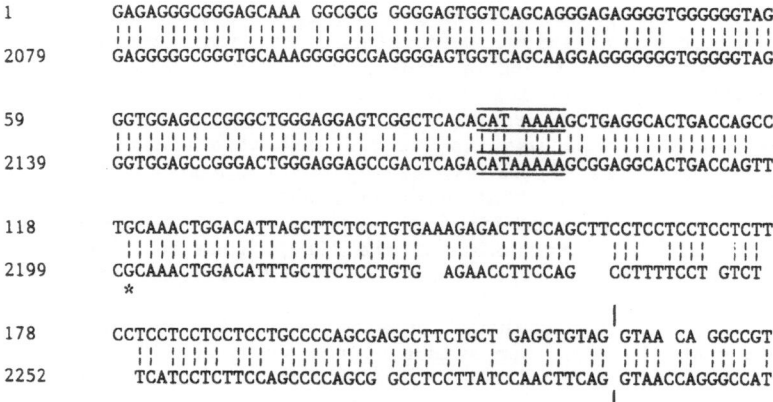

Fig. 5. Comparison of the nucleotide sequences of human IGF-II exon 4B region (upper sequence 1-233) and the corresponding rat sequence (lower sequence 2079-2307) (19). A potential TATA-box is underlined. The start site of transcription in the rat gene is indicated with an asterisk and the splice donor sites in both genes with |.

of qualitative modulation of somatomedin activity. It is not unlikely that the different IGF-I precursors have different biological effects.

In conclusion, it is obvious that further investigation of this gene will yield better insight into eukaryotic regulation of gene expression. Further, it might lead to the identification of development-specific transcription factors and the elucidation of various processes involved in development and differentiation.

ACKNOWLEDGMENTS

The authors thank F. M. A. van Schaik and R. van der Kammen for excellent technical assistance. They gratefully acknowledge Drs. P. Berg and M. McPhaul (Stanford, USA) for the HepG2 cDNA library, Dr. G. J. B. van Ommen (Leiden, The Netherlands) for cosmid libraries, and Dr. G. I. Bell (Emeryville, USA) for communicating unpublished sequence data. This research was supported in part by the Foundation for Medical Research (MEDIGON) with financial aid from the Netherlands Organization for the Advancement of Pure Research (ZWO).

REFERENCES

1. Daughaday WH, Hall K, Raben MS, Salmon WD, Van den Brande JL, Van Wyk JJ. Somatomedin: a proposed designation for the "sulfation factor." Nature 1972; 235:107.
2. Clemmons DR, Van Wyk JJ. Somatomedin C and platelet-derived growth factor stimulate human fibroblast replication. J Cell Physiol 1981; 106:361.
3. Rinderknecht E, Humbel RE. The amino acid sequence of human insulin-like growth factor I and its structural homology with pro-insulin. J Biol Chem 1978; 253:2769.
4. Rinderknecht E, Humbel RE. Primary structure of human insulin-like growth factor II. FEBS Lett 1978; 89:283.
5. Jansen M, Van Schaik FMA, Ricker AT, et al. Sequence of cDNA encoding human insulin-like growth factor I precursor. Nature 1983; 306:609.
6. Jansen M, Van Schaik FMA, Van Tol H, Van den Brande JL, Sussenbach JS. Nucleotide sequence analysis of cDNAs encoding precursors of human insulin-like growth factor II (IGF-II) and an IGF-II variant. FEBS Lett 1985; 179:243.
7. Bell GI, Merryweather JP, Sanchez-Pescador R, et al. Sequence of a cDNA clone encoding human preproinsulin-like growth factor II. Nature 1984; 310:775.
8. LeBouc Y, Dreyer D, Jaeger F, Binoux M, Sondermayer P. Complete characterization of the human insulin-like growth factor I nucleotide sequence isolated from a newly constructed adult liver cDNA library. FEBS Lett 1986; 196:108.
9. Rotwein P. Two insulin-like growth factor I messenger RNAs are expressed in human liver. Proc Natl Acad Sci USA 1986; 83:77.
10. Hoppener JWM, de Pagter-Holthuizen P, Geurts van Kessel AHM, et al. The human gene encoding insulin-like growth factor I is located on chromosome 12. Hum Genet 1985; 69:157.
11. Bell GI, Gerhard DS, Fong NM, Sanchez-Pescador R, Rall LB. Isolation of the human insulin-like growth factor genes: insulin-like growth factor II and insulin genes are contiguous. Proc Natl Acad Sci USA 1985; 82:6450.
12. De Pagter-Holthuizen P, Van Schaik FMA, Verduijn GM, et al. Organization of the human genes for insulin-like growth factors I and II. FEBS Lett 1986; 195:179.

13. Rotwein P, Pollock KM, Didier DK, Krivi GG. Organization and sequence of the human insulin like growth factor I gene. J Biol Chem 1986; 261:4828.

14. De Pagter-Holthuizen P, Hoppener JWM, Jansen M, Geurts van Kessel AHM, Van Ommen GJB, Sussenbach JS. Chromosomal localization and preliminary characterization of the human gene encoding insulin-like growth factor II. Hum Genet 1985; 69:170.

15. De Pagter-Holthuizen P, Jansen M, Van Schaik FMA, et al. The human insulin-like growth factor II gene contains two development-specific promoters. FEBS Lett 1987; 214:259.

16. Dull TJ, Gray A, Hayflick JS, Ullrich A. Insulin-like growth factor II precursor gene organization in relation to insulin gene family. Nature 1984; 310:777.

17. McKnight S, Tjian R. Transcriptional selectivity of viral genes in mammalian cells. Cell 1986; 46:795.

18. Dynan WS. Promoters for housekeeping genes. Trends in Genetics 1986; 2:196.

19. Soares MB, Turken A, Ishii D, et al. The rat insulin-like growth factor II gene: a single gene with two promoters expressing a multi-transcript family. J Mol Biol 1986; 192:737.

20. Frunzio R, Chairotti L, Brown AL, Graham DE, Rechler MM, Bruni CB. Structure and expression of the rat insulin-like growth factor II (rIGF-II) gene. J Biol Chem 1986; 262:17138.

21. Leff SE, Rosenfeld MG, Evans RMA. Complex transcriptional units: diversity in gene expression by alternative RNA processing. Annu Rev Biochem 1986; 55:1091.

22. Bell GI, Pictet R, Cordell B, Tischer E, Goodman HM, Rutter WJ. Sequence of the human insulin gene. Nature 1980; 284:26.

23

SUMMARY OF SESSION IV

GROWTH HORMONE ACTION

A. Joseph D'Ercole, M.D.

Professor of Pediatrics
The University of North Carolina at Chapel Hill
School of Medicine
Chapel Hill, North Carolina

How growth hormone (GH) exerts its growth-promoting actions has been a subject of controversy. The debate has centered on whether these effects of GH result from direct action on target cells or are mediated indirectly by stimulation of production of somatomedins/insulin-like growth factors (Sm/IGFs). Resolution of this question now appears to be coming into sight. A variety of lines of evidence suggest that both GH and the Sm/IGFs act sequentially and in concert to promote growth. While it has not been shown to stimulate cellular proliferation directly (erythroid cell being a possible exception), GH causes differentiation of myoblast and preadipocyte cell lines (1). Once differentiated, these cells proliferate readily in response to somatomedin-C/insulin-like growth factor I (SmC/IGF-I) (2). The data presented by Dr. Isaksson and colleagues in this volume strengthen the belief that the sequential action of GH and SmC/IGF-I may be operative also in the growth of chondrocytes. They have shown that GH increases the abundance of SmC/IGF-I messenger RNA (mRNA) and the appearance of SmC/IGF-I immunoreactive cells in the epiphyseal proliferative zone of hypophysectomized rat cartilage. It is likely that SmC/IGF-I then stimulates cellular proliferation and expansion of the epiphysis. SmC/IGF-I and IGF-II have well-documented mitogenic effects on a wide variety of cultured cells. When administered in vivo to hypophysectomized rats, Sm/IGFs can reproduce GH's growth-promoting actions (see reviews by Doctors Froesch and Hizuka and their co-workers). While SmC/IGF-I seems to mediate the stimulatory effect of GH cellular proliferation, GH probably acts without SmC/IGF-I to stimulate cellular differentiation and a variety of other metabolic events (the latter are reviewed by Dr. Goodman and co-workers).

Even if the above hypothesis of GH's actions proves to be correct, a number of other important questions need to be answered. These include the mechanisms of GH's regulation of Sm/IGF synthesis and the mode of Sm/IGF action. The Sm/IGFs are encoded by single, large complex genes (see reviews by Doctors Sussenbach and Rechler and their respective co-workers) and give rise to multiple transcripts of various sizes. These multiple RNAs may result from regulation of transcription by two or more promoters, alternative splicing of the transcript, and multiple poly-adenylation sites. Although GH regulates the abundance of SmC/IGF-I mRNA (3), it isn't known whether this regulation occurs by stimulation of transcription or by stabilization of preformed transcripts.

Because most, if not all, organs synthesize Sm/IGFs (4,5), it is appealing to speculate that these peptides act locally, either on their cells of synthesis (an autocrine mode of action) or on cells near their sites of synthesis (a paracrine mode of action). The finding that Sm/IGF receptors (a subject reviewed by Dr. Czech) are nearly ubiquitous and that Sm/IGFs act on a wide variety of cell types in culture supports this hypothesis. Nonetheless, an endocrine mode of action is possible, because blood concentrations of the Sm/IGFs are higher than those of any known tissue (suggesting that the growth factor in the circulation has important actions) and because Sm/IGFs administered systemically exert growth-promoting effects. It is possible that these alternative modes of action operate in different physiologic situations and at different developmental stages.

Although progress in understanding the actions of GH has been made in recent years, the puzzle is far from complete. The GH receptor has not yet been characterized completely, and we know virtually nothing about how GH stimulates biologic events after its binding to its receptor. We have only a rudimentary understanding of the regulation of Sm/IGF synthesis, and we are not yet certain of the biochemical nature of the proteins encoded by each of the multiple Sm/IGF transcripts. Questions also remain as to how Sm/IGFs are delivered to their target cells. As with GH, our understanding of how Sm/IGFs exert their actions after they interact with receptors is superficial. Finally, evidence is emerging that Sm/IGFs can induce cellular differentiation, suggesting that our view of Sm/IGFs as mitogens may be too restrictive.

REFERENCES

1. Nixon BT, Green H. Growth hormone promotes the differentiation of myoblasts and preadipocytes generated by azacytidine treatment of 10T cells. Proc Natl Acad Sci USA 1984; 81:3429-32.
2. Zezulak KM, Green H. The generation of insulin-like growth factor-I-sensitive cells by growth hormone action. Science 1986; 233:551-3.
3. Hynes MA, Van Wyk JJ, Brooks PJ, D'Ercole AJ, Jansen M, Lund PK. Growth hormone dependence of somatomedin-C/insulin-like growth factor I and insulin-like growth factor II mRNAs. Mol Endocrinol 1987; 1:233-42.
4. D'Ercole AJ, Stiles AD, Underwood LE. Tissue concentrations of somatomedin-C: further evidence for multiple sites of synthesis and paracrine or autocrine mechanisms of action. Proc Natl Acad Sci USA 1984; 81:935-9.
5. Han VKM, D'Ercole AJ, Lund PK. Cellular localization of somatomedin (insulin-like growth factor) messenger RNA in the human fetus. Science 1987; 236:193-7.

V. THERAPEUTIC EFFECTS OF GROWTH HORMONE

24

ASSESSING SELECTED ASPECTS OF ADEQUACY OF THE GROWTH HORMONE-SOMATOMEDIN AXIS IN SHORT CHILDREN WITH QUANTITATIVELY NORMAL GROWTH HORMONE SECRETION

D. P. Dempsher, S. E. Tollefsen, E. Heath-Monnig,
B. Trivedi, J. R. Gavin III, W. H. Daughaday, and
D. M. Bier

Washington University School of Medicine
St. Louis, Missouri 63110

Conventional approaches for confirming growth hormone adequacy in children with growth failure are the subject of considerable current debate. There is general agreement that individuals who fail repeatedly to secrete growth hormone in response to pharmacological provocation are growth hormone deficient. However, there is no uniform opinion concerning the diagnosis of, or even the presence of, lesser degrees of growth hormone insufficiency including those which might result from structurally abnormal molecules, defects at the growth hormone receptor/postreceptor levels, ineffective mutant somatomedins, or defective IGF-I receptor/postreceptor signal transduction at the cellular level.

Therefore, in an attempt to investigate these issues, we have begun to study the above indices of the growth hormone-IGF-I axis in a selected group of short children with a peak plasma growth hormone response of greater than 10 ng/ml measured by polyclonal RIA following challenge with insulin, clonidine, or both (Table 1).

Table 1. Patient entry classification.

	"Phenotype" of growth hormone deficiency	Delayed growth	Intrinsic short stature
Height	> -2 SD[1]	> -2 SD	> -2 SD
Height velocity	> -2 SD	WNL	WNL
Bone age	> -2 SD	> -2 SD	WNL
Peak [GH][2]	> 10	> 10	> 10
Predicted height	--	WNL	> -2 SD

[1]More than 2 standard deviations below the age appropriate mean value.
[2]Clonidine; insulin (ng/ml).

All were healthy, proportionate, euthyroid prepubertal children more
than two standard deviations below the expected mean height for age. The
girls had a normal peripheral lymphocyte karyotype. For the purposes of
clinical characterization, the children were divided arbitrarily into
three groups. The first we have designated as individuals with the
"phenotype" of growth hormone deficiency since they had the severe bone
age delay and diminished height velocity found in classic growth hormone
deficiency. The second group were those classified as children with
constitutionally delayed growth because their predicted adult height was
in the normal range due to a normal height velocity and delayed bone age.
The third group, on the other hand, were called intrinsically short
because they lacked a bone age delay and, therefore, were predicted to
become short adults (Table 1). To date, 20 individuals with the
"phenotype" of growth hormone deficiency, 13 with delayed growth, and 18
with intrinsic short stature have received all or part of the assessment
described below.

GROWTH HORMONE STRUCTURE

In order to screen for possible abnormalities in the structure of
circulating growth hormone, the plasma samples which contained the peak
growth hormone values measured by polyclonal RIA during the clonidine and
insulin tests were analyzed by IM-9 lymphocyte radioreceptor assay (1) as
well as by a two-site monoclonal antibody assay (Hybridtech, San Diego,
CA). Under the assay conditions used in our laboratory, each of these
methods gives an identical value for purified human growth hormone
preparation No. 4793B supplied by the National Hormone and Pituitary
Program and made up in growth hormone-free human serum as the reference
standard in each assay. Due to inherent intra- and interassay variance in
the analysis of plasma samples, assay ratios of plasma growth hormone
content measured using the three methods are not considered abnormal
unless the ratio is less than 0.5. In the study group, plasma RRA/RIA and
IRMA/RIA growth hormone ratios distributed normally around mean values of
1.04 ± 0.35 (SD) and 1.03 ± 0.41 (SD), respectively. A single subject had
a low IRMA/RIA assayable growth hormone ratio of 0.2 but his RRA/RIA
growth hormone ratio was a normal value of 0.7. The full significance of
this observation is uncertain. However, if this individual has a variant
growth hormone molecule, it is apparently recognized fully by the
receptor.

GROWTH HORMONE RECEPTOR

Recently, Herrington and co-workers (2-4) and Baumann et al. (5)
demonstrated convincingly that serum contained a specific growth hormone
binding protein. The former group suggested that this protein was related
to the growth hormone receptor since it exhibited complete cross
reactivity with a monoclonal antibody raised against the receptor (3). At
the present symposium, Spencer et al. (6) have confirmed the above
hypothesis by reporting that the liver growth hormone receptor and serum
growth hormone binding protein in the rabbit have the same N-terminal
amino acid sequence.

To investigate the clinical application of this discovery, two of us
(WHD and BT) developed a simple, practical method for measuring human
serum growth hormone binding protein (7). In 30 of the 35 study children
tested, the levels of growth hormone binding protein were within the
normal childhood range (Table 2) but this protein was completely absent in
1 child with the characteristics of Laron dwarfism (patient 1, reference
7). Three children had growth hormone binding protein levels below the

current normal range. Whether this finding is causally related to the etiology of their growth failure is not yet known. Clearly, since the number of normal children studied is small, the normal range first needs more accurate definition by expanding the subject number. In addition, 2 short teenagers who were not members of the study groups but who demonstrated the laboratory findings of Laron dwarfism were also found to be completely deficient in serum growth hormone binding protein (subjects 2 and 3, reference 7). Recently, Baumann et al. (8) reported a fourth individual with these findings. We believe these data provide strong evidence that human serum growth hormone binding protein is a derivative of the growth hormone receptor and postulate that study of this easily accessible, circulating protein will permit a fuller understanding of the pathophysiologic role of normal and abnormal growth hormone receptors in children with attenuated growth.

TISSUE RESPONSIVENESS, IN VITRO

Despite several reports (9,10) of children whose growth failure appeared to be secondary to a relative refractoriness of the subject's tissues to the actions of IGF-I, in none was there conclusive demonstration of an aberrant tissue responsiveness to IGF-I at the cellular level. Subsequently, Kaplowitz et al. (12) devised an assay measuring the effect of purified IGF-I on the uptake of α-aminoisubutyric acid (AIB) by cultured human fibroblasts and postulated that this system "might prove useful in determining whether some children with growth failure of unknown etiology have target cell resistance to somatomedins" (12).

Using a slight modification of Kaplowitz's technique (13), we measured the ability of highly pure recombinant (Thr^{59}) human IGF-I to stimulate the uptake of [^{3}H]AIB by fibroblasts of 36 of the short study children. In 35 of these subjects, both the concentration of IGF-I that half-maximally stimulated AIB uptake (ED_{50}) and the magnitude of increase in AIB uptake produced by a maximally stimulating dose of IGF-I were within the normal range (Table 3). In fact, the subjects' cells, as a group, tended to be slightly more responsive to IGF-I than the normal cell lines. However, the fibroblasts from 1 girl (a patient of Dr. Hulda Wohltmann, Charleston, SC) had an ED_{50} of 10.7 ± 1.8 ng IGF-I/ml, a value more than 8 standard deviations above the average value of 3.2 ± 0.9 ng/ml

Table 2. Serum growth hormone binding protein in normal adults, normal children, and children with attenuated growth.

Subjects	Serum growth hormone binding protein[1]
Normal adults (8)[2]	101 ± 9%
Normal children (13)	54 ± 22%
Study children (35)	45 ± 16%
Laron-type dwarfism (3)	0

[1]Expressed as percent ± SD specific binding relative to that of the reference serum (7).
[2]Number in parentheses represents the number of subjects.

in normal fibroblast lines (13) (Table 3). Since this child also had markedly elevated circulating IGF-I levels in vivo, we suggest that her growth attenuation is the result of cellular resistance to the actions of IGF-I. Recently, using a similar approach, Conover et al. (14) reported a child with growth failure secondary to a postreceptor defect in IGF-I effects in target cells.

TISSUE RESPONSIVENESS, IN VIVO

Before the availability of a radioimmunoassay for growth hormone, the metabolic effects of this hormone were used both as an aid in diagnosis of growth hormone deficiency as well as an index of growth hormone responsiveness (15–18). Even after the introduction of an RIA for quantitation of plasma growth hormone, in vivo metabolic responses to growth hormone administration continued to be employed for research purposes (19–27). However, they were soon abandoned since they appeared to offer no diagnostic advantage over the far simpler RIA measurements, and there were conflicting data regarding the usefulness of acute metabolic effects in predicting long-term growth response (19,23,25,27). Over the last several years, however, there has been a rekindled interest in evaluating the potential of quantifying various in vivo metabolic effects of growth hormone as indices of growth hormone sufficiency in short children who appear to secrete adequate amounts of hormone.

Although growth hormone's effects on carbohydrate (28,29) and mineral (30) metabolism have been assessed, metabolic studies in short children have centered principally on growth hormone's role in protein metabolism since a net body protein gain is the sine qua non for growth. Thus, Ballard et al. (31) demonstrated that growth hormone administration reduced the urinary excretion of N^τ-methylhistidine, suggesting that some of growth hormone's net anabolic effects might be explained by a decrease in the rate of myofibrillar protein breakdown. In a series of investigations, Rudman and his co-workers (32–36) showed that a subgroup of short children with apparently normal growth hormone secretion were able to retain nitrogen when treated acutely with growth hormone and, further, that this augmented nitrogen retention was an index of long-term growth response to chronic treatment.

Most intriguing, however, was the recent report by Richter et al. (37) which described the effects of a 2-day challenge with human growth hormone on the retention of an oral dose of $[^{15}N]$ glycine in children with various degrees of growth hormone insufficiency. In this report, children who had classical growth hormone deficiency reduced their excretion of

Table 3. Indices of fibroblast sensitivity to IGF-I.

Fibroblast lines	AIB uptake (ED_{50}) [1]	AIB uptake (Fold stimulation)
Normal subjects (11)	3.2 ± 0.9	2.3 ± 0.5
Study children (35) [2]	2.5 ± 0.7	2.3 ± 0.4
Child with IGF-I resistance [9] [3]	10.7 ± 1.8	2.3 ± 0.2

[1] ng/ml; mean ± SD
[2] Number in parentheses represents number of individuals.
[3] Number in brackets represents number of replicate assays.

urinary ^{15}N by more than 50% when treated with growth hormone, while children with normal growth hormone levels following pharmacologic challenge with insulin and clonidine had no change in their urinary ^{15}N excretion as a function of growth hormone treatment. Furthermore, children who had peak plasma growth hormone responses between 5 and 10 ng/ml to <u>both</u> secretagogues showed a decline in urinary ^{15}N excretion of similar relative magnitude to that seen by the subjects with classical growth hormone deficiency (37). This latter observation in particular suggests that various tracer probes of amino acid-protein metabolism might also serve to identify those children who, despite normal quantitative secretion of growth hormone, are functionally deficient in subsequent steps of the growth hormone-somatomedin axis.

Thus, we have employed a protocol based on that of Richter et al. (37) to study the acute effects of human growth hormone 0.016 mg/kg given subcutaneously every 12 h for 4 days, on the retention of a mixed amino acid "meal" consisting of 5 essential and 6 nonessential amino acids labeled with ^{15}N. Figure 1 shows the time course of total urinary nitrogen-15 excretion in 2 children who were given a mixed ^{15}N amino acid test dose on day 0 and day 4 and begun on twice daily growth hormone injections on day 3. These tracer excretion curves are highly reproducible and can be integrated easily to determine cumulative excretion. In the basal state, 20.0 ± 4.6% of the administered ^{15}N dose was excreted in the urine. During the final 3 days of twice daily growth hormone injections, each of the 18 subjects so far tested improved his/her retention of ^{15}N (Table 4). In 3 children the change was trivial (less than 5%), in 5 others the improvement was substantial (greater than 25%) and, in the remaining children, values were intermediate (Table 4). Since there are, as yet, limited data on the responses of normal-sized children to growth hormone challenge, the ^{15}N results shown in Table 4 are not subject to precise interpretation at this time. However, two points are clear. First, the subject's clinical classification bore no relationship to his/her nitrogen-15 retention response to acute growth hormone chal-

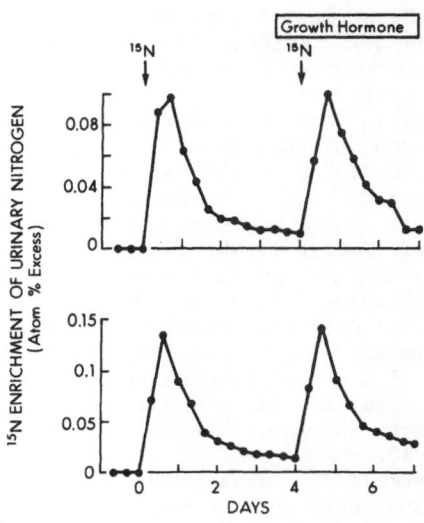

Fig. 1. The time course of total urinary nitrogen-15 excretion in 2 children given a mixed ^{15}N amino acid test dose on day 0 and day 4 and begun on twice daily growth hormone injections on day 3.

Table 4. Percent improvement in [^{15}N] retention during 4 days of rhGH treatment.*

"Phenotype" of GH deficiency	Delayed growth	Intrinsic short stature
1.3	7.3	7.3
2.2	9.1	14.7
3.3	11.1	18.3
15.7	13.5	24.3
27.3	17.9	25.3
34.2	35.7	25.4

*0.016 mg kg^{-1} subcutaneously every 12 h.

lenge. Secondly, some children appeared to demonstrate no positive body protein metabolic effect of short-term growth hormone supplementation, while others conserved nitrogen to a degree previously reported in classically growth hormone deficient subjects. Presumably, there are physiologic reasons for these differences which, if discovered, might lead to an improvement in our understanding of the possible role of growth hormone in the pathophysiology of the subject's growth failure.

Finally, it is also conceivable that a subject's nitrogen-15 retention response during acute growth hormone challenge might be inversely related to the individual's "functional" growth hormone status and, therefore, might reflect the potential for growth under long-term treatment. This hypothesis is currently under investigation.

REFERENCES

1. Gavin JR III, Trivedi B, Daughaday WH. Homologous IM-9 lymphocyte radioreceptor and receptor modulation assays for human serum growth hormone. J Clin Endocrinol Metab 1982; 55:133-8.
2. Ymer SI, Herington AC. Evidence for the specific binding of growth hormone to a receptor-like protein in rabbit serum. Mol Cell Endocrinol 1985; 41:153-61.
3. Herington AC, Ymer S, Roupas P, Stevenson J. Growth hormone-binding proteins in high-speed cytosols of multiple tissues of the rabbit. Biochim Biophys Acta 1986; 881:236-40.
4. Herington AC, Ymer S, Stevenson J. Identification and characterization of specific binding proteins for growth hormone in normal human sera. J Clin Invest 1986; 77:1817-23.
5. Baumann G, Stolar MW, Amburn K, Barsano CP, DeVries BC. A specific growth hormone-binding protein in human plasma: initial characterization. J Clin Endocrinol Metab 1986; 62:134-41.
6. Spencer SA, Hammonds RG, Waters MJ, Wood WI. Purification and characterization of a growth hormone receptor from rabbit liver and a related binding protein from rabbit serum. In: International symposium on growth hormone: basic and clinical aspects. Tampa, June 14-18, 1987:50.
7. Daughaday WH, Trivedi B. Absence of serum growth hormone binding protein in patients with growth hormone receptor deficiency (Laron dwarfism). Proc Natl Acad Sci USA 1987; 84:4636-40.
8. Baumann G, Shaw MA, Winter RJ. Absence of the plasma growth hormone-binding protein in Laron-type dwarfism. J Clin Endocrinol Metab 1987; 65:814-6.
9. Carmina E, LoCoco R, Porcelli P, Lanzara P, Janni A. Dwarfism with high somatomedin activity and delayed bone age: a syndrome of

receptor insensitivity to the somatomedins? In: LaCauza C, Root AW, eds. Problems in pediatric endocrinology. New York: Academic Press, 1980:147–72.

10. Lanes R, Plotnick LP, Spencer EM, Daughaday WH, Kowarski AA. Dwarfism associated with normal serum growth hormone and increased bioassayable, receptorassayable and immunoassayable somatomedin. J Clin Endocrinol Metab 1980; 50:485–90.

11. Bierich JR, Moeller H, Ranke MB, Rosenfeld RG. Pseudopituitary dwarfism due to resistance to somatomedin: a new syndrome. Eur J Pediatr 1984; 142:186–91.

12. Kaplowitz PB, D'Ercole AJ, Underwood LE, Van Wyk JJ. Stimulation by somatomedin-C of aminoisobutyric acid uptake in human fibroblasts: a possible test for cellular responsiveness to somatomedin. J Clin Endocrinol Metab 1984; 58:176–81.

13. Heath-Monnig E, Wohltmann HJ, Mills-Dunlap B, Daughaday WH. Measurement of insulin-like growth factor I (IGF-I) responsiveness of fibroblasts of children with short stature: identification of a patient with IGF-I resistance. J Clin Endocrinol Metab 1987; 64:501–7.

14. Conover CA, Hintz RL, Rosenfeld RG. Impaired synergism between somatomedin C/insulin-like growth factor I and dexamethasone in the growth of fibroblasts from a patient with insulin resistance. Pediatr Res 1987; 22:188–91.

15. Ikkos D, Luft R, Gemzell CA. The effect of human growth hormone in man. Lancet 1958; 1:720–1.

16. Medical Research Council. The effectiveness in man of human growth hormone. Lancet 1959; 1:7–12.

17. Henneman PH, Forbes AP, Moldawer M, Dempsey EF, Carroll EL. Effects of human growth hormone in man. J Clin Invest 1960; 39:1223–8.

18. Shepard TH II, Nielsen RL, Johnson ML, Bernstein N. Human growth hormone. I. Metabolic balances studies carried out in a hypopituitary child. Am J Dis Child 1960; 99:90–6.

19. Prader A, Illig R, Szeky J, Wagner H. The effect of human growth hormone in hypopituitary dwarfism. Arch Dis Child 1964; 39:535–44.

20. Hubble D. Studies with human growth hormone. Arch Dis Child 1966; 41:17–24.

21. Brown GA, Stimmler L, Lines JG. Growth hormone-induced nitrogen retention in children of short stature. Arch Dis Child 1976; 42:239–44.

22. Prader A, Zachmann M, Poley JR, Illig R. The metabolic effect of a small uniform dose of human growth hormone in hypopituitary dwarfs and in control children. Acta Endocrinol (Copenh) 1968; 57:115–28.

23. Clayton BE, Tanner JM, Vince FP. Diagnostic and prognostic value of short-term metabolic response to human growth hormone in short stature. Arch Dis Child 1971; 46:405–13.

24. Rudman D, Chyatte SB, Patterson JH, et al. Observations on the responsiveness of human subjects to human growth hormone. J Clin Invest 1971; 50:1941–9.

25. Grunt JA, Enriquez AR. Acute and long-term responsiveness to growth hormone in children with short stature. Pediatr Res 1972; 6:664–74.

26. August GP, Hung W, Houck JC. The effects of growth hormone therapy on collagen metabolism in children. J Clin Endocrinol Metab 1974; 39:1103–9.

27. Joss EE. Growth hormone deficiency in childhood. In: Falkner F, Kretchmer N, Rossi E, eds. Monographs in paediatrics; vol 5. Basel: S Karger, 1975:1–83.

28. Lippe BM, Kaplan SA, Golden MP, Hendricks SA, Scott ML. Carbohydrate tolerance and insulin receptor binding in children with hypopituitarism: responses after acute and chronic human growth hormone administration. J Clin Endocrinol Metab 1981; 53:507–13.

29. Tamborlane WV, Genel M, Gianfredi S, Gertner JM. The effect of small

but sustained elevations in circulating growth hormone on fuel metabolism in growth hormone deficiency. Pediatr Res 1984; 18:212-5.

30. Gertner JM, Tamborlane WV, Hintz RL, Horst RL, Genel M. The effects on mineral metabolism of overnight growth hormone infusion in growth hormone deficiency. J Clin Endocrinol Metab 1981; 53:818-22.

31. Ballard FJ, Burgoyne JL, Tomas FM, Penfold JL. Growth hormone-induced changes in myofibrillar protein breakdown in hypopituitary children. Clin Sci 1983; 64:315-20.

32. Rudman D, Kutner MH, Fleming GA, et al. Effect of 10-day courses of human growth hormone on height of short children. J Clin Endocrinol Metab 1978; 46:28-35.

33. Rudman D, Kutner MH, Blackston RD, Jansen RD, Patterson JH. Normal variant short stature: subclassification based on responses to exogenous human growth hormone. J Clin Endocrinol Metab 1979; 49:92-9.

34. Rudman D, Kutner MH, Goldsmith MA, Blackston RD. Predicting the response of growth hormone-deficient children to long term treatment with human growth hormone. J Clin Endocrinol Metab 1979; 48:472-7.

35. Rudman D, Kutner MH, Goldsmith MA, Kenny J, Jennings H, Bain RP. Further observations on four subgroups of normal variant short stature. J Clin Endocrinol Metab 1980; 51:1378-84.

36. Rudman D, Kutner MH, Blackston RD. Children with normal-variant short stature: treatment with human growth hormone for six months. N Engl J Med 1981; 305:123-31.

37. Richter I, Heine W, Plath C, Mix M, Wutzke KD, Towe J. [15]N tracer techniques for the differential diagnosis of dwarfism and prediction of growth hormone action in children. J Clin Endocrinol Metab 1987; 65:74-7.

25

THERAPEUTIC EFFECTS OF GROWTH HORMONE RELEASING HORMONE

A. D. Rogol, R. M. Blizzard, P. M. Martha, Jr.,
W. S. Evans, M. L. Vance, C. Brook, P. Smith,
G. Klingensmith, I. Burr, J. Najjar, R. Furlanetto,
J. Rivier, W. Vale, M. O. Thorner

University of Virginia Medical Center, Charlottesville, VA;
The Middlesex Hospital, London, England; The Children's
Hospital, University of Colorado School of Medicine,
Denver, CO; Vanderbilt University School of Medicine,
Nashville, TN; Children's Hospital of Philadelphia, PA;
The Clayton Foundation Laboratories of Peptide Biology,
Salk Institute, San Diego, CA

INTRODUCTION

The existence of hypothalamic-hypophyseal releasing factors was suggested by the pioneering work of Sir Geoffrey Harris (1); Reichlin and co-workers postulated that a specific releasing factor for growth hormone (GH) was present in the hypothalamus (2). Its isolation, purification, and synthesis followed more than three decades of intensive investigation and awaited many refinements in the fields of bioassay, analytic biochemistry and, most importantly, a rich source of the peptide free from "contamination" with somatostatin (SRIH).

The delineation of the chemical structure of GHRH began with several "experiments of nature," in patients in Charlottesville, Virginia, and Lyon, France, who had acromegaly and had not been cured by presumed selective transsphenoidal pituitary surgery. In the Charlottesville patient, an ectopic source of GHRH was sought because the pituitary histology revealed an unusual finding: somatotroph hyperplasia instead of the expected pituitary adenoma (3). A tumor in the tail of the pancreas was demonstrated on CT scan. After the tumor was removed, the biochemical and clinical features of acromegaly abated, and this patient has been well for more than 5 years. From this rich source of hormone, along with that from several other tumors, Drs. Vale and Guilleman, working independently, were able to extract, isolate, purify, sequence, and synthesize a family of peptides with specific growth hormone releasing activity (4,5).

HYPOTHALAMIC-PITUITARY AXIS AND GH SECRETION

The complex system that encompasses the release and action of growth hormone (GH) includes many neurotransmitters, hormones, and organs. Among these are biogenic amines such as dopamine and serotonin in the brain; growth hormone-releasing hormone (GHRH) and somatostatin or somatotropin release-inhibiting hormone (SRIH) in the hypothalamus; somatotropin or GH in the pituitary; and insulin-like growth factors I (IGF-I) and II (IGF-II) in the liver and possibly in other organs. The mechanisms by which this complex system generates growth as a result of GH production and release from the pituitary are rapidly being elucidated.

Growth hormone releasing hormone and somatostatin are transported from the hypothalamus via the portal system to the anterior pituitary, where they bind to their respective receptors on the somatotroph. The three forms of GHRH identified—a 44, a 40 and a 37 amino acid peptide (4,5)—are approximately equipotent in vitro and in vivo. The first two have been identified in the human hypothalamus (6,7).

The synthesis and release of GH in the somatotrophs are under the control of the cAMP system. Both synthesis and release are sensitive to calcium ion fluxes and diacylglycerol. Protein kinase-C, the putative diacylglycerol receptor, also plays an important role in the stimulated secretory pathway for GH, as indicated by marked increases in GH release by anterior pituitary cells of rats following stimulation with the phorbol ester, phorbol-12-myristate-13-acetate (5). Somatostatin, cholera toxin, and forskolin lead to cAMP accumulation in somatotrophs and stimulate GH release; SRIH inhibits both actions of these secretagogues, and thus its mechanism of action is also closely related to the cAMP system. As the pituitary portal blood concentrations of GHRH and SRIH change, the serum levels of GH rise and fall in an intermittent pulsatile fashion.

The feedback mechanisms to control GH release are multiple and complex. For example, GHRH can diminish its own secretion in the rat, as shown by Tannenbaum, who injected GHRH in graded doses into the cerebral ventricles of rats (8). Increasing doses given in this manner led to a dose-dependent inhibition of GH secretion. This profound effect was not due to SRIH secretion, as shown by the inability of the antiserum to SRIH to reverse the suppression of GH release. Thus, GHRH can affect its own secretion by means of an ultra-short negative feedback loop mechanism.

In addition, GHRH produces negative feedback at the somatotroph when there is lengthy exposure to the peptide. Pretreatment of anterior pituitary cell cultures from rats with GHRH resulted in decreased cAMP and GH concentrations in these cells when the cells were re-exposed to GHRH.

Insulin-like growth factors also are involved in the feedback control of GH secretion. When placed in the cerebral ventricles, IGF-I causes a profound decrease in the spontaneous intermittent secretion of GH in rats (9). This action may occur through the release of SRIH; Berelowitz and co-workers demonstrated that IGF-I directly stimulates the acute release of SRIH from rat hypothalamic fragments in culture (10).

CLINICAL STUDIES WITH GHRH

Normal Male Volunteers

Growth hormone-releasing hormone (1 μg/kg) was administered as an intravenous bolus dose to 6 healthy men (mean age 25.2 years, range 21-29) who were all within 15% of ideal body weight. They were studied on two occasions separated by at least 7 days (11).

During the control study, serum GH concentrations were generally less than 2 ng/ml, although a spontaneous pulse of 8 ng/ml occurred in one subject (Fig. 1) (11). After GHRH administration, serum GH concentrations increased in 4 subjects at 5 min (the earliest time studied) and reached a peak between 30 and 60 min of 20.4 ± 6.5 ng/ml versus 2.1 ± 0.1 ng/ml after injection of the vehicle solution (P=0.005). The GH concentrations returned to control levels with 90 min of GHRH injection. The responses of GH to GHRH at this dose were highly variable (Fig. 1).

Twelve additional young men were studied in a similar manner to determine the dose response relationship to varying amounts of GHRH (0.1 to 10 µg/kg). Six subjects were tested at each dose (12). Serum GH levels were generally less than 0.5 ng/ml after the injection of the vehicle solution, although isolated peaks of GH up to 9.7 ng/ml were found in 7 of the 12 subjects. The mean increases in GH concentration for each of the amounts of GHRH injected are shown in Figure 2 (12). Serum GH increased in all after GHRH administration; this increase occurred within 5 min of injection in most subjects, and maximal levels were noted within 1 h in 29 of 30 studies. There was considerable variability in response among subjects who received the same dose. The lower doses, 0.1, 0.3 and 1 µg/kg produced a monophasic response; however, the higher doses of 3.3 and 10 µg/kg resulted in a more prolonged elevation of GH, characterized by a secondary rise at 2 h. Values of integrated GH release over 5 h after the 0.3, 1.0, 3.3 and 10 µg/kg doses of GHRH were significantly greater than those after vehicle treatment (Fig. 3A) (12).

Differences in the integrated hourly GH release after the various doses were compared during the 3 h after GHRH administration (Fig. 3B) (12). During the first hour there was a significant increase in GH levels after all doses of GHRH compared to the administration of the vehicle solution (P<0.05); however, there were no differences in GH release in response to the various doses. During the second hour a significant increase in GH concentrations was produced by the 0.3, 1.0, 3.3 and 10 µg/kg doses compared to those after the administration of vehicle solution (P<0.05). During the third hour, only the 3.3 and 10 µg/kg doses resulted in a significant increase in GH release compared to that following vehicle

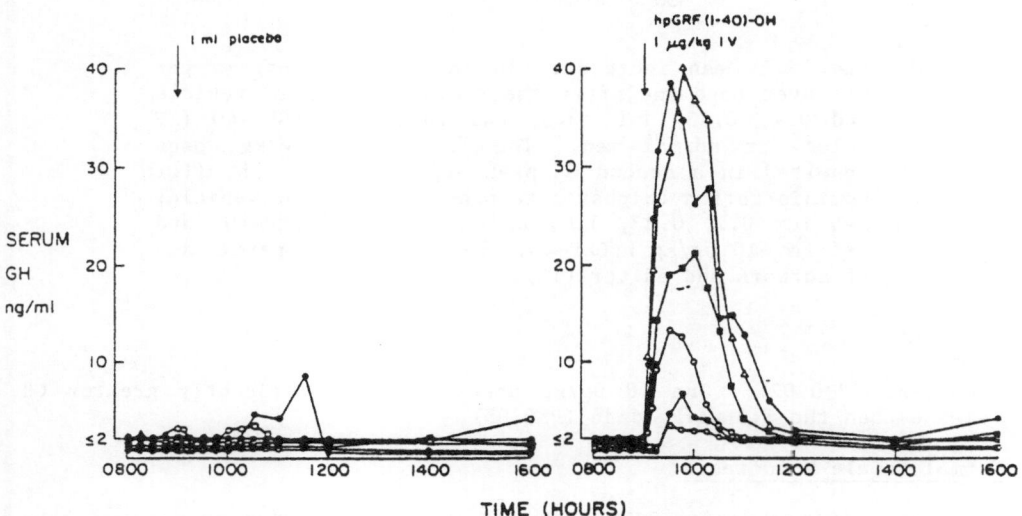

Fig. 1. Serum growth hormone before and after placebo (left panel) and hpGRF (human pancreatic GH releasing hormone or GHRH) (right panel) in 6 normal men. Note the variability of response to hpGRF among the subjects. Reprinted with permission of authors and editor (11).

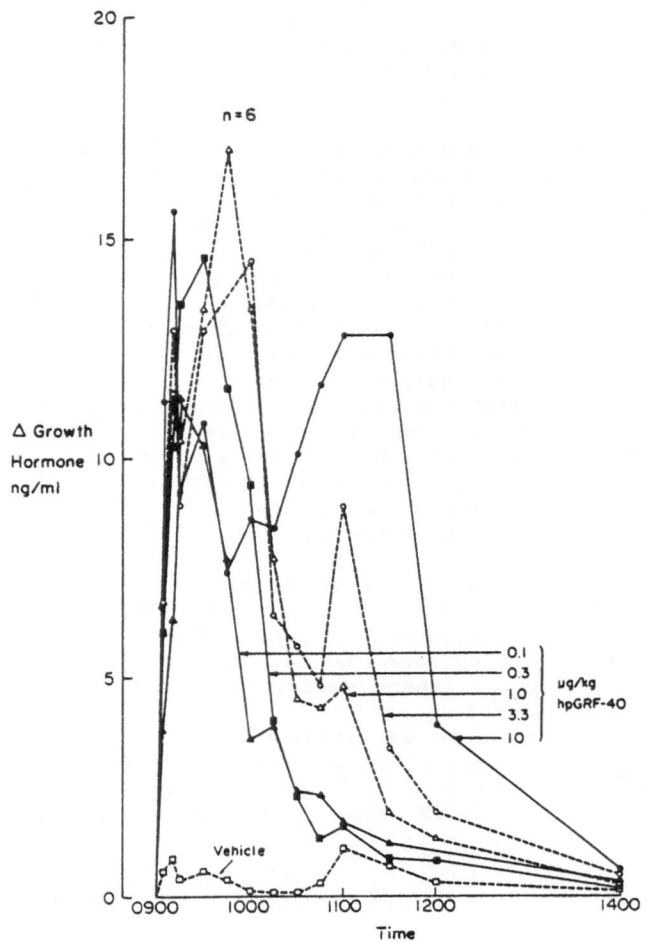

Fig. 2. Mean increments in serum GH (nanograms per ml) over baseline after the administration of vehicle and 0.1, 0.33, 1.0, 3.3, and 10 µg/kg hpGRF-40 (IV bolus) in normal men. The 3.3 and 10 µg/kg doses resulted in a second GH peak approximately 2 h after administration (biphasic response). n=11 for vehicle; n=6 for 0.1, 0.33, 1.0, and 3.3 µg/kg hpGRF-40; and n=5 for 10 µg/kg hpGRF-40. Reprinted with permission of authors and editor (12).

treatment (P<0.02). The 10 µg/kg dose caused significantly greater GH release than the 3.3 µg/kg dose (P<0.05).

Normal Female Volunteers

In a similar manner GHRH (3.3 µg/kg) administration to women in the early follicular phase of the menstrual cycle resulted in increased GH levels (maximal GH 34.9 ± 8.3 ng/ml). No differences in peak GH concentrations were found when the GHRH test was done in the early follicular, late follicular or luteal phases of the menstrual cycle at the single dose of 3.3 µg/kg (13).

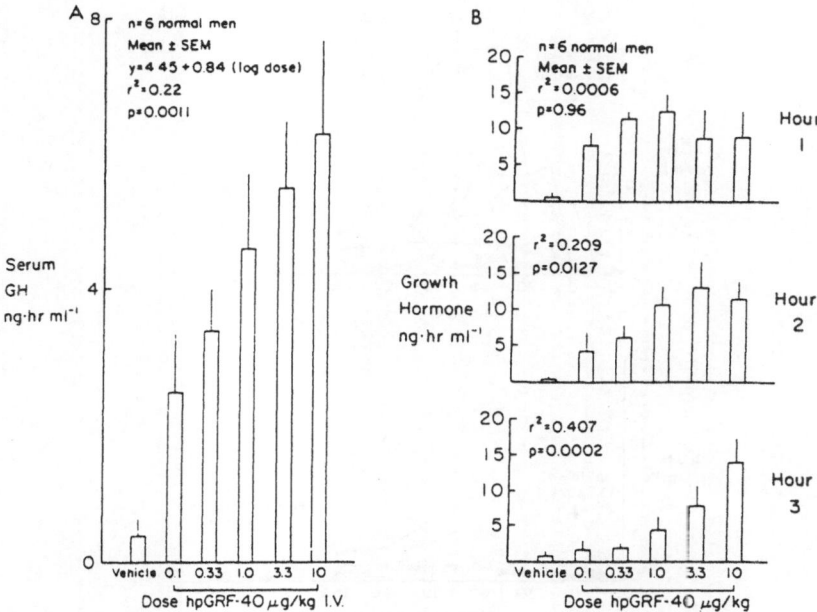

Fig. 3. (A) Mean change (nanograms per h/ml) in serum GH during the 5 h after the administration of vehicle and 0.1, 0.33, 1.0, 3.3, and 10 µg/kg hpGHRH-40 (hpGRF-40). Note the progressive increase in GH release after increasing doses of hpGRF-40. (B) Mean change (nanograms per h/ml) in GH release during hourly intervals after the administration of vehicle and 0.1, 0.33, 1.0, 3.3, and 10 µg/kg hpGRF-40. Reprinted with permission of authors and editor (12).

Growth Hormone Sufficient Children with Short Stature

We evaluated a large series of short children for growth hormone sufficiency by standard pharmacologic tests and by the infusion of a single dose of GHRH. Subjects were tested on 2 consecutive days—on the first a combined test using the IV administration of L-arginine (0.5 g/kg for 30 min) and the oral administration of L-dopa (9 mg/kg). On the following day GHRH, 3.3 µg/kg, was injected as a bolus dose. For both tests blood samples were withdrawn at 15-min intervals for up to 2 h. The responses to the pharmacological tests were normal (peak GH level >7 ng/ml) in those classified as intrauterine growth retardation or constitutional delay of growth and adolescence and/or familial short stature. As shown in Figure 4A and 4B, all GH-sufficient children responded to a single dose of GHRH with an increase in circulating GH levels (14). The vast majority, 19/23, achieved levels of 10 ng/ml or more. These percentages have been confirmed in our now larger series of 71 GH sufficient children. These data are quite similar to those of Takano and co-workers (15).

Multiple Doses of GHRH

A single patient with isolated GH deficiency who had minimal GH responses to GHRH (10 µg/kg) and hypoglycemia (maximal GH levels 0.3 and 1.0 ng/ml, respectively), received GHRH 0.33 µg/kg every 3 h for 5 days (16). Maximal serum GH concentrations 90 min after administration of the 0800 h dose of GHRH were <0.25, 0.7, 0.5, 0.6, 0.4 and 0.4 ng/ml respec-

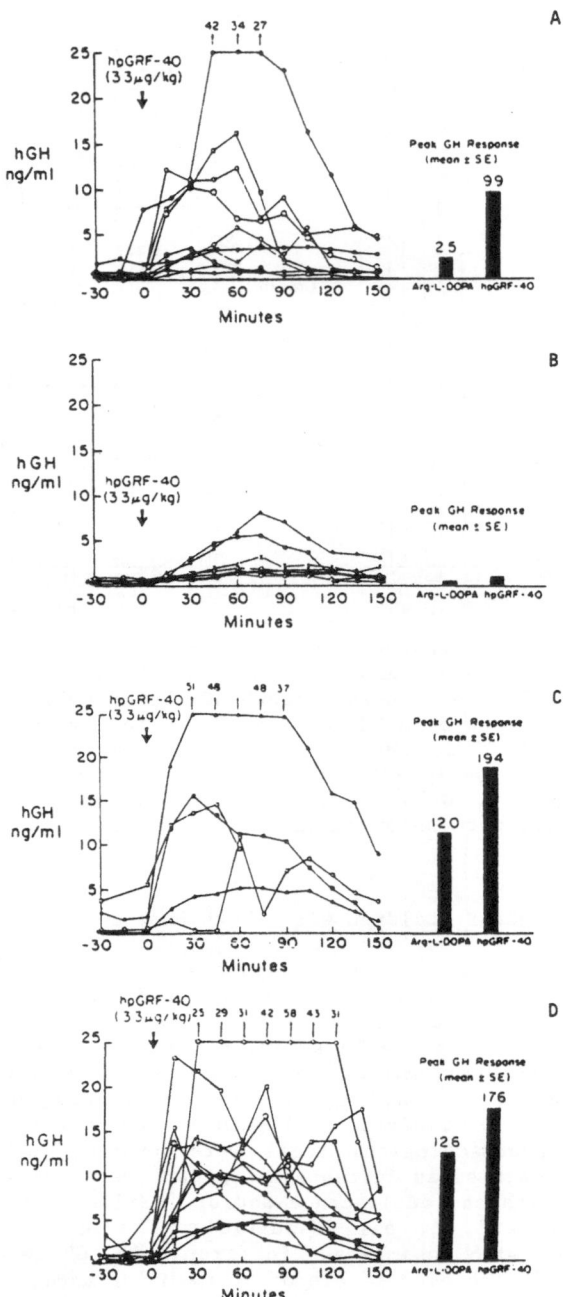

Fig. 4. GH release in response to hpGHRH-40 (hpGRF-40) in children with short stature. The horizontal axis is time (min) before and after the IV injection of hpGRF-40, 3.3 µg/kg as a bolus dose. The vertical axis is GH concentration (nanograms per ml). Each set of symbols represents an individual patient. (A) Isolated GH deficiency; (B) organic hypopituitarism; (C) intrauterine growth retardation; (D) constitutional delay of growth and adolescence and/or familial short stature. Bars at the lower right of each panel are the mean ± SE of the peak responses to the arginine/L-dopa and hpGHRH-40 stimulation tests. Reprinted with permission of authors and editor (14).

tively on days 0-5. On the fifth day, 4 h after administration of the last 0.33 µg/kg GHRH dose, the patient was challenged with GHRH (10 µg/kg). The GH peak response rose to 2.0 ng/ml (Fig. 5).

To assess the biological significance of changes in GH levels, serum somatomedin-C levels were measured every 12 h in the same patient (Fig. 6). Within 12 h of the start of GHRH administration, serum somatomedin-C levels increased from a pretreatment level of 0.06 U/ml on day 0 and peaked at 0.36 U/ml after 72 h, despite the negligible increase in serum GH concentrations.

Six additional adult subjects with idiopathic GH deficiency were studied with a single 10 µg/kg dose of GHRH before and after 40 consecutive 3 hourly doses of GHRH [0.33 µg/kg, IV (17)]. Each morning serum GH concentrations were measured at 15 min intervals for 1 h after administration of the 0800 h dose of GHRH. Serum somatomedin-C concentrations were measured twice daily. Basal serum GH levels were less than 1 ng/ml before administration of vehicle or GHRH. The initial administration of GHRH, 10 µg/kg, resulted in an increase (>1 ng/ml) in maximal serum GH levels compared to baseline levels in 2 of 6 subjects. The maximal serum GH level (above baseline) achieved in response to 0.33 µg/kg GHRH given at 0800 h was higher after 1 day of 3 hourly GHRH administration than after vehicle treatment (P=0.02). In response to the second 10 µg/kg dose of GHRH, 3 of the 4 subjects who had initially failed to respond or had minimal responses (<1 ng/ml) had an increase in maximal GH levels compared to baseline. One of the two remaining subjects had a greater increase in GH after the second 10 µg/kg dose of GHRH compared to that after the first challenge (Fig. 7). Serum somatomedin-C levels rose progressively during the 3 hourly treatment in all patients. The basal and maximal somatomedin-C levels during GHRH treatment are shown in Figure 8. All but 2 reached the normal adult range by the end of the treatment.

Two older female members (ages 85 and 54) of a family with isolated GH deficiency in 4 generations also received multiple doses of GHRH, 0.33 µg/kg, 3 hourly for 30 doses preceded and ended with single 10 µg/kg doses

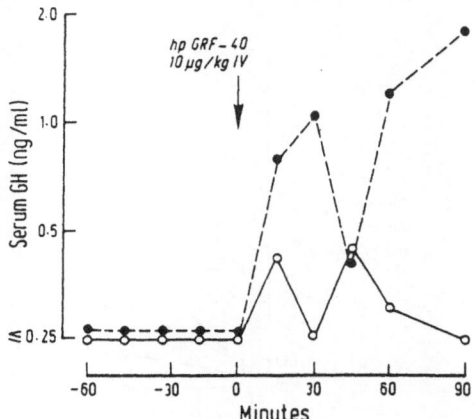

Fig. 5. Serum GH concentrations in 1 patient (2) with isolated GH deficiency in response to hpGRF-40 before (o——o) and after (●---●) 5 days of hpGRF-40 (0.33 µg/kg) administration every 3 h for 5 days. Reprinted with permission of authors and editor (16).

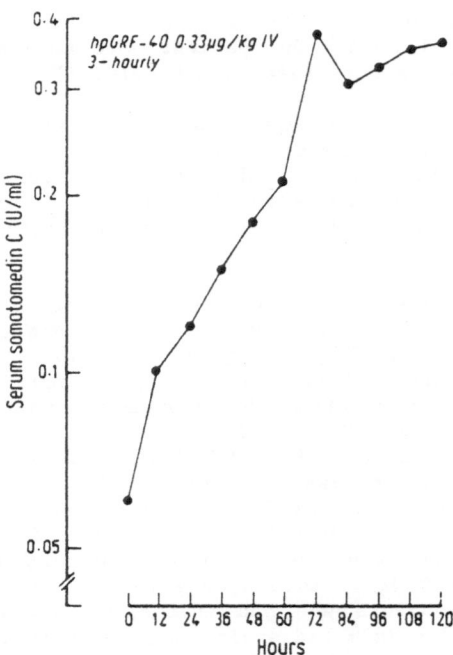

Fig. 6. Serum somatomedin-C concentrations in Patient 2 with isolated GH deficiency during 5 days of treatment with hpGRF-40. Reprinted with permission of authors and editor (16).

of GHRH (18). None of the concentrations exceeded 0.5 ng/ml nor were any somatomedin-C levels above 0.06 U/ml. The lack of increase may indicate that the "priming" protocol used may have been inadequate, or that their somatotrophs could never be stimulated. The latter condition might arise because of the underlying defect or decreased GH secretion with age.

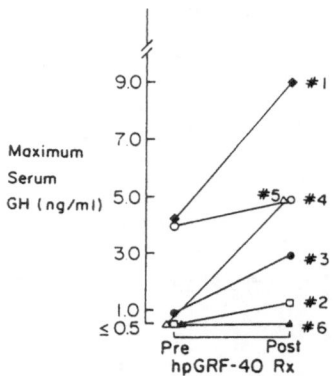

Fig. 7. Maximum serum GH levels (nanograms per ml) in 6 adults with idiopathic GH deficiency after IV bolus hpGRF-40 (10 µg/kg) administration before (Pre) and at the termination of (Post) 5 days of hpGRF-40 treatment (0.33 µg/kg, IV bolus given every 3 h). Reprinted with permission of authors and editor (17).

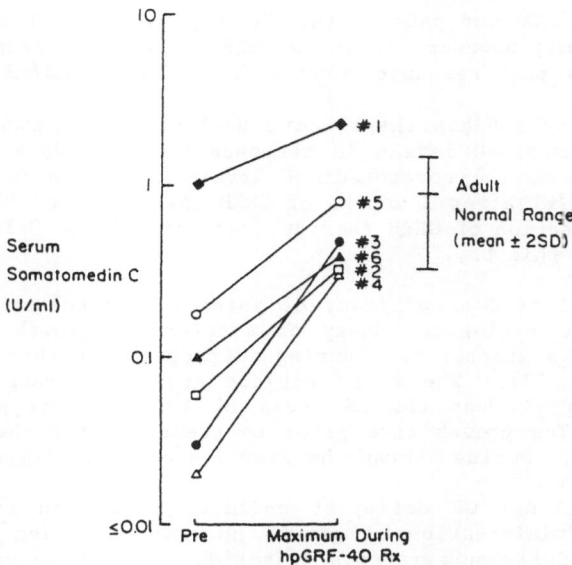

Fig. 8. Serum somatomedin-C levels (units per ml) before (Pre) and maximum levels during 5 days of intermittent pulsatile hpGRF-40 administration. Note the log-arithmic scale. Reprinted with permission of authors and editor (17).

GROWTH HORMONE RELEASING HORMONE THERAPY IN GROWTH HORMONE DEFICIENT CHILDREN

To determine whether GHRH is efficacious in the treatment of certain children with GH deficiency, we administered the peptide every 3 h for 6 months to 2 GH deficient boys (19). The 3 hourly rate was chosen to mimic the physiological secretion of GH of approximately 8 episodes per day (20). The boys received GHRH (1 or 3 µg/kg) subcutaneously via an indwelling catheter (autosyringe Sub-Q Set) placed in the abdominal wall. The peptide was administered over 1 min every 3 h by a Pulsamat® peristaltic pump (Ferring, Inc., Ridgewood, NJ).

Each child was discharged home with a pump after preliminary studies (19) at the Clinical Research Center. The pump had a reservoir with a capacity sufficient to contain peptide solution for at least 14 days. For the first 6 months each child received GHRH 1 or 3 µg/kg every 3 h. Each child's height and somatomedin-C concentration were measured every 2 weeks. Immediately prior to commencing GHRH therapy and at 4-week intervals thereafter, each child underwent a GHRH test (1 µg/kg as an intravenous bolus) 3 h after the previous subcutaneous dose. Both tolerated the 6 months of pump therapy well. The only problem was blockage of pump catheter on a single occasion in each child.

The GH responses to the intravenous bolus administration of GHRH (1 µg/kg) are shown before and during the 6 months of therapy (Fig. 9). Both children responded to the initial dose, but the responses varied greatly during treatment. However, on 6 of 7 and 7 of 8 occasions respectively, the GH responses of the boys were greater than before therapy. After 4 months of therapy we measured the serum GH levels every 20 min for 24 h to demonstrate the efficacy of each subcutaneous pulse of GHRH on GH secretion (Fig. 10). In one patient the GH response to each dose of GHRH was less than 4 ng/ml; however, in the second patient the responses were much greater with the peak response varying from 10 to 50 ng/ml.

In the first subject there was a negligible and inconsistent change in serum somatomedin-C levels in response to GHRH (data not shown). In the other subject, the somatomedin-C levels rose from 0.09 to a maximal value of 0.70 U/ml after 3 months of GHRH therapy (Fig. 11). Three and 4 weeks after cessation of GHRH therapy, the somatomedin-C levels had fallen to 0.17 U/ml in this boy.

The crucial test of efficacy of intermittent pulsatile GHRH therapy is the in vitro biological assay of accelerated growth velocity. Each subject grew at a greater rate during therapy than either before or after treatment (Fig. 12). The first subject grew at a rate of 4.6 cm/year prior to therapy. Over the 28 weeks of treatment he grew 3.8 cm (or 7.1 cm/year). The growth rate prior to treatment for the second subject was 2.1 cm/year. During therapy he grew 7.4 cm (13.7 cm/year).

Five additional GH deficient children have been treated with the intermittent administration of growth hormone releasing hormone. Three received twice daily subcutaneous injections of GHRH (4 µg/kg). All grew at an accelerated rate but there was great variability in the growth rates (Fig. 13, including the original 2 children). Our present experience is that we have administered GHRH to 24 GH deficient children for 28 6-month treatment periods. The children received GHRH subcutaneously either using a mechanical pump (Pulsamat®; Ferring, Inc., Ridgewood, NJ) which deliv-

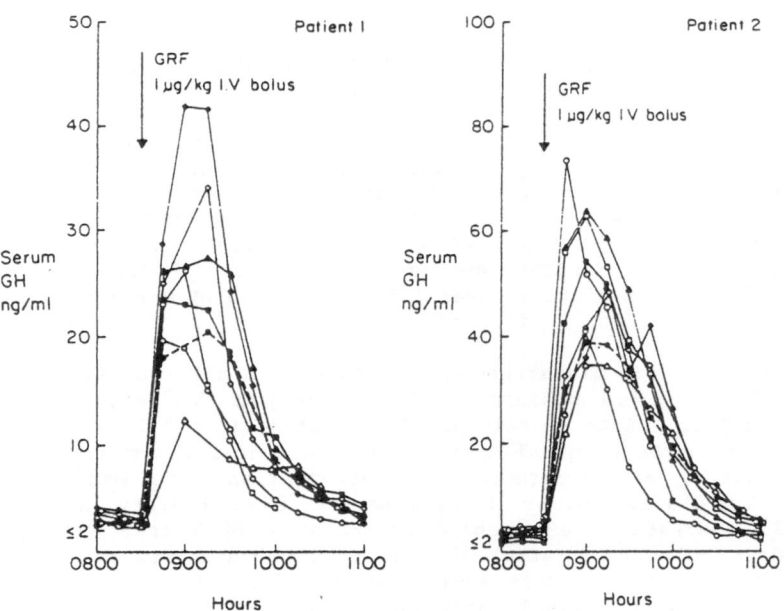

Fig. 9. Serum growth hormone (GH) levels in 2 growth hormone-deficient boys before and after therapy with growth hormone-releasing hormone factor (GRF). An intravenous bolus injection (1 µg per kilogram) was administered for 6 months. Pretreatment values are indicated by dashed lines; values determined at other intervals are indicated as follows: 1 day, 4 weeks, 8 weeks, 12 weeks, 16 weeks, 20 weeks, 24 weeks, and 28 weeks. Reprinted with permission of authors and editor (19).

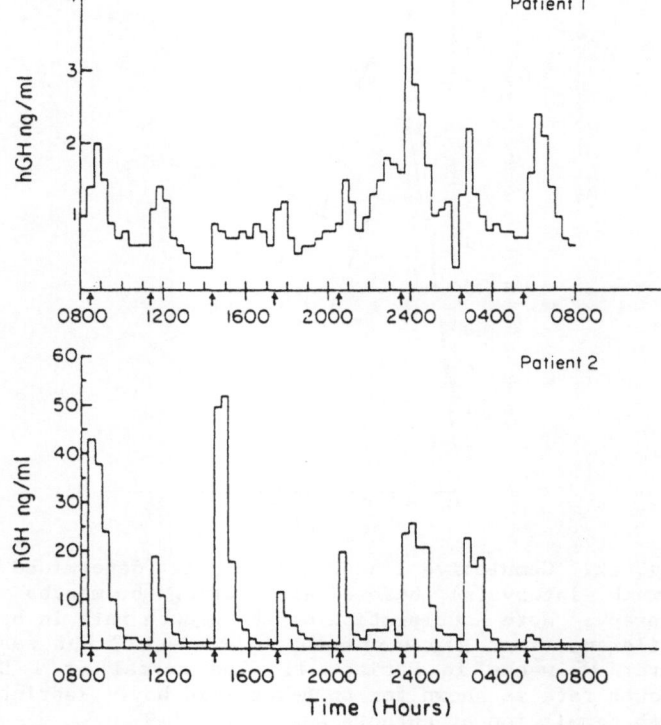

Fig. 10. Serum growth hormone (hGH) levels determined at 20-min intervals for 24 h during which growth hormone-releasing factor was administered every 3 h (arrows). Note the very small increase of growth hormone in Patient 1 in response to the pulses of growth hormone-releasing factor, as compared with the larger increases in Patient 2. In contrast, the responses to the supramaximal intravenous doses were larger in both patients before and during therapy (see Figure 9). The scales on the vertical axes in the two panels are different. Reprinted with permission of authors and editor (19).

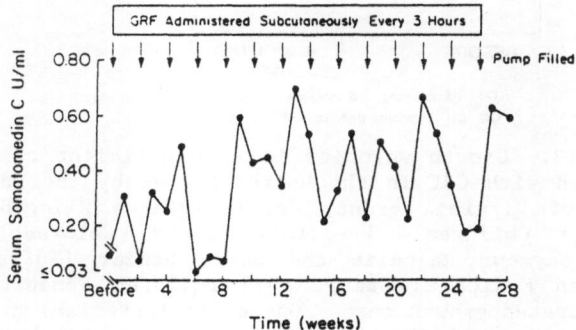

Fig. 11. Serum somatomedin-C levels in Patient 2, determined weekly during 6 months of therapy. Note the levels rose in response to therapy. They were lowest when the pump inadvertently became empty at the end of the sixth and eighth weeks. Note also the marked variability in the levels. Reprinted with permission of authors and editor (19).

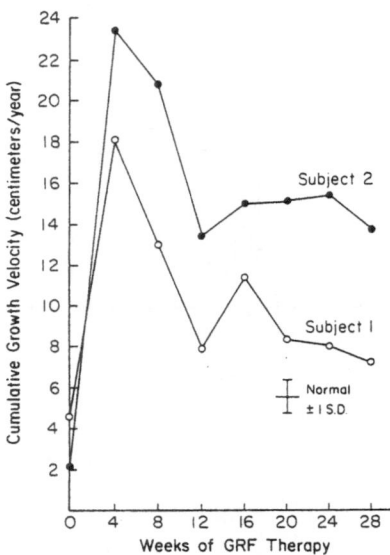

Fig. 12. Cumulative linear growth rate (determined at 4-week intervals) before and during 6 months of therapy. Note acceleration of the growth rate in both children, which was sustained in Patient 2 but waned after 16 weeks in Patient 1. The normal (± 1 SD) growth rate is shown for an 8-year-old boy. Reprinted with permission of authors and editor (19).

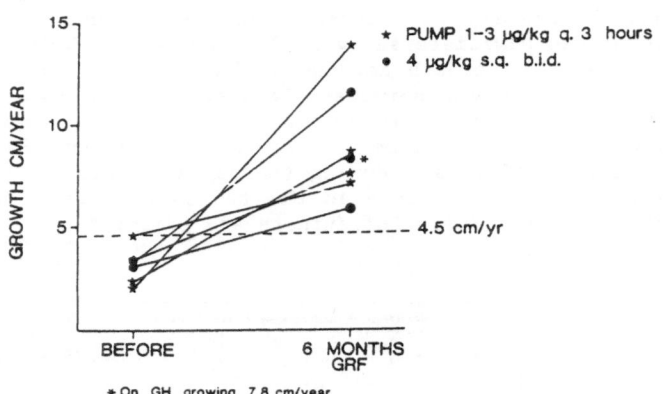

Fig. 13. Growth velocity in 7 GH deficient children treated with GRF in the United States by the University of Virginia group, Dr. Georgeanna Klingensmith (Denver Children's Hospital, Denver, Colorado) and Drs. Seymour Reichlin and Boris Senior (Tufts New England Medical Center). All children demonstrated accelerated growth rate. One child (asterisk) grew at the same rate during GRF therapy as on growth hormone. During the 6 months prior to GRF therapy, this child did not take the growth hormone and did not grow (data not shown). Note that 4 children were treated with subcutaneous injections every 3 h administered by Pulsamat® pump (Ferring) and 3 received GRF, 4 µg/kg, subcutaneously twice daily.

ered a dose every 3 h, or by twice daily injections (4 6-month treatment cycles). Ten cycles were administered by pump overnight only and 14 using the pump throughout the 24 h. All children who received GHRH using the pump throughout 24 h and all receiving twice daily injections had accelerated growth velocity at a rate indistinguishable from GH deficient children receiving GH therapy. Eight of the 10 children receiving GHRH using the pump overnight only had accelerated growth rates.

Five children developed low titers of circulating anti-GHRH antibodies that disappeared either during continuous treatment or after discontinuation of GHRH. There is no evidence to suggest that these antibodies inhibited the GH response to GHRH or impaired the growth velocity.

REFERENCES

1. Green JD, Harris GW. The neurovascular link between the neuro-hypophysis and adenohypophysis. J Endocrinol 1947; 5:136.
2. Reichlin S. Growth hormone content of pituitaries from rats with hypothalamic lesions. Endocrinology 1961; 69:225.
3. Thorner MO, Perryman RL, Cronin MJ, et al. Somatotroph hyperplasia: successful treatment of acromegaly by removal of a pancreatic tumor secreting a growth releasing factor. J Clin Invest 1982; 70:965.
4. Rivier J, Spiess J, Thorner M, Vale W. Sequence analysis of a growth hormone releasing factor from a human pancreatic islet tumor. Biochemistry 1982; 24:6037.
5. Guilleman R, Brazeau P, Bohlen P, et al. Growth hormone-releasing factor from a human pancreatic tumor that caused acromegaly. Science 1982; 218:585.
6. Bohlen P, Brazeau P, Block B, et al. Human hypothalamic growth hormone-releasing factor (GRF): evidence for two forms identical to tumor derived GRF-44-NH$_2$ and GRF-40. Biochem Biophys Res Commun 1983; 114:930.
7. Mayo KE, Vale W, Rivier J, et al. Expression cloning and sequence of cDNA encoding human growth hormone-releasing factor. Nature 1983; 306:86.
8. Tannenbaum GS. Growth hormone-releasing factor: direct effects on growth hormone, glucose and behavior via the brain. Science 1984; 226:464.
9. Tannenbaum GS, Guyda HJ, Posner BI. Insulin-like growth factors: a role in growth hormone negative feedback and body weight regulation via the brain. Science 1983; 220:77.
10. Berelowitz M, Szabo M, Frohman LA, Firestone S, Chu L, Hintz RL. Somatomedin-C mediates growth hormone negative feedback by effects on both the hypothalamus and the pituitary. Science 1981; 212:1279.
11. Thorner M, Rivier J, Spiess J, et al. Human pancreatic growth-hormone-releasing factor selectively stimulates growth-hormone secretion in man. Lancet 1983; 1:24.
12. Vance M, Borges J, Kaiser D, et al. Human pancreatic tumor growth hormone releasing factor (hpGRF-40): dose response relationships in normal man. J Clin Endocrinol Metab 1984; 58:838.
13. Evans WS, Borges JLC, Vance ML, et al. Effect of human pancreatic growth hormone-releasing factor-40 on serum growth hormone, pro-lactin, luteinizing hormone, follicle-stimulating hormone, and somatomedin-C concentrations in normal women throughout the menstrual cycle. J Clin Endocrinol Metab 1984; 59:1006.
14. Rogol AD, Blizzard RM, Johanson AJ, et al. Growth hormone release in response to human pancreatic tumor growth hormone-releasing factor-40 in children with short stature. J Clin Endocrinol Metab 1984; 59:580.

15. Takano K, Hizuka N, Shizume K, et al. Plasma growth hormone (GH) response to GH-releasing factor in normal children with short stature and patients with pituitary dwarfism. J Clin Endocrinol Metab 1984; 58:236.

16. Borges J, Blizzard R, Gelato M, et al. Effects of human pancreatic growth hormone releasing factor on growth hormone and somatomedin C levels in patients with idiopathic growth hormone deficiency. Lancet 1983; ii:119.

17. Borges J, Blizzard R, Evans W, et al. Stimulation of growth hormone (GH) and somatomedin C in idiopathic GH-deficient subjects by intermittent pulsatile administration of synthetic human pancreatic tumor GH-releasing factor. J Clin Endocrinol Metab 1984; 59:1.

18. Rogol AD, Blizzard RM, Foley TP Jr, et al. Growth hormone releasing hormone and growth hormone: genetic studies in familial growth hormone deficiency. Pediatr Res 1985; 19:489.

19. Thorner M, Reschke J, Chitwood J, et al. Acceleration of growth in two children treated with human growth hormone releasing factor. N Engl J Med 1985; 312:4.

20. Spiliotis B, August G, Hung W, Sonis W, Mendelsohn W, Bercu BB. Growth hormone neurosecretory dysfunction: a treatable cause of short stature. JAMA 1984; 152:2223.

26

IMPROVEMENT IN GROWTH RATE AND MEAN PREDICTED HEIGHT DURING LONG-TERM TREATMENT WITH GROWTH HORMONE IN CHILDREN WITH NON-GROWTH HORMONE DEFICIENT SHORT STATURE

Selna L. Kaplan, M.D., Ph.D.

Department of Pediatrics
University of California
San Francisco, CA 94143

INTRODUCTION

Children with short stature, a normal RIA GH response to provocative stimuli, delayed bone age and a decreased growth rate for age comprise a heterogenous group (1-7). An inadequate growth rate in prepubertal children suggests deficits of growth promoting factors and/or hormones or the inability to respond to them (8-20). The term "short normal" children is an inappropriate designation for these children.

In our initial studies, the magnitude of the retardation in the bone age and the height velocity for age correlated significantly with the response to a 6-month trial treatment with growth hormone (6). In most of these patients, serum somatomedin-C was appropriate for bone age. In 60-80% of short children with an inadequate growth rate, an improvement in growth rate has been reported after treatment with growth hormone (1-8,12,21).

This report describes the long-term effect (2-6 years) of growth hormone on growth rate and predicted height in children identified as responders after a 6-month treatment course.

METHODS AND RESULTS

Table 1 lists the characteristics of the 34 children selected for treatment with growth hormone. The age range of the 14 females was 6.5-12.5 years and of the 20 males, 4.0-14.5 years. The initial dose of hGH was 0.1-0.2 U/kg. Historical data on 13 nontreated male prepubertal children with comparable retardation in height, bone age and growth rate were used for comparison.

All selected children had a peak GH response of more than 7 ng/ml to at least one provocative stimulus (1). In 80% of the children, heights and weights were available for 1-3 years prior to treatment.

Bone age was determined by the method of Greulich and Pyle. Height prediction was determined by the Bayley-Pinneau method (22) for bone age 7 years or more and by the RWT method (23) for bone age less than 7 years.

Table 1. Basal data of non-GH deficient children.

	Height (-SD)	BA Retardation (years) (-SD)	Height Velocity for BA (cm)	Deviation from Midparental Height (cm)	Target Height (cm)
Mean ± SD	-3.1 ± 0.5	2.3 ± 0.9	-1.7 ± 1.1	-9.3 ± 1.0	-9.4 ± 1.4
Range	-2.3 to -4.1	1.0 to 4.0	-1 to -4.6	-0.4 to 27	-1.0 to -22

The mean growth before and at intervals after administration of growth hormone is shown on Table 2. Twenty-four of the 34 children had an improved growth rate of 2 cm or more above baseline after 6 months of treatment. Ten patients showed no change or less than 2 cm increment in growth rate. During the 6 months without treatment, reversion to pre-treatment growth rate was observed in 17 patients. In 11 patients, the growth rate was 1-3 cm less. In 6 children who progressed into puberty, the augmented growth rate was sustained.

In 19 of the responders, growth hormone treatment was re-initiated. Eight of these children have maintained an augmented growth rate after 2-6 years of treatment. The advancement in bone age was equivalent to the advancement in chronological age.

The initial mean height prediction was 5 cm or more below the mid-parental or target height in 62.5% of the children. The increase in mean height prediction was 4-10.9 cm in 50% of the patients after 2-6 years of therapy. In the group of 13 nontreated children with short stature, the increment in height prediction was less than 2.5 cm during 2-4 years of observation.

None of the children developed detectable antibodies to either pituitary or methionyl growth hormone during the entire course of treatment. Urinary glucose, 2-h postprandial serum glucose, and Hgb AlC was within normal range during treatment.

DISCUSSION

Prior reports have demonstrated the beneficial effects of short-term therapy with growth hormone in non-growth hormone deficient short children (2-8,14,21). This study provides the first data on long-term treatment of these children. A sustained improvement in growth rate and in mean height prediction was demonstrated in 50% of the children treated for 2-6 years. This effect on predicted height is evident after 1½ years of interrupted treatment or 1 year of continuous therapy. Since potential beneficial effects may be dissipated during 6 months off therapy, we propose that if an increment of 3 cm/year or more above baseline rate is induced during the first 6 months of treatment, long-term therapy should be maintained. The ultimate aim of growth hormone therapy in the child with short stature is to improve final height. At present, 50% of the children of the initial group have maintained an augmented growth rate and height predic-tion. However, final height measurements will be necessary to validate the observed advancement in predicted height (24-27).

None of the current GH secretory pattern or stimulatory tests pro-vides a reliable discriminatory index for selection for response to ther-apy. Thus, it is not clear whether the administered growth hormone is

Table 2. Growth velocity (cm/year ± SD) before and at
intervals after therapy with hGH.

	Pre	6 mos Rx	6 mos no Rx	12-24 mos Rx	24-48 mos Rx
NN	34	34	33	19	8
Mean ± SD	4.4 ± 0.9	7.1 ± 1.9	4.2 ± 1.6	6.7 ± 2.0	8.0 ± 2.2
Range	(2.0-5.8)	(4.6-11.8)	(1.7-9.0)	(5.0-9.4)	(6.0-10.2)

supplemental or replacement therapy. In addition, the appropriate dose per kilogram of body weight may not have been optimal for all the children in this study. At present, the use of higher doses should not be considered until adequate data are available on the toxic dose of growth hormone.

In summary, short children with normal immunoreactive levels of growth hormone, with a growth rate below the fifth percentile for age, a bone age retardation of 2 years or more, and a mean predicted height that is 5 cm less than midparental or target height merit a trial treatment with growth hormone.

REFERENCES

1. Kaplan SL, Abrams CAL, Bell JJ, Conte FA, Grumbach MM. I. Changes in serum level of growth hormone following hypoglycemia in 134 children with growth retardation. Pediatr Res 1960; 2:43-63.
2. Grunt JA, Enriquez AP. Acute and long-term responsiveness to growth hormone in children with short stature. Pediatr Res 1972; 6:664-74.
3. Rudman D, Kutner MH, Blackston RD, Jansen RD, Patterson JH. Normal variant short stature: subclassification based on responses to exogenous human growth hormone. J Clin Endocrinol Metab 1979; 49:92-9.
4. Lenko HL, Leisti S, Perheentupa J. The efficacy of growth hormone in different types of growth failures: analysis of 101 cases. Eur J Pediatr 1982; 138:241-9.
5. Tanner JM, Whitehouse RH, Hughes PCR, Vince FP. Effect of human growth hormone treatment for 1 to 7 years on growth of 100 children with growth hormone deficiency, low birth weight, inherited smallness, Turner's syndrome and other complaints. Arch Dis Child 1971; 46:745-82.
6. Van Vliet G, Styne DM, Kaplan SL, Grumbach MM. Growth hormone treatment for short stature. N Engl J Med 1983; 309:1016-22.
7. Plotnick LP, Van Meter QL, Kowarski AA. Human growth hormone treatment of children with growth failure and normal growth hormone levels by immunoassay. Pediatrics 1983; 71:324-7.
8. Grunt JA, Howard C, Daughaday WH. Comparison of growth and somatomedin responses following growth hormone treatment in children with small-for-date short stature, significant idiopathic short stature, and hypopituitarism. Acta Endocrinol (Copenh) 1984; 106:168-74.
9. Wise PH, Burnet RB, Geary TD, Berriman H. Selective impairment of growth hormone response to pharmacological tests. Arch Dis Child 1975; 50:210-4.
10. Cacciari E, Coccagna G, Cicognani A, et al. Growth hormone release during sleep in growth-retarded children with normal response to pharmacological tests. Arch Dis Child 1978; 53:487-90.

11. Plotnick LP, Lee PA, Migeon CJ, Kowarski AA. Comparison of physiological and pharmacological tests of growth hormone function in children with short statute. J Clin Endocrinol Metab 1979; 48:811-5.

12. Spiliotis B, August G, Hung W, Sonis W, Mendelson W, Bercu BB. Growth hormone neurosecretory dysfunction: a treatable cause of short stature. JAMA 1984; 251:2223-30.

13. Siegel SF, Beeker DJ, Lee PH, Gutai JP, Foley TP, Drash AL. Comparison of physiologic and pharmacologic assessment of growth hormone secretion. Am J Dis Child 1984; 138:540-3.

14. Bercu BB, Shulman D, Root AW, Spiliotis BE. Growth hormone provocative testing frequently does not reflect endogenous growth hormone secretion. J Clin Endocrinol Metab 1986; 63:709-16.

15. Frazier TE, Gavin JR, Daughaday WH, Hillman RE, Weldon VV. Growth hormone-dependent growth failure. J Pediatr 1982; 101:12-5.

16. Blethen SL, Chasalow FI. Use of a two-site immunoradiometric assay for growth hormone (GH) in identifying children with GH dependent growth failure. J Clin Endocrinol Metab 1983; 57:1031-5.

17. Tokuhiro E, Dean HJ, Friesen HG, Rudman D. Comparative study of serum human growth measurements with NB2 lymphoma cell bioassay, IM-9 receptor modulation assay and radioimmunoassay in children with disorders of growth. J Clin Endocrinol Metab 1984; 58:549-54.

18. Kowarski AA, Schnieder J, Ben-Balim E, Weldon VV, Daughaday WH. Growth failure with normal serum RIA-GH and low somatomedin activity: somatomedin restoration and growth acceleration after exogenous GH. J Clin Endocrinol Metab 1978; 47:461-4.

19. Valenta LJ, Siegel MB, Lesniak MA, et al. Pituitary dwarfism in a patient with circulating abnormal growth hormone polymers. N Engl J Med 1985; 312:214-7.

20. Lanes P, Plotnick LP, Spencer ME, Daughaday WH, Kowarski AA. Dwarfism associated with normal serum growth hormone and increase bioassayable receptorassayable and immunoassayable somatomedin. J Clin Endocrinol Metab 1980; 50:485-8.

21. Gertner JM, Genel M, Gianfredi SP, et al. Prospective clinical trial of human growth hormone in short children without growth hormone deficiency. J Pediatr 1984; 104:172-6.

22. Bayley N, Pinneau SR. Tables for predicting adult height from skeletal age: revised for use with Greulich-Pyle hand standards. J Pediatr 1952; 40:423-41.

23. Roche AF, Wainer H, Thissen D. The RWT method for the prediction of adult stature. Pediatrics 1975; 56:1026-33.

24. Tanner JM. Use and abuse of growth standards. In: Falkner F, Tanner JM, eds. Human growth; vol 3. New York: Plenum Press, 1986:95-109.

25. Tanner JM, Whitehouse RH, Marshall WA, Carter BS. Prediction of adult height from height bone age and occurrence of menarche at ages 4 to 16 with allowance for midparent height. Arch Dis Child 1975; 50:14-26.

26. Zachman M, Sobradillo B, Frank M, Frisch H, Prader H. Bayley-Pinneau, Roche-Wainer-Thissen and Tanner height predictions in normal children and in patients with various pathologic conditions. J Pediatr 1978; 93:749-55.

27. Roche AF. Adult stature prediction: a critical review. Acta Med Auxol 1985; 16:5-28.

CONSTITUTIONAL DELAY OF GROWTH AND ADOLESCENT DEVELOPMENT

J. R. Bierich

Universitaetskinderklinik Tuebingen
F.R.G.

Height, height velocity and sexual development are growth parameters with great variations. In the European countries and the USA, numerous systematic investigations with regard to this variability have been carried out during the 1930s and 1940s (1-7). In 1931, Priesel and Wagner demonstrated convincingly this variation in groups of girls of the same age but different stages of maturity (4). The more advanced the sexual development, the taller the girls were. In 1933, Rosenstern reported a series of observations in late maturing adolescents (5). He wrote ". . . that there occur rather considerable retardations of sexual maturation which lie far beyond the normal range and that nevertheless the final result can correspond to the norm." In 1950, Lawson Wilkins added skeletal maturation to the usual growth parameters of height, growth velocity and sexual maturation (8). He considered this information particularly suitable to adequately characterize the general biological maturity of the individual (8). As it turned out, the late maturing children always had a retarded bone age. According to Wilkins, constitutional delay of growth and adolescent development (CDGAD) is characterized by the following symptoms: (1) retarded longitudinal growth, generally from early childhood; (2) retarded skeletal maturation; (3) retarded sexual development; and, (4) consistent family history.

Table 1 shows our experience of the extent of retardation of longitudinal growth and sexual maturation and its correlation to bone age (9).

Table 1. Correlation (coefficient of correlation or r) between bone age (BA) and parameters of development in patients with CDGAD.

	r
Height age/BA	0.92
Testicular development/BA	0.86
Pubic hair/BA	0.83
17 ketosteroids/BA	0.71
Testosterone (urine)/BA	0.86

We are indebted to Lawson Wilkins for the correct interpretation of the disorder under discussion. With respect to the relationship between bone age and sexual maturation, he concluded ". . . that a certain level of general maturity must be reached before the pituitary gonadotropic mechanism is activated" (8). Thus, a new concept emerged that the delayed sexual maturation is a secondary phenomenon, a sequel of the retarded growth.

Combining the two main features of the disorder, Wilkins coined the name "constitutional delay of growth and adolescent development" which is, in fact, to the point and appears much better than any other term, e.g., "idiopathic short stature," "essential growth retardation," or the German designation "constitutional delay of development." Rudman's designation, "normal variant short stature," appears ambiguous as it leaves open whether the disorder is temporary or permanent (10). Spiliotis and co-workers wrote in 1984: "We feel that the children with GH neurosecretory dysfunction may represent a substantial number of short children, some of whom may have been previously diagnosed as having constitutional delay of growth and puberty" (11). In my view, the designation "neurosecretory dysfunction" represents a pathophysiological conception. This kind of dysfunction is found in leukemic children after irradiation by X-rays, in other hypothalamic disorders (e.g., tumors), and also in CDGAD. However, the diagnosis CDGAD describes not only this dysfunction but a factual clinical entity, a genetically determined syndrome. Therefore, the classical designation of Wilkins should be retained.

HEREDITY AND FREQUENCY

With respect to heredity, the family history demonstrates a similar disorder in the majority of cases in one and sometimes in both parents. The children who inherit the predisposition from both parents usually have an even more delayed development. Figure 1 demonstrates a typical pedigree with a dominant inheritance pattern through three generations.

Concerning its prevalence, CDGAD is considered the most frequent growth disorder during childhood and adolescence and is by far the most frequent cause of retarded puberty. Of importance is the fact that the syndrome is often combined with constitutional or familial short stature. Tanner has coined the term "small/delay" to describe the combined problem.

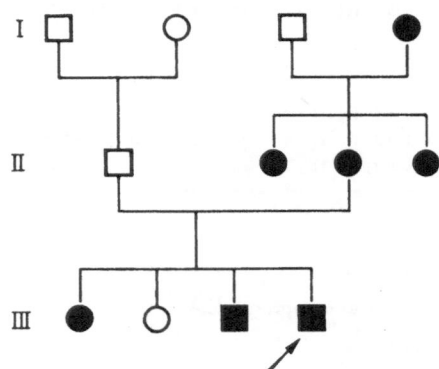

Fig. 1. Pedigree of a representative family. CDGAD (dark symbols) in three generations.

AUXOLOGY

Children who later develop CDGAD are born with normal birth length and weight. Frequently the disorder is manifest in infancy. At the age of entry into school, the children are among the smallest of their peer group. In the linear growth chart, the growth curve lies at or below the third centile of the norm (Fig. 2). At the time of normal age for puberty, growth velocity is markedly diminished. The characteristic nadir of the growth tempo which precedes the beginning of puberty can be less than 3 cm per year. Often, the parents claim their child has ceased growing. At the time of puberty, the growth spurt relative to chronological age is delayed by two or four years, but it occurs at the approximate time relative to bone age.

ENDOCRINOLOGICAL FINDINGS

In accordance with Wilkins' hypothesis that retarded puberty is a secondary phenomenon caused by retarded growth, plasma concentrations of sexual hormones and gonadotropins are low for chronological age but normal for bone age. After stimulation with gonadotropin or luteinizing hormone releasing hormone (LHRH), the peak gonadotropin responses also correspond to bone age rather than to chronological age. On average, the peaks are higher than in true hypogonadal hypogonadism, but there is considerable overlap of the two groups (13-15). HCG stimulation of testosterone secretion is a better diagnostic test, but it is still not entirely reliable. This test has proven beneficial particularly in prepubertal boys (16). Another method for the differentiation of the two groups is the measurement of the spontaneous secretion of the gonadotropins at night. Patients with CDGAD display a pulsatile output of FSH and LH; patients with hypogonadotropic hypogonadism do not (17).

In view of the importance to determine pathologic causes of retarded growth, investigations concerning growth hormone (GH) are of great interest. As a rule, the usual provocative tests with arginine, ornithine, insulin and glucagon render results within the normal range (18-22). In Figure 3, the results of arginine tests in some of our own patients with CDGAD are compared to those of healthy controls. Statistically, there is no difference between the two groups (22). In a minority of children, the GH responses were found within the hypopituitary range. Retesting these patients during puberty usually provided GH peak responses that were considered normal. Thus, the concept of a temporary and transient disorder developed (21,23,24). It is, however, incorrect to compare normal values obtained after the onset of puberty with the same normal values found prior to puberty. The mean stimulated values in normal adolescence are approximately twice those of prepubertal children. After provocative testing, such patients with CDGAD reportedly do not have GH peaks of the same magnitude as normal children in puberty.

In view of the disappointing results of the provocative tests, a number of authors investigated the nonstimulated spontaneous GH secretion during 24 h or during the night (20,25-28). Only in a few instances, low maxima during sleep were recorded, e.g., in 2 of 14 patients of Wise and co-workers (26).

Our own group investigated GH secretion during 5½ h of nocturnal deep sleep (29-32). The patients were compared to healthy controls with equivalent sexual maturation. Figure 4 shows three examples reported in 1979. In the 3 children with constitutional delay (of whom 2 were investigated twice), nocturnal secretion was markedly diminished. During the last 10 years, we have conducted similar investigations in 133 patients with

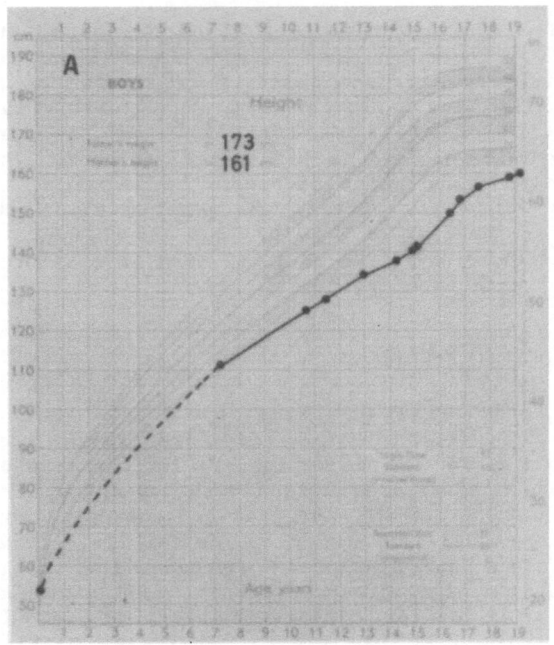

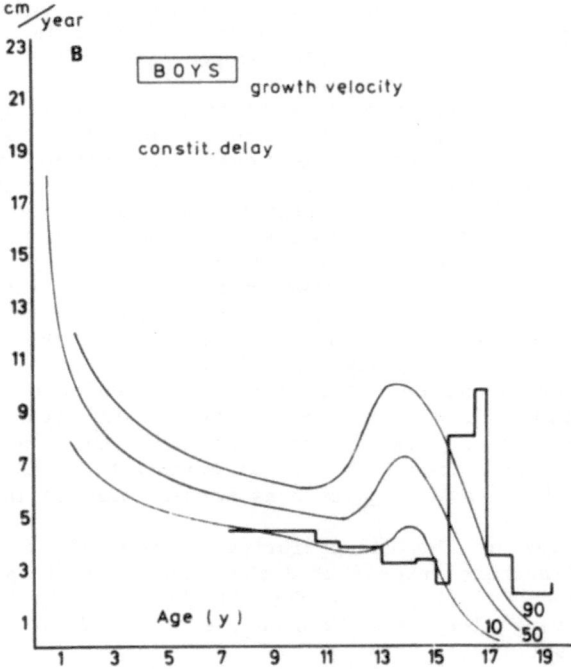

Fig. 2. A 19-year-old boy with CDGAD: (A) longitudinal height measurements; (B) height velocity.

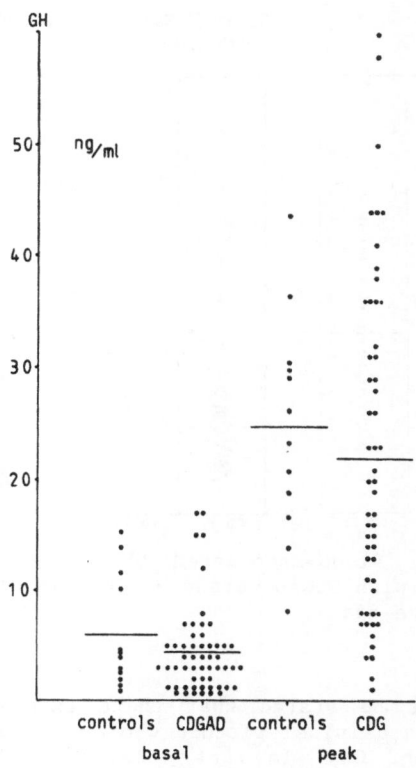

Fig. 3. Basal and peak serum GH levels during arginine testing in patients with CDGAD and control subjects.

constitutional delay (32). Figure 5 demonstrates the results of the 87 children in puberty stage 1. Three parameters were examined in all patients and in healthy controls: (1) the integrated total secretion of the hormone during the testing time interval of 5½ h; (2) the highest peak attained within the 5½-h period; and, (3) the maximum peak following IV arginine.

The integrated total secretion was markedly diminished in CDGAD with a statistical significance of P<0.01. The mean value of the patients was 53% of the mean value of the controls. Also, the highest GH peaks attained were significantly lower in CDGAD compared to controls (mean value of 17 ng/ml versus 37 ng/ml, CDGAD versus controls, respectively). However, with regard to the arginine tests, there were no statistical differences.

Comparable results were obtained in the patients in puberty stage 2 (Fig. 6) and 3/4 (Fig. 7). In the last group, no overlap occurred between patients and controls. This indicates that the basic disorder, i.e., diminished spontaneous GH secretion, is not a transient condition but a permanent feature of the patients. The discrepancy between the diminished spontaneous and the stimulated hormone secretion is noteworthy. It shows clearly that we are not dealing just with simple pituitary GH deficiency but with hypothalamic dysfunction, that is, a cybernetic disorder.

Similar findings to those we first published 10 years ago have been observed during the last 3 years by a great number of authors (11,33-37). The crucial finding, i.e., diminished spontaneous GH secretion, has been confirmed by all authors.

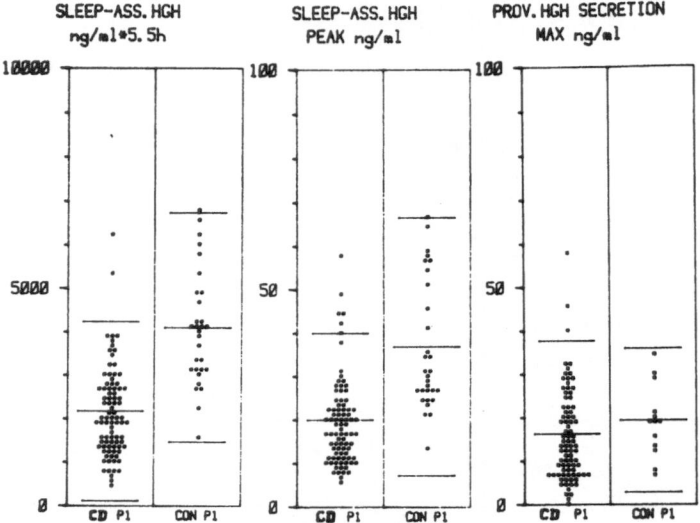

Fig. 4. Sleep-associated GH secretion in 3
patients with CDGAD versus 3 controls with identical bone age.

However, it must be stated that there exists a certain group of
patients with the same clinical picture who do not produce diminished but
have normal amounts of GH. In fact, they have significantly elevated
concentrations of GH but at the same time, low levels of somatomedin-C
(22,32). The first description of such cases were by Hayek et al. and

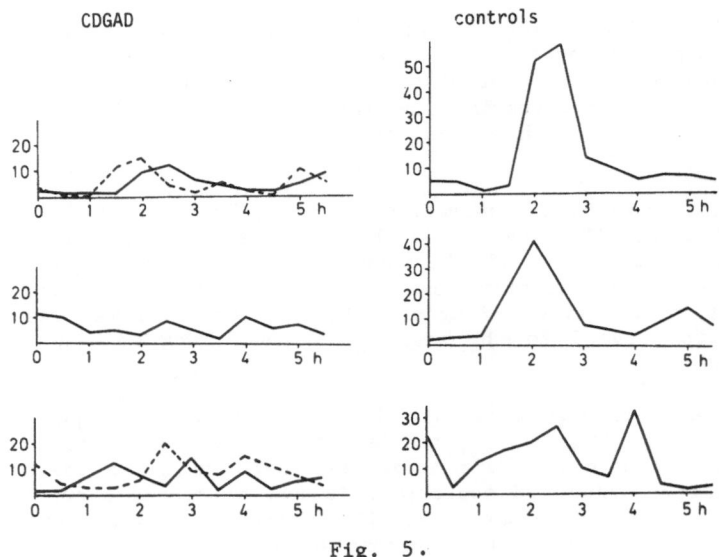

Fig. 5.

Fig. 5-7. Sleep-associated GH secretion and provocative testing with arginine in 3 pubertal-stage
groups (P_1, P_2, $P_{3/4}$) of patients with CDGAD versus
healthy controls. CD = CDGAD, CON = control.

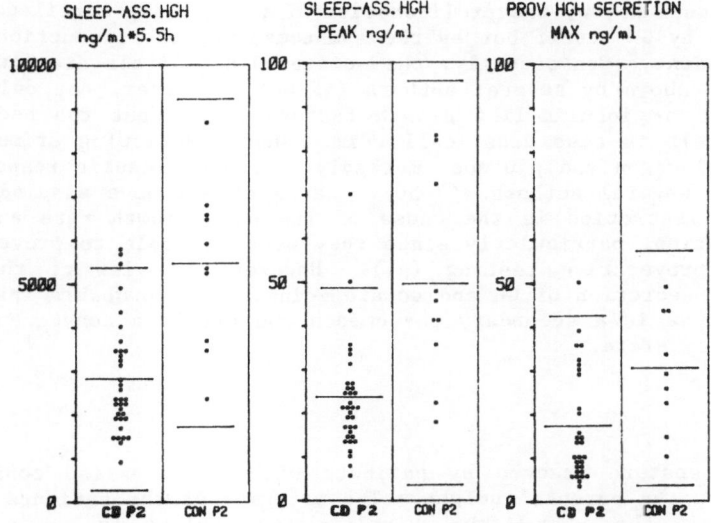

Fig. 6.   See legend, opposite page.

Kowarski et al. in 1978 (38,39).   These authors claimed the existence of a
biologically defective GH since radioreceptor assays gave distinctly lower
GH values than when measured by radioimmunoassay.   Meanwhile, similar
cases have been reported (10,22,40,41).   Recently, Valenta et al. and
Abucham-Filho et al. were able to prove the anticipated abnormal composition of the circulating GH.   Using column chromatography, they demonstrated disproportionately large amounts of polymers and only small
amounts of the physiologically active monomeric forms of GH (40,41).   In
the meantime, similar observations were made in one of our cases by Heinze
and Schleyer (unpublished results).

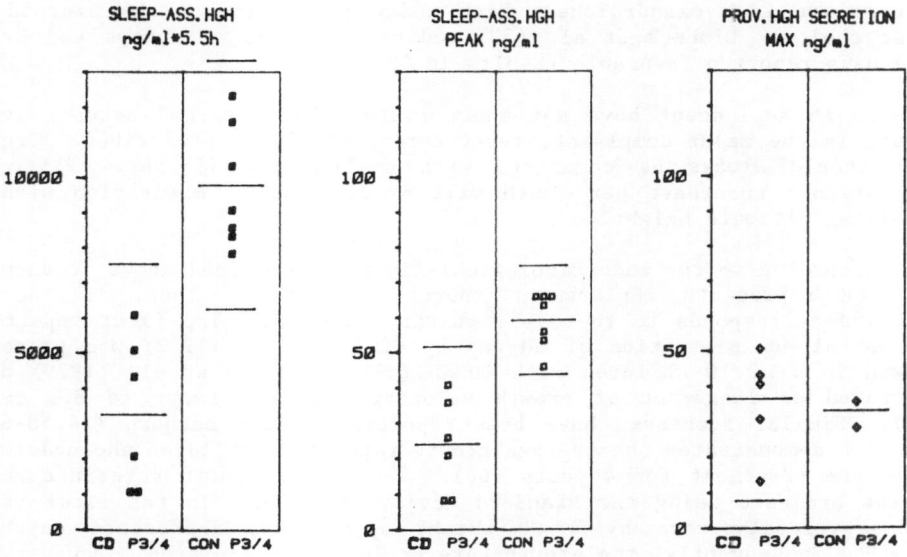

Fig. 7.   See legend, opposite page.

As is well known, the proliferation of the growing cartilage is stimulated less by GH itself but by the somatomedins, the production of which is GH dependent. Consequently, the somatomedin-C levels are low in CDGAD as has been shown by several authors (42-46). However, not only are the somatomedins or insulin-like growth factors lower, but the secretion of insulin itself is also drastically diminished. Following stimulation by arginine, glucagon and glucose, markedly decreased insulin responses were measured by several authors (47-50). Laron et al. have assumed that the low insulin secretion is the cause of the slow growth rate and delayed bone maturation, particularly since they were not able to prove GH deficiency by provocative testing (47). However, in view of the reduced spontaneous secretion of GH and somatomedins, it is probable that the low insulin output is a secondary phenomenon and merely a consequence of the GH deficiency state.

THERAPY

Adult stature reached by patients with CDGAD varies considerably, depending on the parents' height. The majority of the patients achieve a height within the normal limits unless they belong to the small/delay group. Nevertheless, ultimate height is below the mean for the population (51,52). In view of the temporary nature of the growth retardation, one has to ask whether long-term treatment with expensive hormones is justified. Most authors agree that this question can be answered only on an individual basis. Many patients, in particular adolescent boys, suffer considerably from their shortness, delayed sexual maturation and their high-pitched voice. At no other time in their life is the height gap with relation to their peers as great as in early adolescence. Their growth velocity reaches its nadir concurrently with the pubertal growth spurt of their age-matched peers. If severe psychological difficulties and inferiority complexes arise, treatment should be recommended.

In principle, there are two therapeutic possibilities: (1) anabolic drugs or testosterone, and (2) growth hormone. Anabolic steroids have been given to patients with CDGAD for many years. Since they are derived from testosterone, they usually possess weak androgenic properties. In high doses, they can accelerate skeletal maturation. The least side effects are from oxandrolone, which today is considered the steroid of first choice. Limbeck et al. (53) and more recently Stanhope and Brook (54) have reported favorable results in CDGAD.

If in adolescent boys not short stature but retarded sexual development is the major complaint, testosterone should be prescribed. Treatment should always be commenced with small doses (55,56). Fifty mg testosterone enanthate per month will promote sexual maturation without impairing ultimate height.

According to the endocrinological findings described above, treatment with GH represents replacement therapy in CDGAD. Thus, the dosage employed corresponds to that in pituitary dwarfism. The first report of successful administration of GH was by Grunt et al. (1972) who promoted growth in 4 of 10 children with CDGAD (57). Kastrup et al. (1979) demonstrated an increment of growth velocity from 4.1 cm/yr to 8.3 cm/yr (23). Similar successes have been reported by many authors (24,58-64). Figure 8 demonstrates the average growth rate of 16 children who underwent long-term treatment for 4 years (66). The annual growth rates are shown on the ordinate using the standard deviation score. In the first year, growth velocity rose by 4 SD which, apparently, represents catch-up growth. Subsequently, the growth rate gradually decelerated. However, up to the third year it still exceeded the pretreatment velocity.

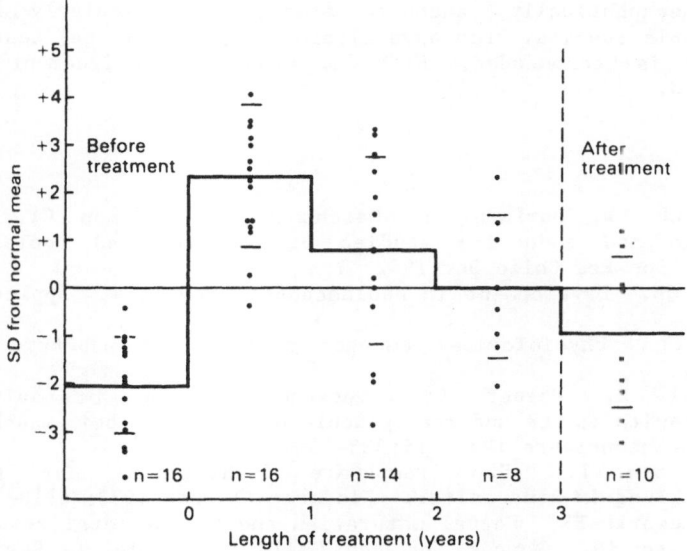

Fig. 8. Treatment with hGH over 4 years in 16 children with hGH. Ordinate: height velocity, standard deviation score.

Preliminary observations suggest that the growth prognosis of most of the children may improve by about 4 or 5 cm, depending on the age at which treatment was begun. However, since none of the patients has reached final height as yet, definite statements cannot be made.

Therapeutic trials with GHRH have not been conducted as yet. Interesting, and perhaps promising, trials are with the α-adrenergic drug clonidine. Pintor et al. administered clonidine over 2 months to 4 patients and ascertained accelerated growth rates concurring with increased values for serum GH and somatomedin (65). However, these investigations are preliminary and require confirmation.

SUMMARY

(1) CDGAD is the most frequent cause of small stature and delayed puberty during childhood. Skeletal maturation is retarded to the same extent as longitudinal growth. The delayed sexual development is a sequel of the retarded total maturation which correlates with bone age.

(2) Birth length and weight are normal. Usually, the disorder is first manifest in infancy. Growth follows the third centile of the norm or is even slower. Puberty ensues with a delay of 2 to 5 years.

(3) Provocative tests for GH secretion are usually normal. Determination of spontaneous GH secretion yields markedly diminished values. Our group measured spontaneous GH in 133 patients through 5½ h of deep sleep and compared the results to those of healthy children. Patients with CDGAD secreted approximately half the amounts of the controls. Also, the highest GH peaks attained during sleep were significantly diminished.

(4) CDGAD is not caused by an organic GH deficiency but is due to a cybernetic disorder at the hypothalamic level.

(5) Therapeutically, anabolic steroids, particularly oxandrolone, give favorable results. For boys already of pubertal age, testosterone in small doses is recommended. With GH, successful replacement therapy can be conducted.

REFERENCES

1. Greulich WW, Dorfman RI, Catchpole HR, Solomon CI, Culota CS. Somatic and endocrine studies of pubertal and adolescent boys. Monogr Soc Res Child Dev 1942; 7.
2. Jones HE. Development in adolescence. New York: Appleton-Century, 1943.
3. Jung ET. Physiological changes incident to puberty. IMJ 1941; 80:477.
4. Priesel R, Wagner R. Gesetzmaßigkeiten im auftreten der extragenitalen sekundaren geschlechtsmerkmale bei madchen. Zschr Konstitutionslehre 1931; 15:333–53.
5. Rosenstern I. Uber temporare disharmonien der korperlichen entwicklung im kindesalter. Kinderarztl Prax 1933; 4:18–31.
6. Shuttleworth FK. Sexual maturation and the skeletal growth of girls age 6 to 19. Monogr Soc Res Child Dev 1938; 3, Series No. 18. Washington, D.C.
7. Stuart HC. Physical growth during adolescence. J Dis Child 1947; 74:495.
8. Wilkins L. The diagnosis and treatment of endocrine disorders in childhood and adolescence. Springfield, IL: C C Thomas, 1950; 1957.
9. Bierich JR. Entwicklungsverzogerung. Monatsschr Kinderheilkd 1975; 123:301–6.
10. Rudman D, Kutner MH, Blackston RD, Cushman RA, Bain RP, Patterson JH. Children with normal variant short stature: treatment with human growth hormone for six months. N Engl J Med 1981; 305:123–31.
11. Spiliotis BE, August GP, Wellington H, Sonis W, Mendelson W, Bercu BB. Growth hormone neurosecretory dysfunction. JAMA 1984; 251:2223–30.
12. Tanner JM. Short stature of pituitary origin: the clinical state of the art. In: Gueriguian JL, ed. Insulin, growth hormone, and recombinant DNA technology. New York: Raven Press, 1981.
13. Roth JC, Kelch RP, Kaplan SL, Grumbach MM. FSH and LH response to luteinizing hormone-releasing factor: prepubertal and pubertal children, adult males and patients with hypogonadotropic and hypergonadotropic hypogonadism. J Clin Endocrinol Metab 1972; 35:926.
14. Job JC, Garnier PE, Chaussain JL, Milhaud G. Elevation of serum gonadotropins (LH and FSH) after releasing hormone (LHRH) injection in normal children and in children with disorders of puberty. J Clin Endocrinol Metab 1972; 35:473–6.
15. Job JC, Garnier PE, Chaussain JL. Effect of synthetic LH-RH on the release of gonadotropins in hypophysiogonadal disorders of children and adolescents. J Pediatr 1976; 88:494.
16. Dunkel L, Perheentupa J, Virtauen M, Maenpaa J. GnRH and hCG tests are both necessary in differential diagnosis of male puberty. Am J Dis Child 1985; 139:494–8.
17. Partsch CJ, Hermanussen M, Sippell WG. Differentiation of male hypogonadotropic hypogonadism and constitutional delay of puberty by pulsatile administration of gonadotropin-releasing hormone. J Clin Endocrinol Metab 1985; 60:1196–203.
18. Root AW, Rosenfield RL, Bongiovanni AM, Eberlein WR. The plasma growth hormone response to insulin-induced hypoglycemia in children with retardation of growth. Pediatrics 1967; 39:844.
19. Kaplan SL, Abramo CAL, Bell JJ, Conte FA, Grumbach MM. Growth and growth hormone. I. Changes in serum level of growth hormone fol-

lowing hypoglycemia in 134 children with growth retardation. Pediatr Res 1968; 2:43.

20. Eastman CJ, Lazarus L, Stuart MC, Casey JH. The effect of puberty on growth hormone secretion in boys with short stature and delayed adolescence. Aust NZ J Med 1971; 2:154.

21. Gourmelen M, Pham-Grung MT, Girard F. Transient partial hGH deficiency in prepubertal children with delay of growth. Pediatr Res 1979; 13:221-4.

22. Bierich JR. Minderwuchs. Monatsschr Kinderheilkd 1983; 131:180-92.

23. Kastrup KW, Andersen H, Eskildsen PC, Jacobsen BB, Krabbe S, Petersen KE. Combined test of hypothalamic-pituitary function in growth retarded children treated with growth hormone. Acta Paediatr Scand 1979; (suppl 277):9-13.

24. Trygstad O. Transitory growth hormone deficiency successfully treated with human growth hormone. Acta Endocrinol (Kbh) 1977; 84:11-22.

25. Blizzard RM, Thomson RG, Baghdassarian A, Kowarski A, Migeon CH, Rodriguez A. In: Grumbach MM, Grave GD, Mayer FE, eds. The control of the onset of puberty. New York: J Wiley & Sons, 1974.

26. Wise PH, Burnet RB, Geary TD, Berriman H. Selective impairment of growth hormone to physiological stimuli. Arch Dis Child 1975; 50:210.

27. Butenandt O, Eder R, Wohlfahrt K, Bidlingmaier F, Knorr D. Mean 24-hour growth hormone and testosterone concentrations in relation to pubertal growth spurts in boys with normal or delayed puberty. Eur J Pediatr 1976; 122:85.

28. Howse PM, Rayner PHW, Williams JW, et al. Nyctohemeral secretion of growth hormone in normal children of short stature and in children with hypopituitarism and intrauterine growth retardation. Clin Endocrinol (Oxf) 1977; 6:347-59.

29. Bierich JR, Potthoff K. Cause of constitutional delay of growth and adolescence: diminished secretion of growth hormone. Ninth Meet Eur Soc Pediatr Res, Venice, September 7-10, 1977.

30. Bierich JR, Potthoff K. Die spontansekretion des wachstumshormons bei der konstitutionellen entwicklungsverzogerung und der fruhnormalen pubertat. Monatsschr Kinderheilkd 1979; 127:561.

31. Bierich JR, Brugmann G, Schippert R. Assessment of sleep-associated hGH secretion in normal children and in endocrine disorders [Abstract]. Pediatr Res 1985; 19:609.

32. Bierich JR. Serum growth hormone levels in provocation tests and during nocturnal spontaneous secretion. Internat Symp Diag Treatm Imp GH Secr, Vienna 1987. Acta Paediatr Scand (in press).

33. Albertsson-Wikland K, Rosberg S, Isaksson O. Secretory pattern of growth hormone in children of different growth rates. Acta Endocrinol (Copenh) 1983; (suppl 256):72.

34. Costin G, Kaufman FR. Growth hormone secretory pattern in children with short stature. J Pediatr 1987; 110:362-8.

35. Hopwood NJ, Bacon GE, Beirins IZ, Hale PM, Mendes TM, Kelch RP. Growth hormone secretory patterns--aid to diagnosis of growth problems [Abstract]. Pediatr Res 1985; 19:608.

36. Rochiccioli P, Sanz MT, Calvet U, et al. Etude de la secretion somatotrope de sommeil dans 60 cas de retards staturaux de l'enfant. Arch Fr Pediat 1985; 42:665-70.

37. Zadik Z, Chalew SA, Raiti S, Kowarski AA. Do short children secrete insufficient growth hormone? Pediatrics 1985; 76:355-60.

38. Hayek A, Peake GT, Greenberg RE. A new syndrome of short stature due to biologically inactive but immunoreactive growth hormone. Pediatr Res 1978; 12:418.

39. Kowarski AA, Schneider J, Ben Galim E, Weldon VV, Daughaday WH. Growth failure with normal serum RIA-GH and low somatomedin activity: somatomedin restoration and growth acceleration after exogenous GH.

J Clin Endocrinol Metab 1978; 47:461.

40. Valenta LJ, Sigel MB, Lesniak MA, et al. Pituitary dwarfism in a patient with circulating abnormal growth hormone polymers. N Engl J Med 1985; 312:214-6.

41. Abucham-Filho JZ, Czepielewski MA, Ribeiro S, et al. Abnormal growth hormone and dwarfism. N Engl J Med 1985; 313:268-9.

42. Hall K, Olin P. Human somatomedin, determination, occurrence, biological activity and purification. Acta Endocrinol (Kbh) 1972; (suppl 163):1-52.

43. Brande L van den, Du Caju MVL. Somatomedin activity in children with growth disturbances. In: Raiti S, ed. Advances in human growth hormone research. DHEW Publ 74-612 (N.J.H.) 1974; 98-115.

44. Lecornu M. Sulfation factor in growth retardation, cerebral gigantism and acromegaly. Arch Fr Pediatr 1973; 30:595.

45. Ranke M, Bierich JR. Somatomedin and sleep-related growth hormone secretion in children with constitutional delay of growth and adolescence. Eur J Pediatr 1980; 133:179.

46. Bala RM, Copatha J, Leung A, McCoy E, McArthur RG. Serum immunoreactive somatomedin levels in normal adults, pregnant women at term, children at various ages, and children with constitutionally delayed growth. J Clin Endocrinol Metab 1981; 52:508-12.

47. Laron Z, Karp M, Pertzelan A, Kauli R. Insulin, growth and growth hormone. Isr J Med Sci 1972; 8:440.

48. Karp M, Laron Z, Doron M. Insulin secretion in children with constitutional familial short stature. J Pediatr 1973; 83:241.

49. Karp M, Laron Z, Doron M. Insulin response to intravenous glucagon in children with familial constitutional short stature. Arch Dis Child 1975; 50:805.

50. Boscherini B, Finocchi G, Lostia O, et al. Insulin secretion in children with growth retardation. Eur J Pediatr 1977; 127:21-6.

51. Preece MA, Greco L, Savage MO, Cameron N, Tanner JM. The auxology of growth delay. Pediatr Res 1980; 15:76.

52. Ranke MB, Schwaderer ML, Bierich JR. Die konstitutionelle entwicklungsverzogerung: eine einfache normvariante des wachstums. Klin Padiatr 1982; 194:289-94.

53. Limbeck GA, Ruvalcaba RHA, Mahoney P, Kelley VC. Studies on anabolic steroids. IV. The effects of oxandrolone on height and skeletal maturation in uncomplicated growth retardation. Clin Pharmacol Ther 1971; 12:798.

54. Stanhope R, Brook CDG. Oxandrolone in low dose for constitutional delay of growth and puberty in boys. Arch Dis Child 1985; 60:379-81.

55. Prader A. Constitutional delay of growth and puberty. In: Chiumello G, Laron Z, eds. Rec Progress of Pediatr Endocrin. Serono Symp 12. London: Academic Press, 1977.

56. Martin MM, Martin ALA, Mossman KL. Testosterone treatment of constitutional delay in growth and development: effect of dose on predicted versus definitive height. Acta Endocrinol (Kbh) 1986; (suppl 279):147-52.

57. Grunt JA, Enriquez AR, Daughaday WH. Acute and longterm responses to hGH in children with idiopathic small for dates dwarfism. J Clin Endocrinol Metab 1972; 35:157.

58. Bierich JR. Treatment of constitutional delay of growth and adolescence with human growth hormone. Klin Padiatr 1983; 195:309-16.

59. Van Vliet G, Styne DM, Kaplan SL, Grumbach MM. HGH therapy can increase height velocity in short children with normal serum somatomedin C and GH by RIA. N Engl J Med 1983; 309:1016-22.

60. Gertner JM, Genel M, Gianfredi SP, et al. Prospective clinical trial of human growth hormone in short children with outgrowth hormone deficiency. J Pediatr 1984; 104:172-6.

61. Underwood LE. Growth hormone treatment for short children. J Pediatr 1984; 104:237-8.

62. Albertsson-Wikland K, Westphal O, Hall K, Lindstedt G. How to predict the growth outcome of growth hormone treatment in short children [Abstract]? Pediatr Res 1985; 19:607.

63. Chalew SA, Armour KM, Raiti S, Kowarski A. Response to growth hormone therapy in children with normal GH by provocative stimulation but deficient integrated concentration of GH [Abstract]. Pediatr Res 1985; 19:195A.

64. Bierich JR. Treatment by hGH of constitutional delay of growth and adolescence. Acta Paediatr Scand 1986; (suppl 325):13-8.

65. Pintor C, Corda R, Puggioni R. Clonidine accelerates growth in children with impaired growth hormone secretion. Lancet 1985; 1482-4.

28

DOSE-RESPONSE RELATIONSHIP OF GROWTH HORMONE THERAPY

S. Douglas Frasier, M.D.

Department of Pediatrics
Olive View Medical Center
14445 Olive View Drive
Sylmar, CA 91342

Although human growth hormone (hGH) has been administered to growth hormone deficient patients for over 25 years (1), minimal data has been published on the relationship of dose to response. This paper will review the dose-response information which is now available for pituitary hGH, based on data derived from the initial year of treatment in growth hormone deficient patients.

While the minimal effective dose of hGH in growth hormone deficiency has been incompletely defined, two studies bear on this point. Rosenbloom (2) found that 0.4 mg (presumed to be 0.4 International Units) hGH daily failed to accelerate linear growth. Frasier et al. (3) found that 0.01 International Units (IU) hGH/kg body weight three times a week (tiw) was ineffective, and 0.03 IU/kg tiw produced a significant acceleration of growth in growth hormone deficient patients. Thus, the minimal effective dose of hGH appears to be no less than 0.03 IU/kg tiw.

There are very few studies in which different doses of hGH were compared without a change in dose schedule. Two of those which are available are shown in Table 1.

The British Medical Research Council trial compared a dose of 5 IU twice a week (biw) with 10 IU biw. As originally reported by Preece et al. (4) and subsequently expanded in the review of Milner et al. (5), there was a significantly greater (P<0.01) effect at the higher dose. The

Table 1. Direct comparisons of the effect of dose of hGH on the linear growth response to an initial year of therapy.

Study	Number of Patients	Dose of hGH		Growth Rate (cm/year)
		IU/Dose	IU/year	
British MRC	2	5 biw	520	7.2 ± 1.4*
	30	10 biw	1040	9.2 ± 2.2
US Collaborative	20	2 tiw	312	9.3 ± 2.2
	9	10 tiw	1560	11.9 ± 2.4

*Mean ± SD

United States Collaborative Project reported similar findings (6). Patients with idiopathic growth hormone deficiency who received 10 IU hGH thrice a week (tiw) showed a significantly greater response (P<0.01) than comparable patients receiving a more conventional dose of 2 IU tiw. The Canadian Medical Research Council Study also reported an increasing response to an increasing dose of hGH expressed as IU/kg body weight (7). It is evident from the British MRC study and the U.S. Collaborative Project data that although increasing the dose leads to a better response, the difference in growth rate is relatively much less than the change in dose. Similar observations were recently reported in a small Spanish study in which doubling the dose of hGH from 4 IU tiw to 8 IU tiw increased the average growth rate during an initial year of therapy from 9.0 ± 1.6 (SD) cm/year to 11.7 ± 0.5 (SD) cm/year (8).

In order to further define these dose-response relationships, we (9) administered varying doses of hGH on the basis of body weight to 93 growth hormone deficient patients over an initial 12 months of treatment. To be included in this analysis, growth hormone deficient patients were required to have a pretreatment growth rate of 5.5 cm/year or less. All patients were tested with insulin-induced hypoglycemia (10), and 60 were also tested with an intravenous infusion of arginine, either as a separate procedure (11), or as part of a sequential arginine-insulin tolerance test (12).

Sixty-five male patients and 28 female patients met the criteria for inclusion. Sixty-three patients had idiopathic growth hormone deficiency, and in 30 there was an underlying intracranial lesion.

The diagnosis of ACTH, TSH and antidiuretic hormone deficiency was made by standard methods, and patients with deficiencies of these pituitary hormones received appropriate replacement therapy. No patient received gonadotropin or gonadal steroid treatment during hGH administration. Forty patients received growth hormone treatment alone and 25 were treated with a combination of hGH and thyroid replacement. Seven patients received hGH, thyroid replacement and glucocorticoid while an additional 7 received this combination and antidiuretic hormone as well. Ten patients received growth hormone, and 4 patients received hGH and only antidiuretic hormone.

Study patients received either 30 (n=27), 60 (n=38), 80 (n=12), or 100 (n=16) milli International Units (mIU) of hGH/kg of pretreatment body weight intramuscularly tiw.

Human growth hormone was obtained from the National Hormone and Pituitary Program and was administered to patients under protocols approved by the appropriate human subjects protection procedures. Treatment was continuous over one year, and the dose was not modified during that time.

Differences between means were compared by the Student's t test. The chi-square statistic and correlation coefficients were calculated using standard methods (13). The statistical analysis of the log-dose response curve was carried out as described by Bliss (14) with the expert assistance of Elliot Landow, M.D., Ph.D., Departments of Biomathematics and Pediatrics, University of California, Los Angeles.

The response to therapy, expressed as absolute growth rate while receiving hGH is shown in Table 2. In each group of patients there was a highly significant difference between the treatment growth rate and the pretreatment growth rate. At each dose of hGH, P was less than 0.001. The growth rate of patients receiving 60 mIU hGH/kg tiw was significantly greater (P<0.01) than that of patients receiving 30 mIU hGH/kg. The growth rate of patients receiving 100 mIU hGH/kg tiw was significantly greater than that of patients receiving either 30 mIU hGH/kg (P<0.01) or 60 mIU hGH/kg (P<0.001). Doubling the dose from 30 to 60 mIU hGH/kg tiw increased the response approximately 1.3 times. A 3.3-fold increase in the dose from 30 to 100 mIU hGH/kg tiw increased the response 1.6 times.

Table 2 also shows the response to therapy expressed as the increase between the pretreatment growth rate and the rate of growth while receiving hGH. When expressed in this way, the response to 60 mIU/kg tiw was significantly greater than the response to 30 mIU hGH/kg (P<0.01). The response to 100 mIU/hGH tiw was significantly greater than the response to either 30 mIU hGH/kg (P<0.01), 60 mIU hGH/kg (P<0.02), or 80 mIU hGH/kg (P<0.001). Doubling the dose from 30 to 60 mIU hGH/kg tiw increased the response 1.3 times. A 3.3-fold increase in the dose from 30 to 100 mIU hGH/kg increased the response 1.6 times.

The calculated log dose-response equation for the absolute growth rate while receiving hGH over the range of doses used in this study is:

$$Y=-3.12 + 5.80 \log X$$

Y is the expected response in cm/year, and log X is the common logarithm of the dose in mIU hGH/kg given three times a week. The log-dose response curve calculated from this equation is shown in Figure 1. The slope of this curve is significantly different from zero (P<0.001), with a 95% confidence interval of 3.5-8.1. The 95% confidence interval for the mean response is 5.5 ± 0.74 cm/year at 30 mIU hGH/kg tiw, 7.2 ± 0.44 cm/year at 60 mIU hGH/kg tiw, and 8.5 ± 0.72 cm/year at 100 mIU hGH/kg tiw.

The calculated log dose-response equation for the increase in growth rate while receiving hGH over the range of doses used in this study is:

$$Y=-6.09 + 5.67 \log X$$

Y is the change in growth rate in cm/year, and log X is the common logarithm of the dose in mIU hGH/kg given three times a week. The log-dose response curve calculated from this equation is shown in Figure 2. The log-dose response curve calculated for this equation is also significantly different from zero (P<0.001). The 95% confidence interval of the slope is 3.4-7.9. The 95% confidence interval for the mean increase in growth rate is 2.3 ± 0.73 cm/year at 30 mIU hGH/kg tiw, 4.0 ± 0.44 cm/year at 60 mIU hGH/kg tiw, and 5.2 ± 0.72 cm/year at mIU hGH/kg tiw.

Table 2. Response to hGH therapy.

Dose of hGH (mIU/kg tiw)	Number of Patients	Absolute Growth Rate (cm/year)	Increase in Growth Rate (cm/year)
30	27	5.59 ± 2.30	2.53 ± 2.26
60	38	7.31 ± 1.75	3.97 ± 1.85
80	12	7.22 ± 3.12	3.79 ± 2.52
100	16	8.94 ± 1.19	5.79 ± 1.35
200*	10	10.08 ± 1.55	6.27 ± 1.96

*See text

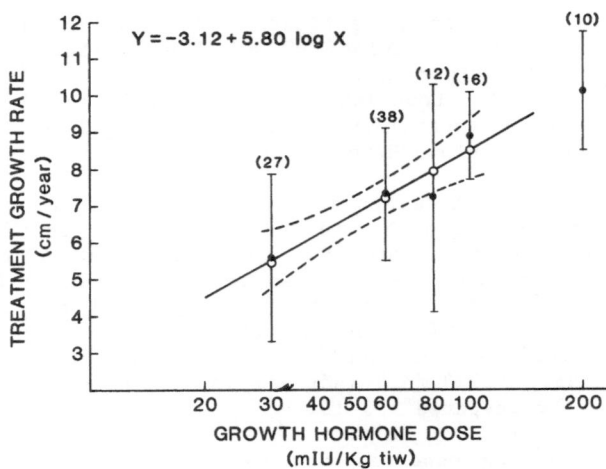

Fig. 1. Log-dose response curve of the annual
growth rate as a function of hGH dose. The
closed circles and vertical bars represent a
mean response plus or minus one standard
deviation at each dose. The numbers of
patients at each dose are shown in the parentheses. The calculated dose-response equation
is shown in the upper left-hand corner. The
open circles show the expected mean response
at each dose as calculated from the dose-
response equation, and the diagonal line is
the calculated log-dose response curve. The
curved lines encompass the 95% confidence
interval for the mean response at each dose.
The response to 200 mIU hGH/k tiw is also
shown (see text).

Initial support for the validity of these equations came from Rudman
and co-workers who administered three doses of hGH to growth hormone
deficient patients for 10 days and followed their growth response over the
next 8 weeks (15). The doses used were 20, 63 and 200 mIU hGH/kg daily
(16). While the design used in this short-term study is quite different
from ours, it is possible to derive a log dose-response equation (Y=0.99 +
3.45 log X) and a dose-response curve from the data provided. The curve
has a shallow slope which is similar to that derived from our data.
Increasing the dose 3.3 times from 60 to 200 mIU hGH/kg increased the
linear growth response only 1.6 times. The validity of our dose-response
curve was also supported by Nugent et al. (17) who found that the
administration of 67 mIU hGH/kg tiw resulted in an average linear growth
response of 6.0 cm/year which is not very different from the 7.5 cm/year
predicted from our equation.

Recent data on the response to pituitary hGH, reported as part of the
Genentech Clinical Trial of methionyl-hGH manufactured by recombinant DNA
technology, allows extension of the dose-response curve to 200 mIU
(0.2 IU) hGH/kg tiw (18-20). As part of that study a control group of 10
patients was treated with this dose of pituitary hGH (Crescormon, Kabi
Vitrum AB). As also shown in Table 2, the growth velocity of these
children was 10.1 ± 1.6 (SD) cm/year during the first year of treatment.
Over that time their growth velocity increased 6.3 ± 2.0 (SD) cm/year.
Our log dose-response equation would have predicted average total linear

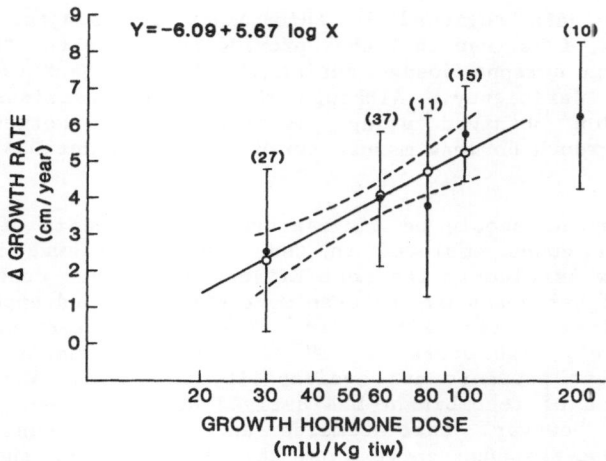

Fig. 2. Log-dose response curve of the change in annual growth rate as a function of hGH dose. The closed circles and vertical bars represent the mean response plus or minus one standard deviation at each dose. The numbers of patients at each dose are shown in the parentheses. The calculated dose-response equation is shown in the upper left-hand corner. The open circles show the expected mean response at each dose as calculated from the dose-response equation, and the diagonal line is the calculated log-dose response curve. The curved lines encompass the 95% confidence interval for the mean response at each dose. The response to 200 mIU hGH/kg tiw is also shown (see text).

growth of 10.3 cm/year and an average increase in growth rate of 7.0 cm/year at this higher dose. Figure 1 also shows the linear growth response to 200 mIU hGH/kg tiw and Figure 2 also shows the increase in growth velocity in response to 200 mIU hGH/kg tiw.

Recent experience with biosynthetic hGH has produced data which adds to the body of information bearing on dose-response relationships. In general, these data corroborate the dose-response curve. The Lilly clinical trial of authentic hGH utilized an hGH dose of 160 mIU/kg tiw. Thirty-six patients have now completed 12 months of therapy with this preparation (Thompson RG, personal communication, 1987). The dose-response equation predicts a response of 9.6 cm/year and a change in growth velocity of 6.4 cm/year at this dose. The observed growth velocity while receiving treatment was 9.1 ± 1.8 cm/year (mean ± SD) and the change in growth velocity was 5.4 ± 2.1 cm/year (mean ± SD) in patients who completed one year of treatment.

The Genentech clinical trial of methionyl-hGH utilized a dose of 200 mIU/kg tiw and treated 35 patients for one year (19,20). As described above, the dose-response curve predicts an average linear growth of 10.3 cm/year and an increase in growth velocity of 7.0 cm/year during treatment with this dose. The observed growth velocity was 10.3 ± 2.5 cm/year (mean ± SD) and the increase in growth velocity was 7.1 ± 2.5 cm/year (mean ± SD) during this year of treatment.

While the data reviewed in this paper are subject to different interpretations, I believe that they provide the basis for recommendations regarding growth hormone dosage during the initial year of treatment of growth hormone deficiency. Although these recommendations are derived from information obtained using pituitary growth hormone, they are applicable to growth hormone manufactured by recombinant DNA technology as well.

Growth hormone should be administered on the basis of body weight. Of the several doses employed in the studies reviewed here, 200 mIU (0.2 IU)/kg tiw is clearly the most efficacious. This dose also appears to be safe. Higher doses may be even more effective and appear to carry a minimal risk of metabolic side effects (21). The factors which limit the use of relatively high doses of hGH as initial treatment in all growth hormone deficient patients are availability and cost. With approval of the distribution of recombinant-DNA derived hGH, the issue of supply has become moot. However, cost remains an important consideration and analysis of dose-response curve from the standpoint of the cost-benefit ratio strongly suggests that a more practical initial dose is 100 mIU (0.1 IU) hGH/kg tiw. This dose provides safe and effective therapy at a reasonable cost. Should the cost become less due to competitive market forces, the cost benefit ratio would favor the use of a higher initial growth hormone dose.

ACKNOWLEDGMENT

The author wishes to acknowledge the expert secretarial assistance of Ms. Maria M. Alagheband.

REFERENCES

1. Raben MS. Treatment of a pituitary dwarf with human growth hormone. J Clin Endocrinol Metab 1958; 18:901-3.
2. Rosenbloom AL. Growth hormone replacement therapy. JAMA 1966; 198:364-8.
3. Frasier SD, Aceto T, Hayles AB, Mikity VG. Collaborative study of the effects of human growth hormone in growth hormone deficiency: IV. Treatment with low doses of human growth hormone based on body weight. J Clin Endocrinol Metab 1977; 44:22-31.
4. Preece MA, Tanner JM, Whitehouse RH, Cameron N. Dose dependence of growth response to human growth hormone in growth hormone deficiency. J Clin Endocrinol Metab 1976; 42:477-83.
5. Milner RDG, Rusell-Fraser T, Brook CGD, et al. Experience with human growth hormone in Great Britain: the report of the MRC working party. Clin Endocrinol (Oxf) 1979; 11:15-38.
6. Aceto T, Frasier SD, Hayles AB, et al. Collaborative study of effects of human growth hormone in growth hormone deficiency. I. First year of therapy. J Clin Endocrinol Metab 1972; 35:483-96.
7. Guyda H, Friesen H, Bailey JD, Leboeuf G, Beck JC. Medical Research Council of Canada therapeutic trial of human growth hormone: first 5 years of therapy. Can Med Assoc J 1975; 112:1301-9.
8. Vicens-Calvet E, Vendrell JM, Albisu M, Potau N, Audi L, Gusine M. The dosage dependency of growth and the maturity in growth hormone deficiency treated with human growth hormone. Acta Paediatr Scand 1984; 73:120-6.
9. Frasier SD, Costin G, Lippe BM, Aceto T, Bunger PF. A dose-response curve for human growth hormone. J Clin Endocrinol Metab 1981; 53:1213-7.
10. Frasier SD. The serum growth-hormone response to hypoglycemia in

dwarfism. J Pediatr 1967; 71:625-38.

11. Parker ML, Hammond JM, Daughaday WH. The arginine provocative test: an aid in the diagnosis of hyposomatotropism. J Clin Endocrinol Metab 1967; 27:1129-36.
12. Penny R, Blizzard RM, Davis WT. Sequential-arginine and insulin tolerance tests on the same day. J Clin Endocrinol Metab 1967; 29:1499-501.
13. Swincoe TDV. Statistics at square one. London: British Medical Association, 1978.
14. Bliss CI. The statistics of bioassay with special reference to the vitamins. New York: Academic Press, 1952:452-71.
15. Rudman D, Kutner MH, Fleming GA, et al. Effect of 10-day courses of human growth hormone on height of short children. J Clin Endocrinol Metab 1978; 46:28-35.
16. Rudman D, Chyatte SB, Patterson JH, et al. Observations on the responsiveness of human subjects to human growth hormone. Effects of endogenous growth hormone deficiency and myotonic dystrophy. J Clin Invest 1971; 50:1941-9.
17. Nugent JN, Moore DC, Ruvalcaba RHA, Kelley VC. Dose response curve for human growth hormone and oxandrolone by weight in children with hypopituitarism. Clin Res 1981; 29:111A.
18. Kaplan SL. Clinical trial of protropin. Meeting of the Endocrinologic and Metabolic Drug Advisory Committee Food and Drug Administration, Bethseda, MD, September 10-11, 1984.
19. Kaplan SL, Underwood LE, August GP, et al. Clinical studies with recombinant-DNA-derived methionyl human growth hormone in growth hormone deficient children. Lancet 1986; 1:697-700.
20. Kaplan SL, Underwood LE, August GP, et al. Clinical studies with recombinant-DNA-derived methionyl-human growth hormone in growth hormone-deficient children. In: Raiti S, Tolman RA, eds. Human growth hormone. New York: Plenum Medical Book Company, 1986:267-77.
21. Gertner JM, Tamborlane WV, Gianfredi SP, Genel M. Renewed catch-up growth with increased replacement doses of human growth hormone. J Pediatr 1987; 110:425-8.

29

EFFECTS OF HUMAN GROWTH HORMONE IN NORMAL SHORT CHILDREN AND IN PATIENTS WITH INTRAUTERINE GROWTH RETARDATION, GLUCOCORTICOID-INDUCED STUNTING OF GROWTH, OSTEOCHONDRODYSTROPHIES AND OTHER DISORDERS

Allen W. Root, M.D., and Frank Diamond, Jr., M.D.

Department of Pediatrics, University of South Florida
College of Medicine, Tampa, and All Children's Hospital,
St. Petersburg, Florida 33731

Human growth hormone (hGH) is of proven value in promoting the growth of hyposomatotropic subjects, but its effects in children with short stature due to other causes is variable. The present communication reviews the reported effects of hGH on linear growth in normal short children and those with "bioinactive" GH and in patients with intrauterine growth retardation (IUGR), the Russell-Silver syndrome, glucocorticoid associated short stature, various osteochondrodystrophies, chromosomal anomalies (other than Turner syndrome) and isolated metabolic disorders. In the children reported, stimulated secretion of immunoreactive hGH was normal when studied. A significant effect of hGH upon growth rate is considered to be an increase in growth rate more than 2.0 cm/year above the pretreatment growth velocity, the limit of normal variation in linear growth velocity (1).

"NORMAL" SHORT CHILDREN

There is a wide spectrum of GH deficiency states, including children in whom the only biochemical manifestation of GH deficiency may be decreased day-to-day secretion of GH. The following narrative reviews the effects of hGH administration to short children with normal GH secretion in response to pharmacologic or physiologic (sleep, exercise) stimuli and in patients with "bioinactive GH" as determined by discrepancies between radioimmunoassayable levels of GH and the biologic activity of endogenous GH expressed by its decreased binding to GH receptors on human monocytes, pregnant rat livers or IM-9 lymphocytes. Thus, within the "normal" category are children who might be classified in groups of patients with constitutional delay in growth and development, GH neurosecretory dysfunction or "bioinactive" GH. However, these children did not have IUGR, malnutrition, congenital malformations, chronic diseases, or other known causes of growth retardation.

Raben (2) first demonstrated that the growth rate of ostensibly normal, small children could be increased by the short-term administration of hGH (Table 1). He treated 5 such children 7.5 to 13 years of age and noted increase in growth rates of +3.3 to +6.8 cm/year over pretreatment growth velocities. In 1964, Soyka et al. (3) reported no significant response to hGH in a group of 10 children with "idiopathic short stature;" nevertheless, in 4/10 children, growth velocity increased >2.0 cm/year during hGH administration. In 1972, Grunt et al. (4) reported an overall 1.6-fold increase in linear growth rate in 10 children with idiopathic short stature during hGH treatment. However, in only 5/10 subjects was the increase in growth velocity >2.0 cm/year. These investigators also treated 4 short, obese children. In only one child did growth rate increase with hGH; whether these children may have had subtle hyperadreno-corticism is uncertain. Hayek and Peake (5) reported that the very short-term linear growth rate of 10 small, but otherwise normal, children increased approximately 2.2-fold after the administration of growth hor-mone for 10 days, measuring growth rate during the ensuing 12 weeks. A similar increase in growth rate was recorded in hyposomatotropic children after the same treatment schedule. Bright and co-workers (6) treated 2 children with hGH for 6 months and recorded a two- to threefold increase in growth rate. In the first child, a second course of hGH again resulted in an increase in growth velocity. However, in both children the post-treatment growth rates were slower than in the control period (i.e., "catch-down" growth occurred). Of interest, both of these children had normal 24-h GH secretory patterns (mean GH concentrations were 13.0 and 12.7 ng/ml respectively). Only 6/15 normal short reported by Van Vliet et al. (7) experienced an increase in linear growth rate >2.0 cm/year) (range 2.2 to 4.2 cm/year) during hGH administration. The responding children were young (7.1 ± 2.9 SD years), with markedly delayed bone ages (-3.7 ± 1.5 years; bone age/chronologic age = 0.48) and extremely slow basal growth rates (5/6 patients had basal growth rates below the third percentile for bone age). In this and other studies (8-10), neither basal nor post-hGH levels of somatomedin-C predicted the linear growth response to hGH.

Plotnick et al. (8) treated 16 short children with growth rates at or below the third percentile for chronologic (and bone) age. In 14 sub-jects, growth rate increased more than 2.0 cm/year during hGH administra-tion. Growth velocities after 4, 8 and 12 months of treatment were 8.6 ± 4.5 (n=16), 7.4 ± 2.9 (n=15) and 7.1 ± 2.3 (n=11) cm/year, respectively. Grunt et al. (11) treated 7 short children with hGH and recorded a 2.1-fold increase in mean growth rate and an increment in growth velocity >2.0 cm/year in 5/7. Gertner and colleagues (9) treated 10 normal short chil-dren (height more than 2.5 SD below mean for age, growth rates ranging between 3.6 and 5.8 cm/year and normal provoked and overnight GH secretory patterns). In 8/10 subjects, growth rate increased more than 2 cm/year during therapy. Albertsson-Wikland (12) treated 31 normal short children with hGH for one year. In 16 of 18 prepubertal children, growth rate increased 1.8-fold during treatment with no adverse effect upon the rate of skeletal maturation. Two prepubertal males, one with food allergies and the other with psychosocial dwarfism, did not respond to hGH. A third child grew but 1.6 cm/year more rapidly while receiving hGH than in the control period. All others recorded an increment in growth rate >2.0 cm/year. In early pubertal subjects, there was a 2.3-fold increase in growth velocity during hGH administration. This investigator noted no relationship between midparental height, previous growth pattern or provoked hGH secretion and the first year linear growth response to hGH. There was an inverse relationship between the growth response to exogenous hGH and the area under the curve of a 24-h GH secretory profile. Basal levels of somatomedin-C/insulin-like growth factor (IGF)-I and IGF-II did not relate to growth response to hGH, but the percentage change in IGF-I and IGF-II after hGH treatment did so relate. Costin and Kaufman (13) treated 17 short children with normal provoked secretion of GH, but mean 24-h GH concentrations <3.0 ng/ml. In 9 prepubertal children, growth rate increased 1.8-fold and in 7 pubertal subjects 1.9-fold during hGH admin-

Table 1. Human growth hormone treatment and "normal" short children.

Ref.	Year	N	Dose	Frequency	Duration	Pre-treatment	Treatment	Post-treatment
			HGH Therapy			**Growth Rate (cm/year)**		
2	1962	5	1-2 U	3-4x/week	4-8 mos	3.9±0.5**	8.0±1.5	—
3	1964	10	1-2 U	3x/week	3-11 mos	5.3±1.0	6.6±1.2	4.7±1.1(9)
4	1972	10	2 U	qod	6-20 mos	4.5±1.6	7.3±1.9	—
16	1981	2	0.08 U/kg	qd	6 mos	(see Table 2)	—	—
5	1981	10	0.13 U/kg	qd	10 days	3*	6.6	—
6	1983	2	0.1 U/kg	3x/week	6 mos	1) 3.4* 2) 4.3	8.0 12.0	<1.0 3.0
7	1983	15	0.1 U/kg	3x/week	6 mos	4.2±0.8	6.1±1.7	3.6±0.8(4)
8	1983	16	0.07-0.18 U/kg	qod	8-19 mos	3.6±1.6	6.8±2.2	—
9	1984	10	0.1 U/kg	3x/week	6 mos	4.3±1.0	7.4±1.6	3.7±1.9(8)
11	1984	7	2 U	qod	6-9 mos	4.1±1.1	8.6±3.2	—
12	1986	31	0.1 U/kg	qd	12 mos	4.1±0.8(16) 3.8±1.1(13)	7.5±1.2 ! 8.9±2.2 !!	— —
13	1987	17	0.05 U/kg	6x/week	6-12 mos	3.9±1.0(9) 5.1±1.3(7)	6.9±0.9 ! 9.5±2.1 !!	— —
10	1987	48	0.1 U/kg	3x/week	6 mos	3.4±0.8	6.9±2.6	4.1±1.8

qd = Daily	* = mean
qod = Every other day	** = mean + 1 standard deviation
3x/week = Three injections per week	(Number)
! = Prepubertal	!! = Pubertal

istration. These findings are similar to those reported in children with GH neurosecretory dysfunction and constitutional delay in growth and development discussed elsewhere in this volume.

In the largest series reported to date, Raiti et al. (10) summarized the results of the National Hormone and Pituitary Program Growth Hormone Subcommittee trial of hGH therapy in 48 GH-sufficient prepubertal children between 4-10 years of age with height below the first percentile (-3 SD), linear growth rate <4 cm/year and bone age more than one year delayed behind chronologic age. In only 3 children did the growth rate not increase during hGH administration. In 20 children who received a second 6-month course of hGH after a 6-month rest period, growth rate again increased almost twofold (3.6 ± 1.3 to 6.7 ± 2.4 cm/year). Bone age increased 0.3 years during the 6 months of hGH administration and 0.9 years in the ensuing 6 months, for an overall increase of 1.2 years in one year. The rate of change in skeletal maturation prior to hGH therapy was not reported. Of the 45 children in the trial whose growth rates increased during hGH therapy, 16 experienced "catch-down" growth after treatment (growth rates of 3.8 → 7.1 → 2.6 cm/year prior to, during and after hGH administration, respectively), and 22 had a "carryover" effect of hGH during the 6 months off treatment (3.2 → 4.4 cm/year before and after therapy). In 7 subjects, the posttreatment growth velocity was similar to the rate recorded during hGH administration (2.9 → 7.3 → 7.0 cm/year, prior to, during and after hGH). The latter observation suggests that there may be a population of children whose growth mechanisms perhaps were "primed" by a brief course of hGH therapy.

It must be emphasized that in the studies cited, the majority of patients were quite small, with delayed bone ages and slow growth rates, the doses of hGH were not uniform and the duration of treatment brief. There are no data to indicate whether hGH treatment will increase adult stature in these or other short children with normal GH secretion.

The concept of a "bioinactive" GH molecule as a cause of short stature was introduced by Kowarski et al. (14) when they described 2 short children with normal immunoreactive GH in response to provocative stimuli, but subnormal GH concentrations when measured in a rat liver radioreceptor assay. Both children responded to exogenous hGH with increase in growth rates (Table 2). Although somatomedin-C levels were low in these and subsequently-described patients, it is clear that basal somatomedin-C values do not predict responsivity to hGH therapy. Frazer et al. (15) described 4 similar patients, one of whom had the Kenny Caffey syndrome of medullary stenosis. In 3/4 patients, growth velocity increased >2.0 cm/year during hGH therapy. In 1980, Rudman et al. (16) described a group of children with subnormal radioreceptor assayable GH compared to immuno-reactive GH in nocturnal samples. These investigators subsequently reported (17) that in 7 such subjects linear growth rates increased in response to hGH administration in a manner quantitatively similar to that of children with classical GH deficiency. In this report, 2 children (Table 1) with normal radioreceptor assayable GH values also responded well to exogenous hGH, but 11 such children did not. Recently, Bistritzer et al. (18) studied the 24-h GH secretory pattern in 6 children with low IM-9 radioreceptor-assayable GH and found it to be normal. There was a 2.8-fold increase in height velocity during hGH administration in these patients. Although decrease in receptor binding of hGH suggests decreased bioactivity, direct measurement has not demonstrated decrease in GH serum bioactivity in a rat Nb2 lymphoma cell division assay (19), nor have there been reports of abnormal structure of DNA, messenger RNA or hGH composition in these patients. Indeed, the frequency of variant forms of hGH in short children is low. Gavin et al. (55) recently found that only 2 of 82 children with non-GH deficient short stature had decreased radioreceptor-assayable GH relative to immunoreactive GH levels.

Rudman et al. (20) administered hGH to 17 persistently hyposomato-medinemic short children with normal sleep-associated and pharmacolog-ically-induced secretion of immunoreactive GH. These children responded to the administration of hGH with increases in growth rates which were 50 to 90% as great as those recorded in hyposomatotropic subjects. With increasing doses of hGH, the growth rates of hyposomatomedinemic patients approached those of GH-deficient children. Valenta et al. (21) described an adolescent with a polymeric form of circulating hGH with decreased radioreceptor activity. Incubation of plasma with urea dissociated dimeric hGH into its monomeric form. The patient's growth rate increased in response to exogenous hGH administration.

INTRAUTERINE GROWTH RETARDATION

IUGR (birth weight and/or length 2 SD or more below the mean for gestational length, sex, maternal size and birth order) may be the result

Table 2. Human growth hormone treatment and "bioinactive" growth hormone.

			HGH Therapy			Growth Rate (cm/year)		
Ref.	Year	N	Dose	Frequency	Duration	Pre-treatment	Treatment	Post-treatment
14	1978	2	2 U	qod	8-12 mos	1) 2	12	—
						2) 4.5	8.3	
16	1981	9*	0.08 U/kg	qd	6 mos			
					NVSS-3(4)**	1.6	8.6	1.7
					NVSS-4(5)	1.8	10.1	2.2
15	1982	4	0.1-0.2 U/kg	3x/week	12 mos	4.2±1.3	7.1±0.7	3.9±0.9
18	1981	6	—	—	—	3.2±0.5	8.8±1.9	—

 * = Includes 2 children with genetic short stature from Table 1.
 ** = "Normal Variant short stature."

of infectious or toxic insults to the fetus, due to placental insufficiency of diverse etiology with consequent suboptimal nutrition of the fetus, associated with chromosomal abnormalities or constellations of congenital anomalies permitting an eponymic classification, or due to unidentified causes. Table 3 summarizes the results of hGH treatment in 101 children with IUGR in 8 reports. Despite the heterogeneity of the patient group and the therapeutic regimens, many investigators have observed an increment in growth rate during hGH administration. Tanner et al. (1) reported that in 17 children with IUGR, 10 of whom had the Russell-Silver syndrome (see below), the mean increment in growth velocity (+1.4 cm) during hGH administration was "barely significant and clinically unimportant." However, within this group several children displayed significant hGH-associated acceleration in growth rate which was maintained for 3 years of treatment. Grunt et al. (22) described 2 children with IUGR who responded to hGH administration with increases in growth rates of +4.2 and +8.7 cm/year, whereas in 4 similar subjects hGH was associated with changes in height velocity of -3.8 to +1.8 cm/year.

Investigators from the Johns Hopkins Hospital have published a series of reports detailing the effects of hGH in IUGR. Foley et al. (23) described 11 children with IUGR who received 1 to 5 U of hGH daily. In all subjects, there was an increase in growth rate (>2.0 cm/year) in response to one or more dosages of hGH. In 2 children treated with 3 different doses of hGH, more rapid growth velocities were observed with increasing hGH dose:

GROWTH RATES

		hGH		
Patient	Pretreatment	1	2	5 U/day
P-2	5.5	7.6	8.9	13.4 cm/year
P-6	4.2	5.5	6.1	11.4

In most patients, growth rates between courses of hGH declined, often to velocities below the pretreatment rate. Lee and co-workers (24) recorded a mean increment in height velocity of 2.3 ± 1.7 (range 0-5.1) cm/year during one year of hGH therapy in 8 children with IUGR. In 5/8 subjects, the increment was >2.0 cm/year. In 1979, Lanes et al. (25) described 19

Table 3. Human growth hormone treatment and intrauterine growth retardation.

Ref.	Year	N	HGH Therapy Dose	Frequency	Duration	Growth Rate (cm/year) Pre-treatment	Treatment	Post-treatment
1	1971	17*	10 IU	2x/week	12 mos	5.3±1.5	6.7±1.6	5.1±0.5
22	1972	6	2 IU	qod	6-10 mos	4.0±1.7	5.0±4.1	-
50	1973	7	-	-	-	-	-	-
23	1974	11	1 U	qd	8-17 mos	4.4±0.8(9)	7.0±1.8	-
			2 U	qd	8-12 mos	4.5±0.9(4)	7.0±1.3	-
			5 U	qd	5-10 mos	4.5±0.7(4)	10.4±2.9	-
24	1974	8	1 U	qd	12 mos	4.7±1.1	7.0±1.2	-
25	1979	19	1-5 U	qd	6-30 mos	4.8±1.4	7.6±2.3	4.2±2.5
26	1982	15**	4.8-8.9 U	2x/week	12 mos	1.9±1.2***	-0.7±1.1	-
11	1984	18	2 U	qod	6-9 mos	3.8±1.2	6.6±1.8	-

     * = 10 with Russell-Silver syndrome.

     ** = 3 with Russell-Silver syndrome (see Table 4), 2 with autosomol chromosomal anomalies (Table 6) and 2 with gonadal dysgenesis.

     *** = Velocity standard deviation score.

full-term neonates with IUGR and normal pituitary function who received two courses of hGH with an intervening nontreatment period. During the first treatment phase, growth rate increased >2.0 cm/year in 9/17 patients for whom data were available (no pretreatment growth rates were recorded for 2 children). During the second hGH course, an increment in growth rate >2.0 cm was recorded in 8/10 children. The authors concluded that many children with IUGR had sustained hGH responsivity over two periods of treatment.

Lenko et al. (26) reported a heterogeneous group of 15 children with "prenatal growth disorders," 8 of whom had IUGR not associated with a defined syndrome. In this group of 15 were 3 children with the Russell-Silver syndrome, 2 with gonadal dysgenesis and 2 with autosomal chromosomal abnormalities. Overall, the hGH response was poor in this group. Grunt et al. (11) documented an increment in growth rate >2.0 cm/year in 11/18 children with IUGR treated with hGH.

Unfortunately, the majority of investigators have not reported the effects of hGH upon skeletal maturation or the relative changes in height age compared to increments in bone age in hGH-treated IUGR children. Tanner et al. (1) reported that the increase in height velocity relative to bone age velocity did not change during or after hGH treatment in IUGR subjects, whereas for hyposomatotrophic children the ratio increased twofold. Thus, no significant "net gain" in growth was apparent in the hGH-treated IUGR patients. Lee et al. (24) noted bone age increments of 0.5 to 1.25 years during one year of hGH treatment, which generally corresponded to the increments in height ages. The data of Foley et al. (23) reveal that the height age/bone age ratio increased from 0.73 ± 0.19 (n=11) at the start of treatment to 0.81 ± 0.16 (n=9) at the end of therapy, an insignificant change again suggesting no overall effect on adult stature.

The studies of hGH treatment of children with IUGR have usually been retrospective, involving children who have been referred to pediatric endocrine units because of short stature. A paired prospective blinded, crossover study of the effect of hGH in young children with IUGR would be useful.

RUSSELL—SILVER SYNDROME

The Russell-Silver syndrome is characterized by low birth weight and IUGR, facial asymmetry with a high forehead, frontal bossing and small mandible (inverted triangular face), low-set ears and downturned corners of the mouth, hemihypertrophy (or hemiatrophy) of the trunk and limbs and postnatal growth retardation. This entity has a variable natural history, but in general the adult stature of these subjects remains below the normal range. Tanner et al. (27) treated 19 such children with hGH (Table 4), all of whom had normal endogenous hGH secretion, with an overall insignificant acceleration of linear growth rate during therapy. Although in 6/19 patients growth rate increased >2.0 cm/year during hGH administration, 3 of these subjects entered puberty during the study. The estimated net gain in height during one year of hGH treatment was +0.53 (±1.9) cm (range −1.4 to +3.5 cm, >2.0 cm in 2/13). The rate of skeletal maturation was not affected by hGH administration. Tanner et al. (27) concluded that hGH therapy was not effective in children with Russell-Silver syndrome. In 2 children with Russell-Silver syndrome, Angehrn et al. (28) observed no growth-promoting effects of hGH. Only 1/3 Russell-Silver syndrome children treated by Lenko et al. (26) experienced an increase in growth rate (+3.0 cm/year) during administration of hGH, but this coincided with attainment of a pubertal bone age. Stahnke (29) reported one child with Russell-Silver syndrome in whom hGH therapy was associated with an increase in growth rate. Partsch et al. (30) studied a boy with Russell-Silver syndrome and normal hGH secretion in whom growth rate increased from 5.4 to 10.4 cm/year during hGH therapy, declined to 5.1 cm/year during 3 months without treatment and increased again to 9.9 cm/year during subsequent administration of biosynthetic hGH.

Eight patients with Russell-Silver syndrome and classical or partial hyposomatotropism have been reported (30-33). In 5 children who received hGH, growth rates of 4.1 to 9.6 cm/year were recorded during treatment.

GLUCOCORTICOID—INDUCED GROWTH RETARDATION

Glucocorticoids inhibit linear growth primarily by antagonizing the anabolic effects of growth hormone mediated by somatomedins at the cellular level (34). They may do so by stimulating the synthesis of inhibitors to somatomedin bioactivity (35). In adults, glucocorticoids also impair stimulated secretion of hGH, but in glucocorticoid-treated children provoked hGH secretion is usually normal (36,37). HGH has been administered to a 16-year-old adolescent female with endogenous Cushing syndrome (38), with a resultant growth spurt of +2.2 cm in 6 months with no further height increment in the next 5 months of therapy. Children receiving glucocorticoids for treatment of asthma, juvenile rheumatoid arthritis, nephrosis and other illnesses have been treated with hGH in an effort to overcome the growth-retarding effects of steroids as well as of the underlying disease itself (Table 5).

The largest group of children to receive hGH is that with juvenile rheumatoid arthritis (JRA). Butenandt (39) administered hGH to 20 patients (3-15 years of age) with JRA. In 15, growth rate increased >2.0 cm during the first 5-7 months of treatment; height velocity increased

Table 4. Human growth hormone treatment and the Russell-Silver syndrome.

| | | | HGH Therapy | | | Growth Rate (cm/year) | | |
| | | | | | | Pre-treatment | Treatment | Post-treatment |
Ref.	Year	N	Dose	Frequency	Duration			
27	1975	19	10 U	2x/week	12 mos	5.5±1.5	6.8±1.4	4.7±1.4(17)
28	1979	2	-	-	-	-	-	-
26	1982	3	-	-	-	-	-	-
29	1984	1	20 U/week	-	36 mos	2.7	5-7	-
30	1986	1	1.4 U	qd	10 mos	5.4	10.4	5.1
Russell-Silver and hyposomatotropism								
32	1978	1	1 U	3x/week	12 mos	-	7.2	-
33	1978	1	8 U	weekly	3 mos	-	9.6	-
31	1986	1	0.1-0.2 U/kg	3x/week	60 mos	3.5	4.1-5.3	-
30	1986	1	3.1 U	qd	9 mos	3.7	7.1	4.6
54	1980	1	-	-	-	2.3	-	-

2.64-fold for the entire group. In 12 patients treated for one year, mean height velocity increased from 2.3 to 6.2 cm/year and there was >2.0 cm/year increment in growth rate in 9/12. Four children were treated with hGH for 2 years. Their growth rates (cm/year) were:

Pretreatment	Year 1	Year 2
2.9 ± 2.0	7.4 ± 1.7	8.6 ± 2.0

Changes in skeletal maturation and height increments were similar in this study. The patients in this report received prednisone 18-60 mg/m^2/week administered on alternate days, while hGH was injected on days when steroids were not given. The majority of other steroid-treated children received daily doses of glucocorticoids. Two of 4 children with JRA reported by Ward et al. (40) and Tanner et al. (1) demonstrated an increase in growth rate during hGH treatment. One patient reported by Root et al. (37) did, and one reported by Morris et al. (41) did not respond to hGH.

In 3/7 children with asthma (37,41,42, Root unpublished data) and in 1/2 patients with nephrosis (37,41), growth rate increased >2.0 cm/year during hGH administration. Individual patients with hypoplastic anemia (42) and iridocyclitis (37) have also responded to hGH. The growth-promoting effects of hGH may be transient. Root et al. (37) reported the most rapid growth rate to occur during the first few months of hGH administration and to wane rapidly thereafter. Butenandt (39), however, noted a sustained response to hGH in children treated with steroids every other day.

In some patients with JRA, hGH seemed to ameliorate the disease. The growth-promoting effects of hGH in such children are difficult to assess and depend upon the severity of the underlying disease and the dose and

Table 5. Human growth hormone treatment and glucocorticoid-induced growth retardation.

Ref.	Year	N	HGH Therapy Dose	Frequency	Duration	Growth Rate (cm/year) Pre-treatment	Treatment	Post-treatment
38	1966	1 *	2 U	4-7x/week	11 mos	—	+2.2	—
40	1966	2**	10 U	2x/week	12 mos	<2	6	—
42	1966	2	3 U	3x/week	15 mos	1) 3.6***	8.5	4.0
			—	—		2) 2.5****	7.0	2.5
41	1968 !	6	20-40 U	2-3x/week	4-8 mos	1.3±1.7	1.6±1.4	-
37	1969 !!	4	5 U	3x/week	6 mos	1.9±2.3	5.5±1.5	2.4±2.6
1	1971	2	10 U	2x/week	—	—	—	—
39	1979	20**	0.18 U/kg	3x/week	5-7 mos	2.2±1.2	5.8±2.9	1.9±1.6(6)
					12 mos	2.3±1.4(12)	6.2±2.4	—

```
   * = Cushing syndrome
  ** = Juvenile rheumatoid arthritis
 *** = Asthma
**** = Hypoplastic anemia
   ! = 4-Asthma, 1-Juvenile rheumatoid arthritis, 1-Nephrosis
  !! = 1-Asthma, 1-Iridocyclitis, 1-Juvenile rheumatoid arthritis, 1-Nephrosis
```

frequency of glucocorticoid administration. Although hGH seems to increase growth rate in many children with glucocorticoid-induced growth retardation, the long-term effects upon adult stature are unknown. Clearly, the most effective therapy of such children is effective treatment of the underlying disease and withdrawal of glucocorticoids.

PSYCHOSOCIAL DEPRIVATION DWARFISM

Growth retardation may be a consequence of disturbing emotional factors. The pathophysiology of this disorder is unclear; pharmacologically-stimulated and sleep-associated secretion of hGH may be abnormal or normal. Studies of endogenous daily hGH secretion in such children have not been reported to date. Tanner et al. (1) observed no effect of therapy with hGH in 4 children with psychosocial short stature (Table 6), the mean increment in growth rate being only +0.35 cm/year. Frasier and Rallison (43) recorded a 3.8-fold increase in growth rate during 18 months of hGH administration in one such child. They commented that the treated growth velocity of this patient (6.9 cm/year) was less than that of 9 hGH-deficient children (8.9-16.0 cm/years, average 11.9 ± 2.0 cm/year). No pretreatment growth rates were mentioned for the hyposomatotropic children. Incidentally, the patient of Frasier and Rallison (43) grew at the rate of 16.1 cm/year when placed in a nonthreatening environment. Albertsson-Wikland (12) commented that one patient with psychosocial dwarfism failed to respond to hGH in her series.

OSTEOCHONDRODYSTROPHY

In 1964, Escamilla and co-workers (44) administered hGH to 2 achondroplastic boys. In the younger boy (case number 2), whose bone age

Table 6. Human growth hormone treatment—miscellaneous.

Reference	Year	N	HGH Therapy			Growth Rate (cm/year)		
			Dose	Frequency	Duration	Pre-treatment	Treatment	Post-treatment
PSYCHOSOCIAL DEPRIVATION								
1	1971	4	10 U	2x/week	12 mos	4.4*	4.8	3.2
43	1972	1	10 U	3x/week	10 mos	1.8	6.9	0.4
12	1986	1	0.1 U/kg	qd	12 mos	–	–	–
OSTEOCHONDRODYSTROPHY								
Achondroplasia								
45	1964	1	3-5 U	3x/week	12 mos	3.8	3.8	–
44	1966	2	5 U	qd	1) 21/33 mos 2) 14/19 mos	2.9 4.5	3.0 6.9	– –
Hypochondroplasia								
3	1964	1	2 U	3x/week	3 mos	5.6	5.2	3.0
Cartilage Hair Hypoplasia								
26	1972	6	24-28 U	3-7x/week	12 mos	-1.9±1.3**	-0.6±1.3	–
Chondrodystrophia Myotonica								
Root (unpublished)		1	2 U	3x/week	6 mos	3.9	6.8	3.6
Morquio Disease								
46	1973	1	5 U	3-7x/week	30/36 mos	2.8	5.1	–
HYPOPHOSPHATEMIC RICKETS								
49	1964	1	2 U	3x/week	4 mos	4.9	3.8	–
1	1971	1	10 U	2x/week	12 mos	–	–	–
50	1973	2	–	–	–	–	–	–
MULIBREY NANISM								
26	1982	8	4-6 U	2x/week	12 mos	-2.0±1.7**	0.8±2.2	–
PRADER WILLI								
52	1979	2	5-10 U	2-3x/week	12 mos	1) 4.0 2) 4.0	7.3 6.0	– –
CHROMOSOMAL ANOMALIES								
Trisomy 21								
53	1986	5	0.5 U/kg	3x/week	6 mos	5.1±0.5	9.2±1.7	5.2±2.0
Ring Chromosome								
26	1982	2	4-6 U	2x/week	12 mos	1) -3.9** 2) -1.9	-1.2 +1.7	– –

* = Mean
** = Velocity standard deviation score

NO EFFECT: Celiac disease   Noonan
              Hypothyroidism   Neurofibromatosis
              Glycogen storage disease   Kenny Caffy syndrome of medullary stenosis (+)

was 4.5 years when initially treated, growth rate increased from 4.5 to 9.2 cm/year during the first 3 months of hGH therapy, but then decelerated to 2.1 cm/year over the next 4 months without treatment (Table 6). During the second 3-month period of hGH administration, growth velocity was 8.8 cm/year and then fell to 4.0 cm/year when hGH was discontinued. Bone age maturation paralleled the increase in chronologic age. In the older boy (case number 1), bone age was 13.5 years. Growth rate was but 3.0 cm/year during the first 3 months of hGH administration and the overall response to hGH poor; during a treatment period of 33 months, bone age increased to 18 years. Gershberg et al. (45) administered hGH to a 15-year-old achondroplastic boy with adult sexual development and noted no significant change in growth rate. A transient increase in growth rate was reported during the first month of treatment.

Escamilla (46) administered hGH to one of twin girls (chronologic age 13, bone age 9.5 years) with "atypical" Morquio's disease and recorded an increase in growth rate from 2.9 to 5.1 cm/year during 36 months of therapy. The bone age advanced to 14 years and sexual maturation coincided with the period of hGH administration. A twin sister of this patient received fluoxymesterone and thyroid hormone while her sister was receiving hGH and experienced a comparable pattern of linear growth, bone and sexual maturation.

Lenko et al. (26) studied the growth-promoting effects of hGH in 6 children with cartilage hair hypoplasia and reported a mean increment in growth velocity standard deviation score of +1.3 ± 1.4 (SD). In 4 of 5 prepubertal children, growth velocity increased by 1.5 to 2.6 SD during hGH administration. Horton et al. (47) described a boy with hypopituitarism and a noncategorized skeletal dysplasia (characterized by absence of chondrocyte differentiation in the endochondral growth plate) in whom treatment with hGH resulted in an increase in growth rate and improvement in the histological appearance of the cartilage growth plate. This author has treated a boy with chondrodystrophia myotonia (48) whose growth rate increased 1.7-fold during 6 months of hGH administration; however, a second 6-month course of hGH after a period without treatment did not increase growth rate substantially (3.6 to 4.2 cm/year).

MISCELLANEOUS

Gershberg et al. (49), Tanner et al. (1), and Crawford et al. (50) have treated 4 patients with hypophophatemic vitamin D-resistant rickets with hGH. In no patient was an acceleration of linear growth rate noted during therapy. However, Gershberg et al. (49) recorded an increase in serum phosphorus concentrations during hGH administration, suggesting that therapy with high doses of hGH might elevate serum phosphorus levels into the therapeutic range. Patients with celiac disease (1), osteogenesis imperfecta (50), glycogen storage disease (1), progeria (50), neurofibromatosis (26), primary hypothyroidism (26), and epidermolysis bullosa (51) have also been treated unsuccessfully with hGH. Two children with the Prader Willi syndrome have received hGH with increases of growth rate of +3.3 and +2.0 cm/year (52). Lenko et al. (24) reported that in children with Mulibrey Nanism, the mean growth velocity standard deviation score increased +2.8 ± 0.5 (range -0.7 to +5.5) during hGH administration. Raben (2) commented that he had treated one child with "bird headed dwarfism" with hGH and recorded almost a twofold increase in growth rate (4.1 to 7.6 cm/year). Soyka et al. (3) had a similar experience.

Lenko et al. (26) reported that in two boys with autosomal ring chromosomes, height velocity standard deviation scores increased +2.7 and +3.6 SD during hGH administration. Anneren et al. (53) administered hGH for 6 months to 5 children (3.5 to 6.5 years of age) with trisomy 21 (Down syndrome) and observed a mean increment in growth rate of +4.1 ± 1.8 cm/year during treatment. Bone age increased 0.6 ± 0.2 years during the 0.5 year of therapy.

Frazer et al. (15) administered hGH to a child with the Kenny Caffey syndrome of medullary stenosis and hypoparathyroidism and recorded an increase in growth rate from 3.4 to 7.9 cm/year during 6 months of treatment, with a posttreatment growth velocity of 4.2 cm/years. In our experience with one such patient, no effect of hGH was observed on linear growth rate. No effect of hGH upon the growth rate of one boy with Noonan syndrome has been observed by the author (Root, unpublished data).

CONCLUSIONS

Not unexpectedly, the administration of hGH to non-hGH deficient subjects has produced variable results. Many children with intrauterine and steroid-induced growth retardation may experience increase in growth rates during initial therapy. Most children with the Russell-Silver syndrome, osteochondrodystrophies and a variety of other diseases do not respond to hGH. Most intriguing is the increase in growth rate reported for children with trisomy 21.

There are no data on the long-term effects of hGH upon adult stature of these children. With the abundant quantity of hGH now available, systematic, prospective, long-term studies of the effects of hGH in well characterized disorders associated with short stature are needed. It is essential that the investigations be conducted in an organized manner so that conclusive data will be available on the dose requirements, efficacy and safety of such therapy.

ACKNOWLEDGMENT

The authors thank Ms. Sue Fine for her competent secretarial assistance.

REFERENCES

1. Tanner JM, Whitehouse RH, Hughes PCR, Vince FP. Effect of human growth hormone for 1 to 7 years on growth of 100 children, with growth hormone deficiency, low birth weight, inherited smallness, Turner's syndrome, other complaints. Arch Dis Child 1971; 46:745-82.
2. Raben MS. Growth hormone. Clinical use of human growth hormone. N Engl J Med 1962; 266:82-6.
3. Soyka LF, Ziskind A, Crawford JD. Treatment of short stature in children and adolescents with human pituitary growth hormone (Raben). N Engl J Med 1964; 754-64.
4. Grunt JA, Enriquez AR. Acute and long-term responsiveness to growth hormone in children with short stature. Pediatr Res 1972; 6:664-74.
5. Hayek A, Peake GT. Growth and somatomedin-C responses to growth hormone in dwarfed children. J Pediatr 1981; 99:868-72.
6. Bright GM, Rogol AD, Johanson AJ, Blizzard RM. Short stature associated with normal growth hormone and decreased somatomedin-C concentrations: response to exogenous growth hormone. Pediatrics 1983; 71:756-8.
7. Van Vliet G, Styne DM, Kaplan SL, Grumbach MM. Growth hormone treatment for short stature. N Engl J Med 1983; 309:1016-22.
8. Plotnick LP, Van Meter QL, Kowarski AA. Human growth hormone treat-

ment of children with growth failure and normal growth hormone levels by immunoassay: lack of correlation with somatomedin generation. Pediatrics 1983; 71:324–7.

9. Gertner JM, Genel M, Gianfredi SP, et al. Prospective clinical trial of human growth hormone in short children without growth hormone deficiency. J Pediatr 1984; 104:172–6.

10. Raiti S, Kaplan SL, Van Vliet G, Moore WV. Short-term treatment of short stature and subnormal growth rate with human growth hormone. J Pediatr 1987; 110:357–61.

11. Grunt JA, Howard CP, Daughaday WH. Comparison of growth hormone treatment in children with small-for-dates short stature, significant idiopathic short stature and hypopituitarism. Acta Endocrinol (Copenh) 1984; 106:168–74.

12. Albertsson-Wikland K. Growth hormone treatment in short children. Acta Paediatr Scand [Suppl] 1986; 325:64–70.

13. Costin G, Kaufman FR. Growth hormone secretory patterns in children with short stature. J Pediatr 1987; 110:362–8.

14. Kowarski AA, Schneider J, Ben-Galim E, Weldon VV, Daughaday WH. Dwarfism due to inactivity of endogenous growth hormone. J Clin Endocrinol Metab 1978; 47:461–4.

15. Frazer T, Gavin JR, Daughaday WH, Hillman RE, Weldon VV. Growth hormone-dependent growth failure. J Pediatr 1982; 101:12–5.

16. Rudman D, Kutner M, Goldsmith MA, Kenny J, Jennings H, Bain RP. Further observations on four subgroups of normal variant short stature. J Clin Endocrinol Metab 1980; 51:1378–84.

17. Rudman D, Kutner MH, Blackston RD, Cushman RA, Bain RP, Patterson JH. Children with normal variant short stature: treatment with human growth hormone for six months. N Engl J Med 1981; 305:123–31.

18. Bistritzer T, Chalew SA, Lovchik JC, Kowarski AA. Decreased growth hormone binding to IM-9 cells in children with biologically inactive GH syndrome. Pediatr Res 1987; 21:244A.

19. Tokuhiro E, Dean NJ, Friesen HG, Rudman D. Comparative study of human growth hormone measurement with NB2 lymphoma cell bioassay, IM-9 receptor modulation assay, and radioimmunoassay in children with disorders of growth. J Clin Endocrinol Metab 1984; 58:549–54.

20. Rudman D, Chawla RK, Heath WP, Berry CJ, Kutner MH. The hyposomato-medinemic short child. In: Raiti S, Tolman RA, eds. Human growth hormone. New York: Plenum Medical Book Co., 1986:135–62.

21. Valenta LJ, Siegel MB, Lesniak MA, et al. Pituitary dwarfism in a patient with circulating abnormal growth hormone polymers. N Engl J Med 1985; 312:214–7.

22. Grunt JA, Enriquez AR, Daughaday WH. Acute and long-term responses to hGH in children with idiopathic small-for-dates dwarfism. J Clin Endocrinol Metab 1972; 35:157–68.

23. Foley TP Jr, Thompson RG, Shaw M, Baghdassariam A, Nissley SP, Blizzard RM. Growth responses to human growth hormone in patients with intrauterine growth retardation. J Pediatr 1974; 84:635–41.

24. Lee PA, Blizzard RM, Cheek DB, Holt AB. Growth and body composition in intrauterine growth retardation (IUGR) before and during human growth hormone administration. Metabolism 1974; 23:913–9.

25. Lanes R, Plotnick LP, Lee PA. Sustained effect of human growth hormone therapy on children with intrauterine growth retardation. Pediatrics 1979; 63:731–5.

26. Lenko HL, Leisti S, Perheentupa J. The efficacy of growth hormone in different types of growth failure. An analysis of 101 cases. Eur J Pediatr 1982; 138:241–9.

27. Tanner JM, Lejapraga H, Cameron N. The natural history of the Silver-Russell syndrome: a longitudinal study of thirty nine cases. Pediatr Res 1975; 9:611–23.

28. Angehrn V, Zachmann M, Prader A. Silver-Russell syndrome. Observations in 20 patients. Helv Paediatr Acta 1979; 34:297–308.

29. Stahnke N. Human growth hormone treatment in short children without growth hormone deficiency. N Engl J Med 1984; 310:925-6.
30. Partsch C-J, Hermanussen M, Sippell WG. Treatment of Silver-Russell type dwarfism with human growth hormone: effects on serum somatomedin C levels and on longitudinal growth studied by knemometry. Acta Endocrinol [suppl] (Copenh) 1986; 279:139-46.
31. Cassidy SB, Blonder O, Courtney VW, Ratzan SK, Carey DE. Russell-Silver syndrome and hypopituitarism. Patient report and literature review. Am J Dis Child 1986; 140:155-9.
32. O'Brien JE, Sadeghi-Nejad A, Feingold M. Growth hormone deficiency in a patient with Silver-Russell syndrome. J Pediatr 1978; 93:152-3.
33. Hall JG. Microphallus, growth hormone deficiency and hypoglycemia in dwarfism. Am J Dis Child 1978; 132:1149.
34. Kappy MS. Regulation of growth in children with chronic illness. Therapeutic implications for the year 2000. Am J Dis Child 1987; 141:489-93.
35. Unterman TG, Phillips LS. Glucocorticoid effect on somatomedins and somatomedin inhibitors. J Clin Endocrinol Metab 1985; 61:618-26.
36. Morris HG, Jorgensen JR, Jenkins SA. Plasma growth hormone concentrations in corticosteroid-treated children. J Clin Invest 1968; 47:427-35.
37. Root AW, Bongiovanni AM, Eberlein WR. Studies of the secretion and metabolic effects of human growth hormone in children with glucocorticoid-induced growth retardation. J Pediatr 1969; 75:826-32.
38. Kunde MM, Marshall RT, Freeman S, Rhoads PS. Metabolic and statural response to human growth hormone in juvenile Cushing's syndrome with dwarfism. JAMA 1966; 21:307-15.
39. Butenandt O. Rheumatoid arthritis and growth retardation in children: treatment with human growth hormone. Eur J Pediatr 1979; 130:15-28.
40. Ward DJ, Hartog M, Ansell BM. Corticosteroid induced dwarfism in Still's disease treated with human growth hormone. Ann Rheum Dis 1966; 26:416-21.
41. Morris HG, Jorgensen JR, Elrick H, Goldsmith RE. Metabolic effects of human growth hormone in corticosteroid-treated children. J Clin Invest 1968; 47:436-51.
42. Matiasevic D, Gershberg H. Studies on hydroxyproline excretion and corticosteroid-induced dwarfism: treatment with human growth hormone. Metabolism 1966; 15:720-9.
43. Frasier SD, Rallison ML. Growth retardation and emotional deprivation: relative resistance to treatment with human growth hormone. J Pediatr 1972; 80:603-9.
44. Escamilla RF, Hutchings JJ, Li CH, Forsham P. Achondroplastic dwarfism. Treatment with human growth hormone. Calif Med 1966; 105:104-10.
45. Gershberg H, Mari S, Hulse M, St Paul H. Long-term treatment of hypopituitary and of achondroplastic dwarfism with human growth hormone. Metabolism 1964; 13:152-60.
46. Escamilla RF. Nonhypopituitary dwarfs and human growth hormone therapy. In: Raiti S, ed. Advances in human growth hormone research. DHEW Publications No. (NIH) 74-612, 1973:765-85.
47. Horton WA, Howard CP, Grunt JA. Skeletal changes following growth hormone treatment in a child with combined hypopituitarism and a skeletal dysplasia. Acta Endocrinol (Copenh) 1983; 103:302-8.
48. Edwards W, Root AW. Chondrodystrophic myotonia (Schwartz-Jampel syndrome). Report of a new case and follow-up of patients initially reported in 1969. Am J Med Genet 1982; 13:51-6.
49. Gershberg H, Neuman LL, Mari S. Studies on vitamin-D-resistant rickets: effects of human growth hormone. Metabolism 1964; 13:636-49.
50. Crawford JD, Bode HH, Botstein PM. Human growth hormone and non-

hypopituitary disorders. In: Raiti S, ed. Advances in human growth hormone research. DHEW Publication No. (NIH) 74-612, 1973:757-64.

51. Zackheim HS. Failure of human growth hormone to benefit dystrophic epidermolysis bullosa. Arch Dermatol 1983; 119:537.

52. Milner RDG, Russell-Fraser T, Brook CGD, et al. Experience with human growth hormone in Great Britain: the report of the MRC working party. Clin Endocrinol (Oxf) 1979; 11:15-38.

53. Anneren G, Sara VR, Hall K, Tuvemo T. Growth and somatomedin responses to growth hormone in Down's syndrome. Arch Dis Child 1986; 61:48-52.

54. Draznin MD, Stelling MW, Johanson AJ. Silver-Russell syndrome and craniopharyngioma. J Pediatr 1980; 96:887-9.

55. Gavin JR, Trived B, Aceto T, Bier DM, Grunt JA. Variant circulating forms of growth hormone constitute an uncommon cause of growth failure in children. Endocrinology 1987; 120:217A.

30

SUMMARY OF SESSION V

THERAPEUTIC EFFECTS OF GROWTH HORMONE

Raymond L. Hintz, M.D.

Department of Pediatrics
Stanford University
Stanford, CA

Most pediatric endocrinologists now in practice were trained during the period of time when the therapeutic use of growth hormone in the United States was perfectly straightforward. Because of the severe limitations of supply, and the centralization of distribution in this country through the National Pituitary Agency, the therapeutic use of growth hormone was restricted to children with severe growth hormone deficiency as defined by rigid and narrowly defined criteria. With the introduction of commercial pituitary growth hormone supplies into this country, and more recently with the introduction of the potentially unlimited supplies of synthetic growth hormone, there has been an increasing number of questions about the use of growth hormone beyond the narrow original definition of growth hormone deficiency.

The original criteria for growth hormone deficiency were never completely validated, and were designed more to choose those patients who had the most severe disorders of growth hormone secretion rather than to include children who might possibly benefit from treatment with growth hormone. Therefore, this questioning of old criteria has been good. However, it has at the same time provided a severe dilemma for pediatric endocrinologists, since they now have no firm criteria by which to diagnose growth hormone deficiency or choose which short child might benefit from treatment. Everyone agrees that there is a subset of children who have severe growth hormone deficiency by every test who are very responsive to growth hormone treatment. However, the issue is whether there is a broader range of children with short stature who have growth limited by their endogenous secretion of growth hormone, and who would respond to the therapeutic administration of moderate doses of growth hormone. We have already seen a change in the criteria used for normal peak response of growth hormone to provocative tests from 6 or 7 ng/ml to 10 ng/ml by most groups in this country. A wide variety of data indicates that there are children who have peak GH responses to stimulatory tests above the 10 ng/ml level who have at least a short-term response to growth hormone therapy.

In this session, Dr. Bier and his co-workers review their studies exploring the diagnosis of short children who might have defects in growth hormone structure, binding protein, or lack of peripheral responsiveness to insulin-like growth factor I. In these studies they have used a variety of radioligand assays, and the stimulation of N15 nitrogen retention by a standard course of human growth hormone given twice a day for 4 days. Dr. Rogol and co-workers report their studies using growth hormone releasing factor as an alternative to treatment with growth hormone in children with growth hormone deficiency. Dr. Kaplan reviews her experience with the long-term treatment of children with severe short stature who are not growth hormone deficient by the classic standard criteria. In this group of patients, she showed that 80% improved their growth rates, and 50% had a >3 cm increase in predicted height. Dr. Bierich reviews the disorder of constitutional delay of growth and adolescent development. He makes the perceptive point that this disorder, initially defined by Lawson Wilkins in 1957, is probably indistinguishable from short patients who are now being proposed for GH treatment under a variety of diagnostic labels. Dr. Frasier reviews the data which suggest that there is a dose responsive curve to GH administration in patients with GH deficiency. Finally, Dr. Root gives a comprehensive review of the past use of growth hormone treatment in a variety of non-growth hormone deficient individuals. Taken as a whole, these papers provide a comprehensive review of the therapeutic use of growth hormone in 1987, and a glimpse of future directions that will be taken in exploring new therapeutic uses of growth hormone in the next few years. Whatever the outcome of these and similar studies, it seems unlikely that we will ever again have a situation where the therapeutic use of growth hormone is dictated by a set of rigid criteria. Rather, we face an era in which the individual merits and potential risks of growth hormone therapy in each case will have to be weighed carefully. Indeed, we may have come full circle back to the era before the widespread use of growth hormone immunoassay, where the ultimate test of potential response to growth hormone treatment was to administer a therapeutic trial of growth hormone.

VI. NEW APPLICATIONS OF GROWTH HORMONE TREATMENT

31

GROWTH HORMONE THERAPY IN TURNER'S SYNDROME

Ron G. Rosenfeld, Raymond L. Hintz, Ann J. Johanson,
Barry Sherman, and the Genentech Collaborative Group*

Department of Pediatrics, Stanford University Medical
Center, Stanford, CA 94305, and Genentech, Inc., South
San Francisco, CA 94080

The estimated incidence of Turner's syndrome in live-born, phenotypic females varies between 1/2,000 and 1/10,000 (1). As such, it is a major cause of growth retardation, and, in many pediatric endocrine centers, is as common a diagnosis as classical growth hormone deficiency. Although significant variability in phenotypic expression exists, all major reviews of spontaneous growth in Turner's syndrome demonstrate significant reduction in final adult heights (2-7). In Ranke's 1983 review of growth in German girls with Turner's syndrome (7), final adult height averaged 146.8 cm (-2.57 standard deviations), while previous reviews reported mean adult heights ranging from 140.2-146.3 cm.

Because of the frequency of growth failure in Turner's syndrome, numerous investigators have studied the use of exogenous androgens and estrogens in such patients. Although these studies have generally been small and retrospective, the consensus has been that both androgen and estrogen therapy stimulate short-term growth, with little positive effect upon final adult height. Studies by Urban et al. (8) using fluoxymesterone and/or oxandrolone, Lenko et al. (9) using fluoxymesterone, and Joss and Zuppinger (10) employing oxandrolone have indicated that androgen therapy may result in a positive effect upon final height. However, Sybert (6) reported that a retrospective review of 66 patients revealed that androgen therapy resulted in no significant increment in adult height.

BACKGROUND

Although the limited supplies of pituitary-derived human growth hormone generally precluded large-scale studies in Turner's syndrome, short-

---

*Investigators in the Genentech Collaborative Group: Jo Anne Brasel, M.D., Stephen Burstein, M.D., Ph.D., Steven Chernausek, M.D., James Frane, Ph.D., Ronald W. Gotlin, M.D., Raymond L. Hintz, M.D., Ann J. Johanson, M.D., Joyce Kuntze, Barbara M. Lippe, M.D., Patrick C. Mahoney, M.D., Wayne V. Moore, M.D., Ph.D., Maria I. New, M.D., Ron G. Rosenfeld, M.D., Paul Saenger, M.D., Barry Sherman, M.D., and Virginia Sybert, M.D.

term studies by Almqvist et al. (25) and Forbes et al. (26) in the early 1960s demonstrated that patients with Turner's syndrome responded to hGH by increasing sulphation factor activity and retention of nitrogen, phosphorus, magnesium, sodium, potassium, and chloride. However, sporadic reports of individual cases treated with hGH were initially discouraging. Soyka et al. (11) and Tanner et al. (15) reported increases in annual growth rate averaging only 1.2 and 1.0 cm/year, respectively. On the other hand, in a total of 5 subjects described in three individual reports, mean annual growth rate increased from 3.1 cm/year to 6.2 cm/year following short-term hGH therapy (12-14). More recently, Butenandt (17) reported an increase in growth rate from 2.0 to 4.1 cm/year in a girl with Turner's syndrome and growth hormone deficiency (peak provocative plasma GH level of 2 ng/ml). However, 4 girls with Turner's syndrome, normal plasma GH levels, and bone ages between 10 and 11 years had virtually no change in growth rates. Similarly, Stahnke (18) reported that 2 of 8 Turner patients responded to hGH with an increase in growth rate to 7-8 cm/year. In 6 additional patients, no improvement in growth rate was observed, although it should be pointed out that the mean chronological age of this group was 16.0 years, and the mean bone age 11.8 years.

LARGE-SCALE STUDIES OF GH THERAPY IN TURNER'S SYNDROME

It has only been in recent years that increased supplies of pituitary-hGH and, subsequently, recombinant DNA-derived hGH have permitted a more thorough evaluation of the efficacy of hGH in Turner's syndrome. Raiti et al. (22) have recently reported results in 52 patients, ages 4.5-14.5 years, with peak plasma GH levels of at least 6 ng/ml following provocative testing. Pituitary-derived hGH was administered at a dose of 0.2 IU/kg three times per week (approximately 0.3 mg/kg/week). During the first year of therapy, the mean annual growth rate increased from 3.2 ± 0.8 cm/year to 5.9 ± 1.4 cm/year, with an accompanying increase in bone age of 1.1 ± 0.9 years. During a subsequent 6-month period off treatment, the annual growth rate decreased to 3.1 ± 1.9 cm/year. When 31 subjects were then given a second course of hGH, for a period of 6 months, the annual growth rate returned to 5.9 ± 1.4 cm/year.

Takano et al. (20,21) have reported the results of recombinant DNA--derived hGH in a total of 25 subjects with Turner's syndrome. In the first study, the mean annual growth rate increased from a pretreatment value of 3.7 cm/year to 5.7 cm/year (based upon 6-month growth data). In the second study, growth rates increased from pretreatment values of 3.6 ± 0.8 cm/year (range: 2.0-5.0 cm/year) to 5.5 ± 1.2 cm/year (range: 3.4-7.8 cm/year). All but one subject showed an increase in annual growth rate, ranging from 0.1-3.9 cm/year. Bone age increased only 0.9 years over the one-year treatment period. During a second year of treatment with hGH, 8 subjects demonstrated an average annual growth rate of 5.1 ± 0.6 cm/year. It is important to note that this study group included 4 subjects who were receiving concomitant anabolic steroids.

GENENTECH COLLABORATIVE STUDY OF GH THERAPY IN TURNER'S SYNDROME

In a prospective, randomized study of the efficacy of hGH, alone or in combination with oxandrolone, in Turner's syndrome, a multi-center investigation was initiated in the summer of 1983 (23,24). Seventy girls, ranging in age from 4.7-12.4 years, from 11 medical centers were enrolled. All subjects were prepubertal, had baseline heights at least 1 SD below the mean for normal females of comparable age (cumulative growth charts, US Public Health Service), had documented pretreatment growth rates below 6 cm/year, and had provocative plasma growth hormone levels of at least

Table 1. Growth hormone therapy in Turner's syndrome.

Author (Reference)	Number of Subjects	Age (years)	Average dose of hGH/wk†	Pre-Rx Growth (cm/yr)††	On-Rx Growth (cm/yr)††
Soyka (11)	2	13.9, 11	13.5 mg	3.1	4.3
Wright (12)	2	12, 15.9	17.0 mg	3.2	5.7
Hutchings (13)	2	12.5, 13	35.0 mg	3.2	6.8
Tzagournis (14)	1	14	10.0 mg	2.7	6.0
Tanner (15)	5		10.0 mg	2.9	3.9
Rudman (16)	6	12.8 (11-15)	0.25 mg/kg	2.0	3.8 7.6*
Butenandt (17)	4	(11-12.5)	11.3 mg	3.3	3.7
Stahnke (18)	8	16	6-12 mg	2.6	2.2**
Singer-Granick (19)	8	11.8 (9.2-14.8)	0.25 mg/kg (0.09-0.32)	3.3	4.9
Takano (20)	20	12.3 (8.4-16.1)	0.27 mg/kg (0.20-0.42)	3.7	5.7
Takano*** (21)	21	11.5 (7.4-13.8)	0.28 mg/kg (0.11-0.47)	3.6	5.5
Raiti (22)	52	(4.5-14.5)	0.30 mg/kg	3.2	5.9
Rosenfeld (23,24)	70	9.3 (4.7-12.4)	0.375 mg/kg	4.2	6.6 9.8*

†Determinations of hGH dose are based upon a potency of 2 U/mg. This may not be true for all hGH preparations, especially the earlier ones.

††Growth rates are expressed as cm/year, although actual periods of study may have been as short as 3 months.

*hGH in combination with oxandrolone.

**Stahnke reported that 2/8 Turner patients responded to hGH, with growth rates as high as 7-8 cm/year. For the 6 nonresponders, the growth rate on treatment was 2.2 cm/year.

***16/20 subjects from the first Takano study are included in the second Takano study.

7 ng/ml. After a pretreatment observation period of at least 6 months, subjects were randomly assigned to 1 of 4 study arms, with balance established with respect to pretreatment growth rate, chronologic age and karyotype. The 4 study groups consisted of: Group 1, control (no treatment); Group 2, oxandrolone (Searle Pharmaceuticals, Chicago), 0.125 mg/kg/day p.o.; Group 3, met-hGH (Protropin®, Genentech, South San Francisco), 0.125 mg/kg IM 3 times/week; and Group 4, combination oxandrolone and met-hGH at the above dose regimen. Table 2 compares the baseline characteristics of the 4 groups.

The first phase of the study last 12-20 months. In the second phase, patients receiving met-hGH alone continued on that regimen; all other subjects were treated with met-hGH plus oxandrolone (at a dose of 0.0625 mg/kg/day). The study arms are summarized in Table 3.

Although all subjects had provocative plasma GH levels of at least 7 ng/ml, 24/70 (34.3%) girls had baseline plasma insulin-like growth factor-I (IGF-I) levels below the 95% confidence limits for age. During the first study year, subjects treated with oxandrolone alone showed no significant change in IGF-I levels. Subjects receiving met-hGH, either alone or in combination with oxandrolone, had a two- to threefold increase in plasma IGF-I levels. This increase was sustained during the second year of met-hGH therapy.

Table 2. Comparison of study groups at baseline.

	Control	Oxandrolone	Met-hGH	Combination
Age (years)	9.3 ± 2.3 (18)	9.6 ± 2.0 (18)	9.1 ± 2.1 (17)	8.9 ± 2.5 (17)
Height (cm)	114.4 ± 10.7 (18)	115.3 ± 9.9 (18)	114.6 ± 9.5 (17)	113.8 ± 10 (17)
Weight (kg)	23.7 ± 9.3 (18)	24.7 ± 7.0 (18)	23.6 ± 7.2 (17)	23.4 ± 6.2 (17)
Growth rate (cm/year)	4.2 ± 1.1 (18)	4.1 ± 1.0 (18)	4.5 ± 0.8 (17)	4.3 ± 0.9 (17)
Bone age (years)	8.3 ± 2.3 (17)	8.5 ± 2.1 (17)	7.7 ± 1.9 (17)	7.7 ± 2.2 (17)
Karyotype				
45,X	15	12	13	13
Other	3	6	4	4

Data are presented as mean ± SD for each group of (n) subjects. There were no statistically significant differences between groups in mean age, height, weight, prerandomization growth rate or bone age. From Rosenfeld et al., Acta Paediatr Scand [Suppl] 1987; 331:59-66 (24).

As shown in Table 5, met-hGH treatment resulted in significant increases in growth velocity during the first 2 years. Compared to a control growth rate of 3.8 cm/year, subjects treated with met-hGH alone grew 6.6 cm during the first year of therapy, and 5.4 cm during the second year. Even greater increases in growth velocity were found in subjects treated with combination met-hGH and oxandrolone. Subjects in Group 4 grew 9.8 cm during year 1 and 7.4 cm during year 2. When the initial control group was started on combination therapy using the lower dose of oxandrolone (0.0625 mg/kg/day), a significant increase in growth velocity was still observed (from 4.0 to 8.8 cm/year). These results are even more impressive when the data are expressed in terms of the growth velocity data for Turner's syndrome, published by Ranke (7). While the control group had a mean growth velocity Z-score of -0.1, patients treated with met-hGH alone had scores of +3.0 during year 1 and +2.0 during year 2. Similarly, Group 4 (combination) had a mean growth velocity Z-score of +6.6 during year 1 and +4.2 during year 2.

Table 3. Study arms.

Group	Phase 1*	Phase 2
1	No treatment	met-hGH, 0.125 mg/kg, 3x/week + oxandrolone, 0.0625 mg/kg/day
2	oxandrolone, 0.125 mg/kg/day	met-hGH, 0.125 mg/kg, 3x/week + oxandrolone, 0.0625 mg/kg/day
3	met-hGH, 0.125 mg/kg, 3x/week	met-hGH, 0.125 mg/kg, 3x/week
4	met-hGH, 0.125 mg/kg, 3x/week + oxandrolone, 0.125 mg/kg/day	met-hGH, 0.125 mg/kg, 3x/week + oxandrolone, 0.0625 mg/kg/day

*Phase 1 consisted of a 12-20 month period.

Table 4. Plasma IGF-I levels.

	Control	Oxandrolone	Met-hGH	Combination
			IGF-I (units/ml)	
Year 1	0.63 ± 0.26	0.68 ± 0.42	1.86 ± 0.85*	1.40 ± 0.74*
Year 2			1.74 ± 0.68*	1.80 ± 0.67*

*Significantly greater than control during year 1 (P<0.05).

UNANSWERED QUESTIONS CONCERNING GH AND TURNER'S SYNDROME

Although the recent studies by Raiti et al. (22), Takano et al. (20,21), and Rosenfeld et al. (23,24) convincingly demonstrate that hGH is capable of accelerating growth in girls with Turner's syndrome, it is important to point out that at this time, no subjects have been continuously treated with hGH for longer than 3.5 years. Thus, several important questions concerning the pathogenesis of short stature in Turner's syndrome, as well as its optimal management, remain:

(1) Are Turner's syndrome patients partially growth hormone deficient? If so, does this merely represent estrogen deficiency, or, rather, an underlying abnormality at the hypothalamic/pituitary level?

(2) Is Turner's syndrome a form of skeletal dysplasia?

(3) What is the effect of hGH therapy upon final adult height? While the data to date are consistent with potential increases in final height, longer follow-up will be required to definitively establish this point.

(4) Does the addition of low-dose androgens and/or estrogens to hGH significantly improve either short-term or long-term growth response to hGH? What are the optimal ages at which these agents should be added, and at what doses?

(5) What is the optimal dose of hGH in girls with Turner's syndrome? Can the dose be increased, or therapy switched to every day, without resulting in significant glucose intolerance or other side effects?

It has certainly been the authors' impression that girls with Turner's syndrome have significant impairment of their self-images,

Table 5. Growth rates (cm/year).

Group	Year 1	Year 2
1 Control	3.8 ± 1.0 (17)	
2 Oxandrolone	7.9 ± 1.0* (17)	
3 Met-hGH	6.6 ± 1.2* (17)	5.4 ± 1.1* (17)
4 Combination	9.8 ± 1.4* (17)	7.4 ± 1.4* (16)
	Phase 1**	Phase 2**
1 control/combination	4.0 ± 0.7 (17)	8.8 ± 4.3* (16)
2 oxand./combination	7.2 ± 1.2* (18)	6.5 ± 1.8* (17)

*Significantly greater than control during year 1 (P<0.05).
**Phase 1 varied from 12-20 months for individual subjects.

frequently resulting in social immaturity, delays in progression through school, and difficulties in assuming normal adolescent and adult roles. While this is certainly due, in part, to gonadal failure, the resulting pubertal delay is readily managed by reassurance and replacement sex steroids. The issues surrounding growth retardation in Turner's syndrome have been more difficult to approach and manage. The overwhelming majority of girls with Turner's syndrome fall off the normal growth curves before adolescence, and, consequently, the management of their short stature must deal not only with their final adult heights, but also with the normalization of growth during childhood. The data to date indicate that early and judicious use of hGH, either alone or in combination with anabolic steroids, may contribute significantly to normalization of growth during childhood, and, potentially, to the attainment of normal final adult heights.

REFERENCES

1. Gerald PS. Sex chromosome disorders. N Engl J Med 1976; 294:706.
2. Palmer CG, Reichmann A. Chromosomal and clinical findings in 110 females with Turner syndrome. Hum Genet 1976; 35:35.
3. Park E, Bailey JD, Cowell CA. Growth and maturation of patients with Turner's syndrome. Pediatr Res 1983; 17:1.
4. Brook CGD, Murset G, Zachmann M, Prader A. Growth in children with 45,XO Turner's syndrome. Arch Dis Child 1974; 49:789.
5. Lev-Ran A. Androgens, estrogens, and the ultimate height in XO gonadal dysgenesis. Am J Dis Child 1977; 131:648.
6. Sybert VP. Adult height in Turner syndrome with and without androgen therapy. J Pediatr 1984; 104:365.
7. Ranke MB, Pfluger H, Rosendahl W, et al. Turner syndrome: spontaneous growth in 150 cases and review of the literature. Eur J Pediatr 1983; 141:81.
8. Urban MD, Lee PA, Dorst JP, Plotnick LP, Migeon CJ. Oxandrolone therapy in patients with Turner syndrome. J Pediatr 1979; 94:823.
9. Lenko HL, Perheentupa J, Soderholm A. Growth in Turner's syndrome: spontaneous and fluoxymesterone stimulated. Acta Paediatr Scand [Suppl] 1979; 277:57.
10. Joss E, Zuppinger K. Oxandrolone in girls with Turner's syndrome: a pair-matched controlled study up to final height. Acta Paediatr Scand 1984; 73:674.
11. Soyka LF, Ziskind A, Crawford JD. Treatment of short stature in children and adolescents with human pituitary hormone (Raben). N Engl J Med 1964; 271:754.
12. Wright JC, Brasel JA, Aceto T Jr, et al. Studies with human growth hormone. Am J Med 1965; 38:499.
13. Hutchings JJ, Escamilla RF, Li CH, Forsham PH. Li human growth hormone administration in gonadal dysgenesis. Am J Dis Child; 109:318.
14. Tzagournis M. Response to long-term administration of human growth hormone in Turner's syndrome. JAMA 1969; 210:2373.
15. Tanner JM, Whitehouse RH, Hughes PCR, Vince FP. Effect of human growth hormone treatment for 1 to 7 years on growth of 100 children, with growth hormone deficiency, low birth weight, inherited smallness, Turner's syndrome and other complaints. Arch Dis Child 1971; 46:745.
16. Rudman D, Goldsmith M, Kutner M, Blackston D. Effect of growth hormone and oxandrolone singly and together on growth rate in girls with X chromosome abnormalities. J Pediatr 1980; 96:132.
17. Butenandt O. Growth hormone deficiency and growth hormone therapy in Ullrich-Turner syndrome. Klin Wochenschr 1980; 58:99.
18. Stahnke N. Human growth hormone treatment in short children without

growth hormone deficiency. N Engl J Med 1984; 310:925.

19. Singer-Granick C, Lee PA, Foley TP Jr, Becker DJ. Growth hormone therapy for patients with Turner's syndrome. Horm Res 1986; 24:246.

20. Takano K, Hizuka N, Shizume K. Treatment of Turner's syndrome with methionyl human growth hormone for six months. Acta Endocrinol (Copenh) 1986; 112:130.

21. Takano K, Hizuka N, Shizume K. Growth hormone treatment in Turner's syndrome. Acta Paediatr Scand [Suppl] 1986; 325:58.

22. Raiti S, Moore WV, Van Vliet G, Kaplan SL, The National Hormone and Pituitary Program. Growth-stimulating effects of human growth hormone therapy in patients with Turner syndrome. J Pediatr 1986; 109:944.

23. Rosenfeld RG, Hintz RL, Johanson AJ, et al. Methionyl human growth hormone and oxandrolone in Turner syndrome: preliminary results of a prospective randomized trial. J Pediatr 1986; 109:936.

24. Rosenfeld RG, Hintz RL, Johanson AJ, Sherman B, The Genentech Collaborative Group. Results from the first 2 years of a clinical trial with recombinant DNA-derived human growth hormone (Somatrem) in Turner's syndrome. Acta Paediatr Scand [Suppl] 1987; 331:59.

25. Almqvist S, Hall K, Lindstedt S, Lindsten J, Luft R, Sjoberg HE. Effects of short term administration of physiological doses of human growth hormone in three patients with Turner's syndrome. Acta Endocrinol (Copenh) 1964; 46:451.

26. Forbes AP, Jacobsen JG, Carroll EL, Pechet MM. Studies of growth arrest in gonadal dysgenesis: response to exogenous human growth hormone. Metabolism 1962; 11:56.

32

USE OF GROWTH HORMONE IN SURGERY

James McK. Manson and Douglas W. Wilmore

Brigham and Women's Hospital
Harvard Medical School
Boston, Mass.

THE METABOLIC RESPONSE TO STRESS

An organism's reaction to injury, including surgery, or infection involves not merely a local healing process, but also a systemic metabolic response. One feature of the adaptation seen is the mobilization of amino acids from muscle and their transport to visceral tissue, primarily liver, to take part in biochemical processes including the synthesis of acute phase proteins and formation of new glucose molecules. The nitrogen released from the amino acids forms urea and appears in the urine. Nitrogen loss is a consistent feature of the metabolic response to stress states, and the amount lost is generally proportional to the severity of the insult.

Although the events outlined above occur following any form of physical stress, if the patient is healthy, the insult not overwhelming and the recovery uncomplicated, the protein losses are usually small, short-lived and well tolerated. However, following major burns, multiple trauma and especially in sepsis, the continued erosion of body protein can, independently of the primary pathology, compromise the ability to fight infection, heal wounds, and ultimately recover.

For nearly 20 years conventional nutritional support, either by enteral or parenteral routes, has formed a part of the care of severely ill, catabolic patients. Exogenous provision of amino acids and calories can decrease net protein losses and improve nitrogen balance. Attempts to demonstrate the efficacy of nutritional support in surgical patients have not always been successful (1,2), but this may well be due, in part, to the difficulty of constructing controlled trials involving patients as ill as those likely to benefit from such treatment. However, there can be little doubt that nutritional support does not provide the complete answer. Its provision, particularly by central venous infusion, carries its own set of complications; such provision does not always result in nitrogen equilibrium, and, on a more philosophical note, it is not directly influencing the metabolic adaptations resulting in protein loss.

The concept of modifying the metabolic response to stress, a response evolved when man lived and hunted like a wild animal and which is perhaps no longer completely appropriate in the era of modern medicine, is not a new one. The mechanisms underlying the metabolic adaptations seen are complex and by no means fully understood. The whole response is orchestrated by the central nervous system and neurological messages are probably of predominant importance in the very early stages postinjury. Changes in the production of hormones undoubtedly play a major part, and recently much attention has been paid to the role of substances released from circulating blood cells, particularly interleukin I.

The hormonal balance in the posttraumatic state is tilted towards catabolism, with high circulating levels of the "counter-regulatory" hormones: glucagon, cortisol and the catecholamines. Although insulin levels are normal or slightly high, peripheral tissues, particularly muscle, exhibit insulin resistance and its anabolic properties are blunted (3). Exogenous insulin has been used in an attempt to decrease nitrogen losses after injury (4,5) and anabolic steroids have also been employed (6,7). Use of both these agents was associated with limited success in terms of nitrogen retention, but there were allied problems including hypoglycemia with insulin and fluid retention with steroids. Neither agent has achieved a widespread clinical use in this context. In many ways, the most attractive candidate for use in the attempt to modify the metabolic response to stress was always growth hormone (GH).

GROWTH HORMONE—PHYSIOLOGICAL PROPERTIES AND CHANGES IN PRODUCTION FOLLOWING STRESS

GH is a potent stimulator of protein synthesis, whether assessed by stimulation of labeled amino acid uptake into cells in vitro (8), turnover studies using labeled glycine (9), or body composition studies performed over long periods of time (10,11). It is now clear that the action of GH on protein metabolism is affected via an intermediary, Insulin-like Growth Factor I (IGF-I) (12). In addition, GH has a "pancreatotropic" effect, stimulating insulin production, first reported by Anselmino et al. in 1933 (13) and since confirmed by many other workers. Insulin is a potent anabolic agent in its own right and there can be little doubt that the effects associated with growth hormone are in part due to the induction of insulin elaboration. Further, GH stimulates lipolysis, as evidenced by raised serum levels of lipid substrates (14) and preferential use of fat as a fuel source (15,16). GH also has a ketogenic action which may be specific, and not merely a result of its lipolytic properties (17,18). Animal experiments have consistently shown that chronic administration of GH spares protein at the expense of fat stores (11,19).

GH release from the anterior pituitary is precipitated by traumatic injury (20), burn trauma (21), surgical operations (22,23), infectious disease (24), and administration of endotoxin (25). Several investigators have shown that the rise in GH production following physical insult is short-lived with normal levels returning in about 5 days (22,23); moreover, the rise is proportional to the severity of the surgery in elective operation (22). The GH response to stress is not consistent, and Dahn et al. have suggested the ability to mount a significant increase in GH elaboration may be associated with improved immune function and decreased peripheral proteolysis (26).

The normal close association between GH elaboration and IGF-I production is lost following physical stress. IGF-I levels fall in the immediate posttraumatic state and return to normal at 1-2 weeks (27,28). The reason for this dissociation of the normal relationship is not entirely clear, but it may be a physiological mechanism acting in an environment where protein conservation is not a priority for the organism, but high levels of GH are useful to maintain circulating glucose levels and aid in the mobilization of fat.

GH production and GH response to standard stimuli decrease with age (29,30). In addition, IGF-I levels are similarly low and respond to exogenous GH provision (31). It might be concluded, although to date no studies have investigated the question, that GH responses to stress are blunted by advancing age and hence exogenous administration of GH may be of particular benefit in the elderly population, who constitute the majority of patients undergoing major elective surgery.

RESULTS OF EXOGENOUS ADMINISTRATION OF GROWTH HORMONE

The potential application of GH therapy in catabolic patients has been realized for many years. The lack of available hormone clearly vitiated against enthusiastic research efforts in the field and the recent availability, due to recombinant DNA techniques, of potentially unlimited quantities of GH has precipitated new interest in defining possible therapeutic roles for this potent anabolic agent.

Since 1941, when Cuthbertson and colleagues in Glasgow showed that treatment of rats, following femoral fracture, with crude anterior pituitary extract lowered both urinary nitrogen losses and posttraumatic weight loss, the effects of GH in the posttraumatic state have been the subject of study (32). The early work on burn patients by Prudden et al. (33) utilized bovine GH, now known to be of exceedingly variable activity in humans, and led to the formation of the "critical level theory." This stated that GH administration was only effective in improving nitrogen balance above a "critical" level of nitrogen intake—below this level GH caused a deterioration in nitrogen balance. Allied to this theory was the suggestion that GH was only effective during the later stages of recovery from burn injury, when the phase of severe catabolism was over. This would coincide with low or normal production of endogenous GH. Work with burn patients by Soroff et al. (34) in 1967 confirmed that the anabolic properties of GH were confined to the later stages of recovery.

The length of the recovery period after burn trauma allows construction of consecutive control and treatment periods and makes this patient group particularly suitable for study. Liljedahl et al. (35) and Wilmore et al. (36) also investigated the effects of human GH on recovering burn patients—both finding that treatment was associated with significantly improved nitrogen balance, irrespective of the time elapsed since injury. Liljedahl allowed ad libitum intake and Wilmore's patients received adequate calories and nitrogen, so no comment could be made on the "critical level theory." Wilmore particularly drew attention to the insulinotropic effect of GH in mediating nitrogen retention and was able to demonstrate a statistically significant relationship between nitrogen intake, nitrogen balance and basal insulin levels.

The effect of exogenous GH therapy after elective surgery has not been widely studied. Ward et al. (37) gave biosynthetic GH to patients following major gastrointestinal surgery, who were receiving only 400 Kcal/day as dextrose infusion, and no nitrogen. GH mediated significant nitrogen retention, and this finding contradicts the "critical level theory" alluded to above. These workers also showed that GH caused a significant increase in IGF-I levels, and furthermore caused protein turnover (estimated using N15 glycine) to increase postoperatively, in marked contrast to control patients where it decreased.

The prospect of potentially unlimited quantities of available GH prompted us to perform further studies to elucidate the actions and possible role of GH in catabolic patients. In a preliminary pilot study we investigated normal volunteers—the advantages of such a group are great, most notably the ability to construct tightly controlled paired studies which were identical except for whether GH or placebo was given. All nutrition was administered intravenously, both because this allows meticulous control of intake and because the combination of GH and intravenous nutrition had not previously been examined. Lingering doubts about the "critical level theory" led us to examine the effect of GH at varying levels of calorie intake (adequate calories, 50% adequate and 30% adequate); nitrogen intake was constant and adequate in all studies. This has more relevance to the clinical situation where adequate nitrogen can be provided by peripheral infusion, but central infusions (or enteral therapy) are usually needed to provide adequate calories. Our 50% and 30% calorie diets were provided by peripheral infusion (16).

Results showed that GH administration was consistently associated with positive nitrogen balance, at all levels of calorie intake. Potassium and phosphorus balance were altered in a similar manner to nitrogen, and, moreover, these three elements were retained in proportions corresponding extremely closely to their relative proportions in skeletal muscle, strongly suggesting that the nitrogen was retained in the form of muscle tissue. The effect of GH on protein metabolism was also investigated by estimating protein turnover using N15 glycine. Results clearly indicated that GH acted by increasing protein synthesis, rather than by decreasing breakdown. Three-methyl-histidine excretion, a mark of myofibrillar protein breakdown, was not altered by GH, and this serves to confirm that no changes in protein breakdown occurred. Since net protein loss following trauma or elective surgery is most commonly the result of a decrease in protein synthesis, GH, which we have shown acts by promoting protein synthesis, might be expected to have a particular role in improving nitrogen balance in these patients.

We also demonstrated that nitrogen retention was associated with increased basal insulin levels and insulin production as assessed by C-peptide excretion, increased ketone production and serum levels of lipid substrates, and increased serum levels of IGF-I.

Armed with this information, we moved on to a patient population. Six adults with acute fistulae of the gastrointestinal tract were studied in a blinded crossover design, where they received GH (10 mg s.q.) daily for one week and placebo the second week or vice versa, receiving placebo the first week and GH the second week. Patients received adequate nitrogen and approximately 50% of adequate calories via the parenteral route (38). Essentially, results obtained were remarkably similar to those seen in normal volunteers, namely consistent GH-mediated retention of nitrogen, phosphorus and potassium in proportions similar to those found in skeletal muscle. If GH was given during the first week, the nitrogen retention, and to a lesser extent that of phosphorus and potassium, seemed to carry over into the second week. Serum levels of glucose and insulin rose with GH treatment (but not significantly so) and there was an increase in serum IGF-I. Despite the anabolic environment, serum free fatty acid (FFA) levels did not change, suggesting continuing lipolysis. As in our study on volunteers, administration of GH was not attended by any ill effects.

GROWTH HORMONE IN THE SURGICAL PATIENT—PROBLEMS AND POSSIBILITIES

Examination of the accumulated evidence now available leaves little doubt that GH can significantly reduce net protein losses in both volunteers and catabolic patients, and, moreover, that this effect does not appear to depend on provision of adequate calories. However, similar effects can be achieved with conventional nutritional support—does GH therapy have any advantages over traditional management and are there specific areas where GH treatment may be indicated?

The ability of GH to produce positive nitrogen balance in volunteers and patients receiving only hypocaloric, peripheral intravenous nutrient infusions is significant. There is a body of patients, including those with sepsis and those with problems of access (either due to repeated line placement or central vein thrombosis), where central line placement is difficult or dangerous. The combination of GH and peripheral nutrient infusions offers a viable alternative. Many of these patients will have malignant disease, and as yet we have not entered such patients in our studies, because of the potential danger of stimulating tumor growth. If and when GH is produced in large quantities, the large costs inherent in the placement and maintenance of central lines may provide an economic argument in favor of peripheral infusion together with GH.

Further, in severely catabolic patients, even hyperalimentation via central infusion may not be successful in achieving nitrogen equilibrium. Available data suggests that the addition of GH can improve utilization of provided nutrients and mediate nitrogen retention.

Conventional nutritional support has therapeutic limitations inasmuch as nutrients are provided, but their utilization cannot be effectively controlled other than by administering appropriate proportions of calories and nitrogen. The tendency is, particularly in relatively immobile patients fed for long periods, for provided nutrients to be converted to fat stores which are of little or no therapeutic value. The lipolytic actions of GH are well known, and have been referred to several times above. Perhaps the most exciting potential application of GH is in directing administered amino acids and carbohydrate toward protein replenishment, and promoting use of administered lipid as an energy source. In patients who already have significant fat stores, no exogenous lipid need be given and GH will favor mobilization and utilization of endogenous fat stores.

As might be expected of an agent with its properties, GH is a potent stimulator of wound healing, both in terms of time to reach a certain wound strength and the final strength of the resulting wound (39,40). Hence, GH may find a role in the catabolic, hypoproteinemic patient who is failing to heal wounds.

On a more practical level, the optimum dose, route and timing of administration of GH are not established and will require controlled studies, probably on normal volunteers, to determine. In no studies of GH administration to volunteers or patients has such treatment been associated with significant side effects, with the exception of obese volunteers fasted for many days (41). GH causes glucose intolerance but has not been associated with significant elevation of serum glucose levels in the studies conducted. However, it would seem prudent to recommend close monitoring of serum levels, especially when GH therapy is initiated.

The widespread adoption of GH therapy in surgical patients will result, not from repeated demonstration of its metabolic effects, but rather from demonstration of its ability to improve the clinical course of a patient after major surgery or injury, as assessed by mortality, morbidity and days in intensive care or days in hospital. The construction of clinical trials to demonstrate such effects is notoriously difficult, largely because of the problems in achieving meaningful controls or control periods. Such difficulties may have contributed to the not entirely successful efforts to demonstrate unequivocally the efficacy of nutritional support. In this latter field, investigators have tended to settle on a patient population undergoing major elective surgery, a reproducible physical insult, but this is almost certainly not the most appropriate group to study. There is little doubt that such a population could be used to show that GH mediates significant nitrogen retention, as indeed Ward et al. have done (37), but differences in clinical criteria would be more difficult to expose.

One fruitful area might be the study of patients, particularly the elderly and obese, recovering from femoral fracture and subsequent operative fixation, in whom GH together with peripheral infusion of amino acids and carbohydrate might be expected to reduce both postoperative complications and time spent in hospital.

The nutritional management of surgical patients has entered a relatively static phase with relation to advancement and improvement. Perhaps the real importance of GH treatment is that it may point the way forward, to a situation where specific polypeptide hormones can be manufactured (by recombinant-DNA techniques) and then used to control the utilization of administered nutrients in a desired manner by stimulating or inhibiting specific metabolic processes, and eventually targeting individual organs for nutritional support.

ACKNOWLEDGMENTS

This work was supported in part by an NIH Trauma Center Grant P50 G.M. 29327-05, and Clinical Research Center Grants 29-9299, AM 15191 and AI 15614.

REFERENCES

1. Holter AR, Rosen HM, Fischer JE. The effects of hyperalimentation on major surgery in patients with malignant disease: a prospective study. Acta Chir Scand 1977; 466(suppl):86-7.
2. Cerra FB, Siegel JH, Coleman B, et al. Septic autocannibalism. A failure of exogenous nutritional support. Ann Surg 1980; 192:570-80.
3. Brooks DC, Bessey PQ, Black PR, Aoki TT, Wilmore DW. Posttraumatic insulin resistance in uninjured forearm tissue. J Surg Res 1984; 37:100-7.
4. Hinton P, Allison SP, Littlejohn S, Lloyd J. Insulin and glucose to reduce catabolic response to injury in burned patients. Lancet 1971; i:767-9.
5. Woolfson AMJ, Heatley RV, Allison SP. Insulin to inhibit protein catabolism after injury. N Engl J Med 1979; 300:14-7.
6. Tweedle D, Walton C, Johnson IDA. The effect of an anabolic steroid on post-operative nitrogen balance. Br J Clin Pract 1973; 27:130-2.
7. Michelsen CB, Askanasi J, Kinney JM, et al. Effect of an anabolic steroid on nitrogen balance and amino acid patterns after total hip replacement. J Trauma 1982; 22:410-3.
8. Kostyo JL. In vitro effects of growth hormone and corticotropin on amino acid transport in muscle. Acta Endocrinol [suppl] (Copenh) 1960; 51:943.
9. Crispell KR, Parson W, Hollifield G. The effect of growth hormone on the amino acid pool and protein synthesis rate in a pituitary dwarf. J Clin Invest 1954; 33:924-5.
10. Collipp PJ, Curti V, Thomas J, et al. Body composition changes in children receiving human growth hormone. Metabolism 1973; 22:589.
11. Korenchevsky V. The influence of the hypophysis on metabolism, growth and sexual organs of male rats and rabbits. Biochem J 1930; 24:383-93.

12. Salmon WD Jr, Daughaday WH. A hormonally controlled serum factor which stimulates sulphate incorporation by cartilage in vitro. J Lab Clin Med 1957; 49:825-35.

13. Anselmino KJ, Herold L, Hoffmann FR. Uber die pankreatrope witkung von hypophysenvorderlappenextrakten. Klin Wirch 1933; 12.2:1245-7.

14. Raben MS, Hollenberg CH. Effect of growth hormone on plasma free fatty acids. J Clin Invest 1959; 38:484-8.

15. Gaebler OH. Some effects of anterior pituitary extracts on nitrogen metabolism, water balance and energy metabolism. J Exp Med 1933; 57:349-63.

16. Manson J McK, Wilmore DW. Positive nitrogen balance with human growth hormone and hypocaloric intravenous feeding. Surgery 1986; 100:188-97.

17. Greenbaum AL, McLean P. The influence of pituitary growth hormone on the catabolism of fat. Biochem J 1953; 54:413-24.

18. Shipley RA, Long CNH. Studies on the ketogenic activity of the anterior pituitary. J Biochem (Tokyo) 1938; 22:2242-56.

19. Greenbaum AL. Changes in body composition and respiratory quotient of adult female rats treated with purified growth hormone. Biochem J 1953; 54:400-7.

20. Carey LC, Cloutier CT, Lowery BD. Growth hormone and adrenocortical response to shock and trauma in the human. Ann Surg 1971; 174:451-60.

21. Wilmore DW, Orcutt TW, Mason AD, Pruitt BA Jr. Alterations in hypothalamic function following thermal injury. J Trauma 1975; 15:697-703.

22. Wright PD, Johnson IDA. The effect of surgical operation on growth hormone levels in plasma. Surgery 1975; 77:479-86.

23. Aarima M, Syvalahti E, Viikari J, Ovaska J. Insulin, growth hormone and catecholamines as regulators of energy metabolism in the course of surgery. Acta Chir Scand 1978; 144:411-22.

24. Beisel WR, Woeber KA, Bartelloni PJ, Ingbar SH. Growth hormone response during sandfly fever. J Clin Endocrinol Metab 1968; 28:1220-1.

25. Frohman LA, Horton ES, Lebowitz HE. Growth hormone releasing action of a pseudomonas endotoxin. Metabolism 1967; 16:57-67.

26. Dahn MS, Mitchell RA, Smith S, et al. Altered immunologic function and nitrogen metabolism associated with depression of plasma growth hormone. JPEN 1984; 8:690-4.

27. Coates CL, Burwell RJ, Carlin SA, et al. The somatomedin activity in plasma from patients with multiple mechanical injuries: with observations on plasma cortisol. Injury 1981; 13:100-7.

28. Frayn KN, Price DA, Maycock PF, Carroll SM. Plasma somatomedin activity after injury in man and its relationship to other hormonal and metabolic changes. Clin Endocrinol (Oxf) 1984; 20:179-87.

29. Bazzare TL, et al. Human growth changes with age. Proceedings of the third international symposium on growth hormone and related peptides. Milan, 1975. Amsterdam: Exerpta Medica, 1976.

30. Finkelstein JW, Roffwarg HP, Boyar RM, et al. Age-related change in the 24 hour spontaneous secretion of growth hormone. J Clin Endocrinol Metab 1972; 35:665.

31. Johanson AJ, Blizzard RM. Low somatomedin-C levels in older men rise in response to growth hormone administration. Johns Hopkins Med J 1981; 149:115-7.

32. Cuthbertson DP, Shaw GB, Young FG. The influence of anterior pituitary extract on the metabolic response of the rat to injury. J Endocrinol 1941; 2:468-74.

33. Prudden JF, Pearson E, Soroff HS. Studies on growth hormone. II: The effect on the nitrogen metabolism of severely burned patients. Surg Gynecol Obstet 1956; 102:695-701.

34. Soroff HS, Rozin RR, Mooty JM, et al. Role of human growth hormone

in the response to trauma. I: Metabolic effects following burns. Ann Surg 1967; 166:739-52.

35. Liljedahl S-O, Gemzell C-A, Plantin L-O, Birke G. Effect of human growth hormone in patients with severe burns. Acta Chir Scand 1961; 122:1-14.

36. Wilmore DW, Moylan JA, Bristow BF, Mason AD, Pruitt BA Jr. Anabolic effects of human growth hormone and high caloric feedings following thermal injury. Surg Gynecol Obstet 1974; 138:875-84.

37. Ward HC, Halliday D, Sim AJW. Protein and energy metabolism with biosynthetic human growth hormone after gastro-intestinal surgery. Presented at ESPEN meeting, Milan 1984 (unpublished data).

38. Young LS, Ziegler TR, Manson J McK, Wilmore DW. The effects of growth hormone in patients receiving nutrition support. JPEN (in press).

39. Prudden JF, Nishihara G, Ocampo L. Studies on growth hormone. III: The effect on wound tensile strength of marked post-operative anabolism induced with growth hormone. Surg Gynecol Obstet 1958; 107:481-2.

40. Barbul A, Rettura G, Prior E, Levenson SM, Seifter E. Supplemental arginine, wound healing and thymus: arginine-pituitary interaction. Surg Forum 1978; 29:93.

41. Felig P, Marliss EB, Cahill GF Jr. Metabolic response to growth hormone during prolonged starvation. J Clin Invest 1971; 50:411-21.

33

INTERACTION OF GROWTH HORMONE AND NUTRITIONAL INTAKE IN FACILITATING NITROGEN CONSERVATION AND PROMOTING LIPOLYSIS

David R. Clemmons, David K. Snyder, and
Louis E. Underwood

Departments of Medicine and Pediatrics
University of North Carolina School of Medicine
Chapel Hill, NC 27514

INTRODUCTION

Growth hormone (GH) has multiple actions on target tissues that are coordinated to promote somatic growth. To provide adequate substrate for growth, GH has significant effects on carbohydrate, lipid and protein metabolism. While the effects on lipid and carbohydrate metabolism are believed to be direct or to be mediated through increased insulin secretion, the effects on protein synthesis are indirect, being mediated through the synthesis and secretion of somatomedin-C/insulin-like growth factor I (SmC/IGF-I), a potent stimulator of protein synthesis. The metabolic processes that coordinate the direct effects of GH with its indirect growth-promoting actions are incompletely understood.

EFFECTS OF GH ON LIPID AND CARBOHYDRATE METABOLISM

Early research on GH revealed that it stimulates lipolysis. Specifically, GH decreases carcass fat content of hypophysectomized or pituitary intact animals that are injected with GH for 3-5 weeks (1). GH subsequently was shown to inhibit the synthesis of lipids from radiolabeled glucose precursors (2). Further studies showed that GH causes a rapid increase in plasma-free fatty acids and glycerol in rats and humans (3,4). Stimulation of fatty acid release in vitro by GH also occurs but requires incubation with other hormones such as dexamethasone or epinephrine (5). Initially, it was believed that the lipolytic effects attributed to GH might be due to contamination of GH preparations with a lipolytic substance (6). However, studies with recombinant GH that is devoid of other pituitary hormones has shown that pure GH retains its lipid mobilizing properties (7). Stimulation of fatty acid oxidation by GH has also been detected in vitro and in whole animals (8). GH, therefore, appears to coordinate several lipolytic reactions, some of which may be counterbalanced by secondary hyperinsulinism, which would shift the equilibrium back toward lipid synthesis and fat retention (9).

The effects of GH on carbohydrate metabolism are more complex than those on lipids. Initially, GH stimulates insulin-like effects that result in an acute lowering of blood glucose within 20 min of injection. This effect is not due to stimulation of insulin secretion (10). After a delay, GH increases the test animal's resistance to insulin's effects (11). The secondary hyperinsulinism that follows GH administration is thought to result from a rise in blood glucose, which occurs as a result of decreased glucose utilization (12), possibly secondary to increased utilization of free fatty acids. These effects on carbohydrate balance, therefore, appear to be coordinated with the effects of GH on lipid metabolism.

EFFECTS OF GH ON PROTEIN METABOLISM

The effects of GH on protein metabolism are also diverse. Following injection of GH into hypophysectomized rats, there is increased incorporation of radiolabeled amino acids into muscle and increased albumin synthesis by the liver. Such actions have been difficult to demonstrate in vitro as direct actions of GH, and it is assumed that they are mediated by SmC/IGF-I. Injections of GH into rats causes positive nitrogen balance and increases muscle protein content. Recent studies in pigs have confirmed that GH has a major protein anabolic effect, even in young growing animals. Specifically, Chung et al. have demonstrated a 6-10% increase in muscle mass after injection of GH for 6 weeks (13).

Prolonged semistarvation regimes used in the treatment of obesity are accompanied by significant losses of total body nitrogen. It is possible that the symptoms of weakness and fatigue that accompany long-term weight loss are related to loss of muscle mass that is reflected in loss of nitrogen. There is, therefore, a need for an anabolic agent that will result in protein sparing. GH might be a useful therapeutic agent in this regard because of its nitrogen sparing and lipid mobilizing properties. The hypothesis that GH might be a useful adjunct to diet therapy for obesity has been difficult to test because of the scarcity of pituitary GH. A few studies, however, have examined the effect of GH on nitrogen retention in obese subjects that were undergoing short-term caloric restriction. Bray observed that injections of GH caused increased fatty acid oxidation when calorie intake was restricted to 500 calories/day (14). Likewise, when T3 was administered to diet-restricted subjects (900 calories/day), there was increased fat oxidation, but also increased nitrogen wasting. When GH was added to the T3 regimen, lipolysis was enhanced and conservation of nitrogen was improved (15). GH used therapeutically, therefore, offers the potential to aid in the mobilization of lipids during caloric restriction, yet preserve sufficient nitrogen to prevent excessive protein catabolism. Since long-term diet therapy is accompanied by an obligatory loss of muscle mass, injections of GH have the potential to counteract this effect and preserve protein stores.

Although GH might be a useful adjunct for treating obesity, dietary restriction remains the cornerstone of therapy. In defining the optimum diet to facilitate lipolysis yet cause maximum protein sparing, precise measurements of protein sparing are needed. In our laboratory, we have used measurements of plasma SmC/IGF-I as one of the indicators of protein sparing. Blood concentrations of SmC/IGF-I increase three- to fivefold after injection of GH into hypopituitary patients (16). Furthermore, SmC/IGF-I has direct stimulatory effects on protein synthesis in vitro and following the infusion of SmC/IGF-I into hypophysectomized animals, there is an increase in muscle protein content (17). Most importantly, the plasma concentrations of this growth factor are not only GH dependent but also reflect changes in nutritional status (18). The measurement of plasma SmC/IGF concentrations, therefore, provides an index of the interaction between GH administration and test diets in promoting nitrogen sparing.

348

To determine the efficacy of SmC/IGF in monitoring the response to nutritional intervention, we fasted 7 obese adult subjects for 10 days. Plasma SmC/IGF-I fell from a mean control value of 0.83 ± 0.26 U/ml (± 1 SD) to 0.21 ± 0.11 U/ml by the end of the fast (19). This change correlated with alterations in mean daily nitrogen balance (r=0.74). This study was extended by the observation of Merrimee et al. who showed that following a 3-day fast, the mean basal SmC/IGF-I concentration of lean adult volunteers did not increase in response to injections of GH (20). This suggested that there is a minimum caloric intake that is required for SmC/IGF-I levels to increase in response to injections of GH.

To determine the dietary components that are required to maintain normal plasma SmC/IGF-I concentrations, we fasted normal weight volunteers for 5 days, then refed one of three test diets. These diets were of the following composition: 1.3 gm protein and 35 Kcal/kg ideal body weight (IBW); 0.4 gm protein and 35 Kcal/kg IBW; or 0.4 gm protein and 11 Kcal/kg IBW. Following 5 days of fasting, there was a 64% decline in plasma SmC/IGF-I concentrations, and ingestion of the control diet led to an increase in SmC/IGF-I to 72% of the control level by the fifth day of refeeding (21) (Fig. 1). The normal calorie, protein-deficient diet resulted in an increase to 55% of the control values, whereas the diet that was restricted in protein and calories led to a further decline in SmC/IGF-I. Both protein and calories, therefore, appear to be required to restore plasma SmC/IGF-I to normal after fasting, although the caloric content of the diet appears to be the more important variable. There was a strongly positive correlation (r=0.90) in these subjects between the change in plasma SmC/IGF-I for each diet interval and the mean daily nitrogen balance for that interval, suggesting that changes in plasma SmC/IGF-I may be linked to changes in protein metabolism.

Because plasma SmC/IGF-I concentrations continued to fall on the protein and calorie restricted diet, we carried out another study in human volunteers to determine whether there is a threshold of calorie or protein intake that is required for any detectable increase in SmC/IGF-I concentrations to occur. To determine the effects of caloric restriction, 6 adult volunteers were fasted for 5 days, then refed in succession diets containing 11, 18 and 25 Kcal with 1.0 gm protein/kg IBW. To determine the effects of protein restriction, these subjects were fasted again, then fed 3 consecutive diets containing 0.2, 0.4 and 1.0 gm protein and 35 Kcal/kg IBW. The results showed that despite normal protein intake, a calorie intake between 11 and 18 Kcal/kg was required for any increase in plasma SmC/IGF-I to occur. The subjects did not reach control SmC/IGF-I values until 25 Kcal/kg was ingested (22). In contrast, if control energy intake (35 Kcal/kg) was maintained, even severe protein restriction (0.2 gm/kg) resulted in a significant increase in SmC/IGF-I, although 1.0 gm protein was required to reach basal prefast SmC/IGF-I concentrations. In this study, as in others, the changes in SmC/IGF-I correlated with changes in nitrogen balance (r=0.88). It appeared that ingestion of between 11-18 Kcal of energy would be required to effect an increase in SmC/IGF-I. More recent studies suggest that this basal caloric requirement may be lower in obesity or during chronic adaptation to calorie-deficient diets. Our results also suggested that SmC/IGF-I may be useful in defining the amounts of protein and energy that are necessary to maintain adequate nitrogen balance during the treatment of obesity by calorie restriction.

To determine the component of dietary protein that is responsible for the effect of protein on plasma SmC/IGF-I, we fasted 6 subjects for two 5-day intervals, then refed one of two diets that were deficient in total nitrogen (48% of control) but contained adequate energy (35 Kcal/kg IBW).

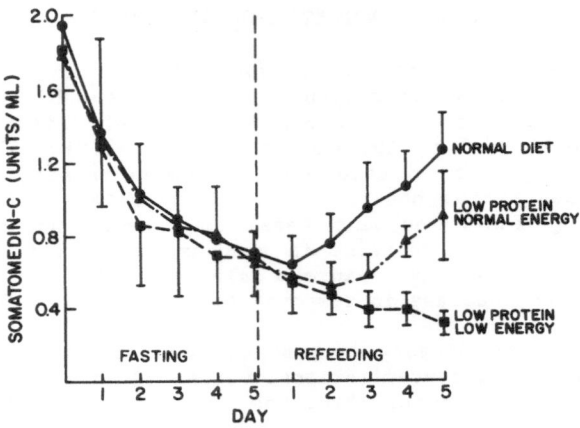

Fig. 1. Change in plasma SmC/IGF-I levels in response to test diets of defined composition. Five normal weight volunteers were fasted for 5-day intervals, then refed one of three test diets. The dietary compositions are indicated in the text. The results represent the mean ± 1 SE. Reproduced from Isley et al. (21).

One diet was further restricted by supplying 80% of the nitrogen as non-essential amino acids (NEAA), whereas the companion diet contained 80% of nitrogen as essential amino acids (EAA). The EAA-supplemented diet caused a greater increase in plasma SmC/IGF-I values (to 1.41 ± 0.19 U/ml by day 10), whereas the NEAA-supplemented diet allowed values to increase to 1.15 ± 0.15 U/ml (P<0.02) (23) (Fig. 2). Therefore, the ratio of EAA to total nitrogen appears to be an important variable in controlling the SmC/IGF-I response to refeeding. Based on these observations, we believe that a calorie-restricted diet enriched in protein and essential amino acids will be optimal for preservation of nitrogen stores, and that measurement of plasma SmC/IGF-I will be useful in monitoring this response.

To test this supposition, we studied 6 obese volunteers who were 30-70% over ideal body weight for two 14-day intervals. During one study interval, they received an isocaloric diet that was deficient in total calories (32% control) but was supplemented with 1.0 gm protein/kg IBW. In the other interval, the diet contained only 0.34 gm protein/kg and the same degree of caloric restriction. Plasma SmC/IGF-I concentrations fell on both diets, but by day 10 the values were 0.63 ± 0.27 U/ml on the nonsupplemented diet and 0.79 ± 0.42 U/ml on the protein-supplemented diet. SmC/IGF-I values in the subjects receiving protein supplementation remained significantly higher through day 14. Nitrogen balance data also reflected these differences, since the subjects on the nonsupplemented diet lost a mean of -5.40 ± 0.98 gm nitrogen/day compared to -3.44 ± 0.56 gm/day on the supplemented diet (P<0.01). Protein supplementation, therefore, resulted in higher plasma SmC/IGF-I concentrations and nitrogen conservation. Both groups of subjects remained in net negative nitrogen balance, however, even with optimization of diet therapy.

GH AS AN ADJUNCT TO DIET RESTRICTION

In the past, studies on the effects of GH on protein sparing and lipolysis have been impeded by the limited supplies of pituitary GH avail-

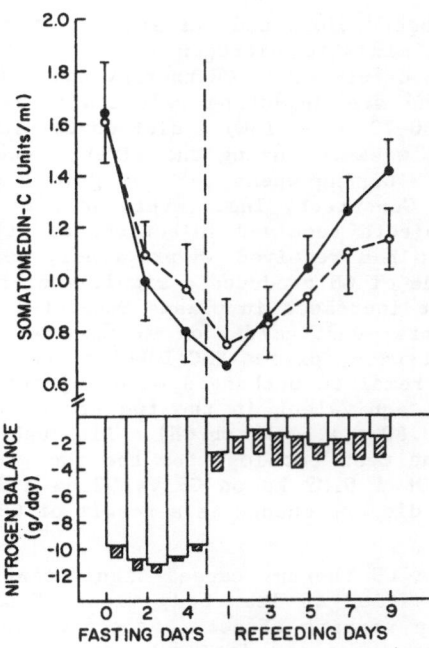

Fig. 2. SmC/IGF-I response to refeeding
test diets of different essential amino
acid content. Six volunteers (normal
weight) were fasted for 5-day intervals,
then refed one of two test diets, both
of which were deficient in total nitrogen (48% of control). The supplemented
diet (•—•; open bars) contained 80% of
the nitrogen as essential amino acids,
whereas the nonsupplemented diet (o--o;
cross-hatched bars) contained 80% of the
nitrogen as nonessential amino acids.
The results represent the mean ± 1 SE.
From Clemmons et al. (23).

able. Bray fed 8 obese adults a diet containing 450 calories for periods
ranging from 11-16 days (14). During the last 4 days of diet restriction,
8 mg of GH was administered each day. Oxygen consumption was increased
from 21.8 to 24.5 (L/min) by GH treatment. In a later study, Bray et al.
(15) fed 8 obese subjects 900 calories/day while administering 200 mcg of
triiodothyronine. This led to significant negative nitrogen balance. Six
of the subjects also received GH (5 mg/day) for 8 days. GH caused significant nitrogen retention in 4 and an additional increase in oxygen consumption. Two subjects, however, did not have improved nitrogen retention
with GH treatment. In another study in which there was total caloric
deprivation for 12 days, nitrogen retention improved in response to GH in
3 of 6 subjects. The mean daily nitrogen balance of control subjects was
-6.2 gm/day, and this increased to -3.5 gm/day with GH therapy (24).
Serum-free fatty acids also increased in response to GH injections. Felig
et al. fasted 5 obese subjects for 31 days, then administered GH (5 mg)
daily for 3 days (25). Although urea nitrogen was retained compared to
the control period, ammonia excretion increased and total urinary nitrogen
remained unchanged.

Based on these observations and our studies of dietary interventions that are designed to minimize nitrogen wasting, we have conducted two preliminary studies to determine if GH therapy can induce nitrogen conservation in subjects who are ingesting calorically restricted diets. We gave 8 obese adults (30-70% over IBW) a diet containing 24 Kcal and 1.0 gm protein/kg IBW for 11 weeks. During the first 2 weeks, we assessed the effect of diet alone. During weeks 3-5, we gave 4 subjects recombinant human GH (Protropin®; Genentech, Inc.) every 48 h at a dose of 0.1 mg/kg IBW. The other 4 subjects received injections of vehicle. During weeks 8-10, the subjects who had received GH previously were given vehicle and vice versa. Injections of GH produced a significant reduction in nitrogen losses and significant increases in plasma SmC/IGF-I values. Specifically, nitrogen losses were -0.35 gm/day on GH compared to -2.21 gm/day with vehicle (Fig. 3). Likewise, plasma SmC/IGF-I increased to 3.2 ± 1.6 U/ml by day 8, whereas it remained unchanged with injections of vehicle (26). Total weight loss was equivalent in the two groups (3.01 ± 1.32 kg with vehicle, compared to 3.80 ± 1.12 kg on GH). Although 3 subjects lost more fat on GH therapy, the mean fat loss for the two groups was not statistically different (3.06 ± 0.39 kg on GH vs. 2.64 ± 1.08 kg on vehicle). Fasting blood glucose did not change as a result of GH treatment.

We concluded that GH therapy caused significant short-term nitrogen retention with preservation of lean body mass. Plasma SmC/IGF-I values reflected this protein sparing effect. Selective fat loss was not documented. However, the treatment interval was short, the GH dosage was near physiologic replacement and the diet was not markedly restrictive. Of interest was the observation that plasma SmC/IGF-I values of control subjects did not decrease with this degree of calorie restriction. When a group of lean volunteers ingested an identical diet, their plasma SmC/-IGF-I values fell to 64% of control after 7 days (27). Therefore, obese and lean individuals differ in their response to caloric restriction.

To determine the effect of GH treatment on fat loss and nitrogen balance over a longer period of time, we selected 20 subjects (16 women, 4 men) who were between 30-70% over ideal body weight and between 23 and 54 years of age. The subjects were fed a diet consisting of 1.2 gm protein and 18 Kcal/kg IBW throughout the study and were given GH or saline from weeks 2-12. Ten subjects received recombinant methionyl GH (Protropin® 0.1 mg/kg IBW) IM every other day, and 10 received vehicle. In the GH-treated subjects, plasma SmC/IGF-I concentrations rose from 1.61 ± 0.81 to 2.92 ± 1.16 U/ml within 48 h. The mean SmC/IGF-I level in the GH-treated group was maximal after 10 days of therapy (4.9 ± 1.3 U/ml), and remained consistently greater than 3.18 ± 1.27 U/ml for the duration of the study. The control group had no change in mean plasma SmC/IGF-I. Likewise, nitrogen conservation began immediately in the subjects receiving GH, with nitrogen balance increasing to +2.3 ± 0.6 gms/day by day 9 of GH injections compared to -3.6 ± 0.8 gms/day in the subjects who received vehicle in conjunction with diet restriction. This difference between GH-treated and control subjects narrowed as the study progressed so that by day 35 there were no significant differences between the GH- and saline-treated groups. The mean nitrogen balance was significantly more positive for the first 33 days of GH administration compared to vehicle (saline, -1.91 ± 1.1 gm/day, compared to GH, +0.07 ± 1.82 gm/day; P<0.001). In contrast, nitrogen balance values were not different during the last 42 days of injections (saline -1.09 ± 0.97 gm/day, compared to GH -1.00 ± 1.67 gm/day, NS). GH, therefore, was able to maintain elevations in plasma SmC/IGF for the entire 11 weeks without attenuation, whereas the nitrogen balance response to GH attenuated significantly after 6 weeks. These results suggest that there is a time-dependent attenuation of the action of SmC/IGF with respect to retention of nitrogen.

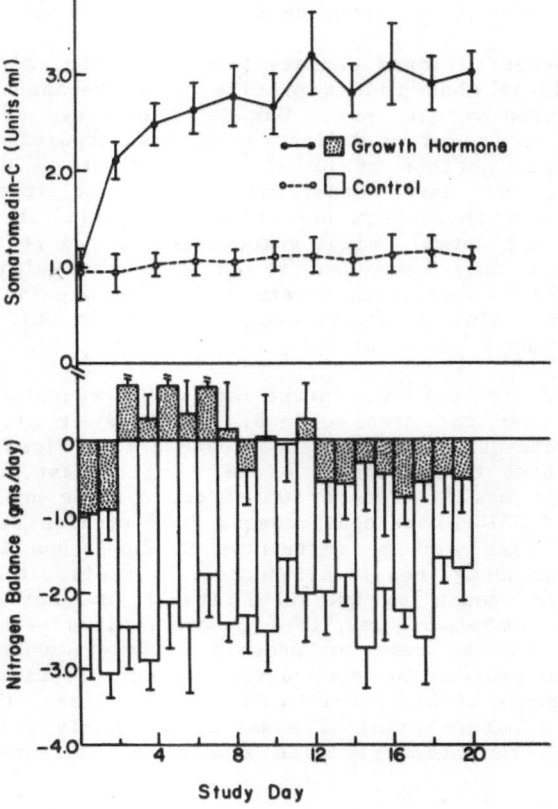

Fig. 3. Changes in plasma SmC/IGF-I and nitrogen balance in response to dietary restriction and GH administration. Eight obese volunteers were placed on a calorically restricted diet containing 24 Kcal/kg. They received Protropin® 0.1 mg/kg every other day or vehicle injections. The results are expressed as the mean ± 1 SD. Reprinted from Clemmons et al. (26).

In contrast to the pronounced effects on protein metabolism, GH did not accelerate the loss of body fat. Specifically, there was no signif-icant difference in total weight loss (GH, 13.9 ± 1.1 kg compared to saline, 15.2 ± 0.8 kg) or percentage body fat loss by hydrostatic weighing (GH, 8.1 ± 2.4% compared to saline, 7.5 ± 1.5%, NS). This failure to lose fat selectively was not due entirely to the development of refractoriness to GH because the increment in plasma free fatty acids (FFA) was not completely lost as GH treatment was prolonged. At the beginning of the study, the increment in FFA that had occurred 4 h after GH was 0.86 ± 0.37 meq/ml. This declined to 0.35 ± 0.41 meq/ml by day 35 of GH injection, but the response was never lost and remained significantly greater than the response of subjects injected with saline. Because net fat loss did not occur, it seems probable that some of the free fatty acids released by GH must have undergone reesterification and synthesis into lipid. We observed no signs of carbohydrate intolerance as a result of GH therapy. Specifically, fasting blood glucose and 2-hr postprandial glucose concentrations were not increased significantly. Likewise, we observed no significant change in urinary C-peptide excretion.

Because GH causes nitrogen conservation even when caloric intake is restricted, we believe that it has promise as a therapeutic adjunct in prolonged diet-induced weight loss. Our data, however, do not yet show this and more work is needed to define the optimal conditions for expression of the biologic actions of GH in such patients. GH also may be useful in patients who have borderline capacity to ingest or absorb nutrients and require short-term nutritional support. In this regard, Wilmore has shown that normal weight volunteers who are restricted to 50% of a normal caloric intake respond to GH with a significant positive nitrogen balance (28). Therefore, treatment with GH may increase nitrogen conservation in the thin, undernourished patients as well as those are dieting to lose weight.

The breakpoint in caloric intake at which resistance to GH or SmC/IGF-I develops has not been defined. Merrimee et al. (20) starved normal weight volunteers for 3 days and showed a significant reduction in the SmC/IGF-I response to injections of GH. In contrast, obese subjects whose caloric intake was limited to 50% of control for prolonged periods maintained normal SmC/IGF-I responsiveness. Our studies suggest that in obese subjects calories must be restricted to less than 18 Kcal/kg IBW before SmC/IGF-I responsiveness is attenuated. Likewise, the factors that might determine resistance to SmC/IGF-I itself are not well defined. Because changes in the plasma SmC/IGF-I concentrations seem to correlate well with changes in the rate of protein turnover, understanding the factors that reduce protein turnover during caloric deprivation may help to predict the response of SmC/IGF-I to diet restriction. These questions should be addressed before clinical studies on acutely ill patients are undertaken in order to rationally plan studies in patients with complex metabolic problems.

ACKNOWLEDGMENTS

The authors gratefully acknowledge the technical assistance of Eyvonne Bruton and Karen Koerber. We thank Emilia Richichi for her help in preparing the manuscript. These studies were supported by Grants AG-02331, HL-36313, HD-08299 and AM-01022 from the National Institutes of Health. These studies were conducted on the Clinical Research Unit that is supported by grant No. RR-00031.

REFERENCES

1. Young FG. Growth and diabetes in normal animals treated with pituitary (anterior lobe) diabetogenic extract. Biochem J 1945; 39:515.
2. Engel F, Engel M, McPherson H. Ketogenic and adipokinetic activities of pituitary hormones. Endocrinology 1957; 61:713.
3. Goodman HM, Knobil E. Growth hormone and fatty acid mobilization: the role of the pituitary, adrenal, and thyroid. Endocrinology 1961; 69:187.
4. Raben MS, Hollenberg CH. Effect of growth hormone plasma fatty acids. J Clin Invest 1959; 38:484.
5. Goodman HM. Permissive effects of hormones on lipolysis. Endocrinology 1970; 86:1064.
6. Frigeri LG. Absence of in vitro dexamethasone dependent lipolytic activity from highly purified growth hormone. Endocrinology 1980; 107:738.
7. Goodman HM, Grichting G. Growth hormone and lipolysis: a reevalua-

tion. Endocrinology 1983; 113:1697.

8. Goldman JK, Bressler R. Growth hormone stimulation of fatty acid utilization by adipose tissue. Endocrinology 1968; 811:306.

9. Mendel VJ. Influence of insulin to growth hormone ratio on body composition of mice. Am J Physiol 1979; 238:E231.

10. Freiberg SE, Merrimee TJ. Acute metabolic effects of human growth hormone. Diabetes 1979; 23:499.

11. Hollobaugh SC, Tzagourinis M, Folk RL, Kruger FA, Hamiur C. The diabetogenic action of human growth hormone; glucose-fatty acid interrelationships. Metabolism 1968; 17:485.

12. Russell JA. Effects of growth hormone on protein and carbohydrate metabolism. Am J Clin Nutr 1957; 5:404.

13. Chung C, Etherton T, Wiggins J. Stimulation of swine growth by porcine growth hormone. J Anim Sci 1985; 60:118.

14. Bray GA. Calorigenic effect of human growth hormone obesity. J Clin Endocrinol Metab 1969; 29:119.

15. Bray GA, Raben MS, Londono J, Gallagher TF Jr. Effect of triiodothyronine, growth hormone, and anabolic steroids on nitrogen excretion and oxygen consumption in obese patients. J Clin Endocrinol Metab 1971; 33:293.

16. Copeland KC, Underwood LE, Van Wyk JJ. Induction of immunoreactive somatomedin-C in human serum by growth hormone: dose response relationships and effect on chromatographic profiles. J Clin Endocrinol Metab 1980; 50:690.

17. Schoenle E, Zapf J, Humbel RE, Froesch ER. Insulin-like growth factor I stimulates growth in hypophysectomized rats. Nature 1982; 296:252.

18. Clemmons DR, Van Wyk JJ. Factors controlling blood concentration of somatomedin-C. Clin Endocrinol Metab 1983; 13:113.

19. Clemmons DR, Kilbanski A, Underwood LE, et al. Reduction in immunoreactive somatomedin-C during fasting in humans. J Clin Endocrinol Metab 1981; 53:1247.

20. Merrimee TJ, Zapf J, Froesch ER. Insulin-like growth factors in the fed and fasted states. J Clin Endocrinol Metab 1982; 55:999.

21. Isley WL, Underwood LE, Clemmons DR. Dietary components that regulate serum somatomedin-C concentrations in humans. J Clin Invest 1983; 71:175.

22. Isley WL, Underwood LE, Clemmons DR. Change in plasma somatomedin-C in response to ingestion of diets with variable protein and energy content. JPEN 1984; 8:407.

23. Clemmons DR, Seek MM, Underwood LE. Supplemental essential amino acids augment the somatomedin-C/IGF-I response to refeeding after fasting. Metabolism 1985; 34:391.

24. Schwartz F, Der Kinderen HG, Van Riet JH, Thijssen H, Van Wayjen GA. Influence of exogenous human growth hormone on the metabolism of fasting obese patients. Metabolism 1972; 21:297.

25. Cahill GF Jr. Metabolic response of human growth hormone during prolonged starvation. J Clin Invest 1971; 50:411.

26. Clemmons DR, Snyder DK, Williams R, Underwood LE. Growth hormone administration conserves lean body mass during dietary restriction of obese subjects. J Clin Endocrinol Metab 1987; 64:878.

27. Smith AT, Clemmons DR, Ben Ezra V, McMurray R, UnderWood LE. Exercise modulates the response of somatomedin-C to dietary restriction. Metabolism (in press).

28. Manson JMcK, Wilmore DW. Positive nitrogen balance with human growth hormone and hypocaloric intravenous feeding. Surgery 1986; 100:188.

34

ASSESSMENT OF THE RISKS OF TREATMENT WITH

HUMAN GROWTH HORMONE

Louis E. Underwood, M.D.

Professor of Pediatrics
University of North Carolina at Chapel Hill
Chapel Hill, North Carolina

Human growth hormone (GH) has an unusual history as a drug, having been used therapeutically for 30 years, but having its distribution limited to relatively few patients, most of whom were GH deficient. Although GH has had remarkably few observable side effects and is accepted as safe when used as replacement therapy (1), this experience provides little insight into the risks of using GH therapeutically in patients who are not GH deficient. Because we now accept that injections of pituitary GH place patients at risk for infection with the agent causing Creutzfeldt-Jakob disease (2), it is likely that GH used therapeutically in the future will be obtained through recombinant DNA techniques. In this presentation, I will draw on data derived from studies of pituitary GH and try to assess the risks of using recombinant GH to treat conditions other than GH deficiency.

RELATIONSHIPS BETWEEN ENDOGENOUS PRODUCTION OF GH AND DOSES USED FOR THERAPY

As with virtually all drugs, it is likely that if too much GH is given, undesirable side effects will result. The GH excess of acromegaly causes bony and soft tissue overgrowth, carbohydrate intolerance, hypertension, and a variety of other harmful effects. On the other hand, no harmful effects have been observed when certain doses of GH are administered to hypopituitary patients for long periods of time. The questions are: What doses of GH are safe? What role does the duration and schedule of therapy play in the occurrence of side effects? To what extent is the patient's endogenous GH involved in determining risk?

The amounts of GH most frequently given in the United States have been 0.05-0.1 mg/kg every other day. Because dosages used in most therapeutic regimens have been based on units of biological activity, this assigns an activity of 2 U of GH/mg. Most GH deficient patients, therefore, have received the equivalent of 25-50 µg GH/kg/day. Using continuous infusions of radiolabeled hGH, several investigators have determined the metabolic clearance rates of this hormone in normal adults and in patients with acromegaly (3-7). Production rates of GH are calculated by relating endogenous concentrations with metabolic clearance rates. Using these techniques, the mean production rates of GH in normal adults are

estimated to be 5.5–17.4 µg/kg/day (Table 1). In patients with acromegaly, production rates are estimated to be 50 to >1,000 µg/kg/day, but
exhibit considerable variability from patient to patient and from the
studies of one group of investigators to another (3–7). The amounts used
for therapy, therefore, are at or above the total daily GH production in
normal individuals and lower than the amounts produced by most patients
with active acromegaly.

These comparisons are problematic because of possible differences in
biological effectiveness between the multiple daily bursts of endogenous
growth hormone and the once daily (or once every other day) injections of
exogenous GH. Indeed, in rats it has been observed that variable growth
rates are obtained when the frequency of administering a fixed total daily
dose of GH is varied (8). Specifically, 50 µg of GH given 4 times daily
produces significantly more linear bone growth and weight gain than 200 µg
administered once daily or 25 µg given 8 times/day. In studies on obese
adults receiving a modestly restricted caloric intake, we have observed
that the injection of the equivalent of 50 µg GH/kg/day produces a plasma
somatomedin–C/insulin–like growth factor I (SmC/IGF–I) concentration of
approximately 3 units/ml, a value that is above the normal range for
adults and is equal to that observed in patients with mild acromegaly (9).

Another important question in determining how much exogenous GH can
be administered safely is whether injections of GH cause suppression of
endogenous GH secretion. Studies in monkeys (10) and in man (11–12)
suggest that infusions or injections of GH suppress GH secretion in
response to provocative stimuli. Likewise, as little as 2 units (~1 mg)
of GH given to normal adults twice daily for 5 days causes significant
suppression of sleep–related GH secretion (13) (Fig. 1). This suppression
of GH secretion might be due to a direct effect of GH, an indirect effect
mediated through SmC/IGF–I, or both. In support of indirect suppression
mediated via SmC/IGF–I are observations that SmC/IGF–I inhibits GH secretion by pituitary explants (14), stimulates somatomedin production in
hypothalamic explants (14), inhibits the GH releasing effect of GH releas-

Table 1. Growth hormone production rates.

Reference number	n	Sex	Production rate (µg/kg/d)
In Normal Adults:			
3	9	M	17.4
3	8	F	15.8
4	6	M	5.5
6	22	M/F	7.1
7	22	F	11.7
7	16	M	17.0
In Acromegaly:			
3	3	M/F	16–1500
5	5	M/F	75 (49–105)
6	4	M/F	60–900
7	3	M/F	207–255

GH Therapy

0.1 Units/kg 3 times weekly = 25 µg/kg/day

ing hormone (GHRH) on cultured pituitary cells (15) and inhibits GH secretion in vivo when infused into the cerebral ventricles of rats (16).

We conclude from these studies that it is likely that exogenous GH suppresses the secretion of endogenous GH, and that in estimating the total amount of GH available to a patient, it may not be necessary to add the amount of GH secreted normally to the amount given by injection. It also seems likely that at least in adults, doses of GH greater than 50 μg/kg/day might exceed safe limits, particularly if given for prolonged periods. Although only speculation, we should consider the possibility that the mechanisms involved in suppression of GH secretion might be activated at lower doses of GH than those that promote growth and other biological effects. If this were the case, injection of modest amounts of GH might not only not have the desired therapeutic effect, but might produce a relative GH deficiency.

RISK OF ANTIBODIES TO GH

With the exception of rare patients with deletions of the GH gene, the principal factor responsible for the formation of antibodies to GH is the purity of the preparation used for therapy. With the first recombinant GH preparations, development of antibodies was the rule. As greater purity has been achieved, however, the percentage of patients developing antibodies has fallen and is now on the order of 5-30%, depending on the patient's previous experience with GH therapy, the duration of treatment, the assay method used to detect the antibodies and the criteria used to establish that antibodies are present. Although development of antibodies to GH in the serum of treated patients is believed to be of no clinical significance, it is often used as an indicator of the overall quality of the GH preparation and of the likelihood that patients will develop antibodies sufficient to attenuate growth. Growth attenuation because of such antibodies is rarely observed with recombinant preparations.

Concern has been expressed that the development of antibodies might be more consequential in individuals who secrete GH normally than in GH deficient patients, because endogenous GH in the former might continue to stimulate the immune response. As a result, antibodies might persist once therapy is stopped, inducing a condition in which serum antibodies continue to bind GH and limit availability of the hormone for biological

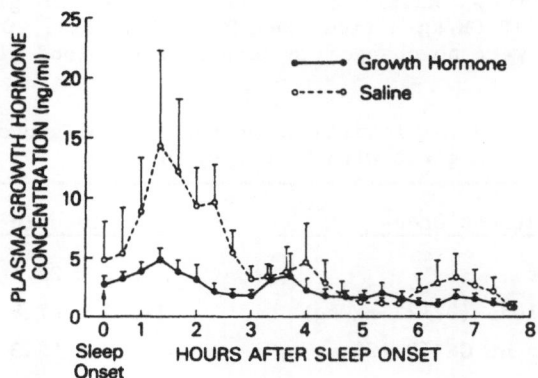

Fig. 1. Effect of GH injections (1 mg twice daily) for 5 days on nocturnal GH secretion in normal adults. From reference 13.

actions. On the basis of experience in hypopituitary children, it seems unlikely that this will occur because antibodies produced in response to one GH preparation often do not persist when another GH preparation is substituted (17). This leads to the conclusion that antibodies to GH are formed because of alterations in the GH molecule or impurities in the GH preparation that serve as adjuvants. It seems unlikely, therefore, that endogenous GH will continue to stimulate the formation of antibodies.

In summary, there is little risk that recombinant GH preparations will stimulate the production of GH antibodies that attenuate the biological effects of exogenous GH. Even if this occurs, there is little reason to believe that the antibodies will persist once therapy is stopped or that antibodies will inhibit the biological actions of endogenous GH.

RISK OF CARBOHYDRATE INTOLERANCE

The observations that 25-50% of patients with acromegaly have carbohydrate intolerance and approximately 10% are diabetic (18) underlies the concern that therapy with GH might have significant adverse effects on carbohydrate metabolism. Adding to this concern are the results from several early studies in which treatment with GH was shown to cause impairment of glucose tolerance (19), to induce hyperglycemia and ketosis in hypophysectomized diabetic patients (20), and to be diabetogenic when given in high doses to young diabetics on a fixed dietary and insulin regimen (21). However, many investigators treating thousands of GH deficient children have observed that GH is not diabetogenic when used as replacement therapy to stimulate growth.

The studies that may provide the best answer to the question of risks of carbohydrate intolerance are those in which prolonged GH therapy is given to short children who are not deficient in GH. Rosenfeld et al. have reported the results of a one-year controlled trial in girls 4-12 years of age with Turner syndrome (22). Seventy girls were assigned randomly to receive either no treatment, methionyl GH (0.125 mg/kg 3 times weekly), oxandrolone (0.125 mg/kg/day) or GH combined with oxandrolone. GH caused no significant change in fasting blood glucose, serum glucose following ingestion of 1.75 gm glucose/kg orally, or in fasting serum insulin concentrations. The only evidence that GH antagonized the action of insulin was significant increases in serum insulin concentrations 60 min after oral glucose loading (Table 2).

In another study, Raiti et al. (23) treated 52 girls with Turner syndrome with 0.2 IU GH/kg 3 times weekly (2.4 IU/mg). Over 18 months of observation there were no changes in mean fasting blood glucose concentra-

Table 2. Serum insulin responses to oral glucose in girls with Turner syndrome.*

Patient Group	Serum Insulin (uU/ml)
Controls	42.2 ± 25.4 (1 SD)
Oxandrolone (0.125 mg/kg)	110.7 ± 87.8
Recombinant GH (0.125 mg/kg)	77.2 ± 52.3
Both oxandrolone and GH	92.2 ± 52.4

*Samples drawn 60 min after oral glucose loading. All treatments were for 1 year. From reference 22.

tions or in blood glucose concentrations obtained 30, 60, 120 and 180 min after oral glucose loading. Three patients had glucose intolerance before GH therapy (1 h glucose >200 mg/dl, and 2 or 3 h glucoses >180 mg/dl). The glucose intolerance of these patients was not worsened by GH therapy. Unfortunately, serum insulin concentrations were not measured in this study.

We have administered recombinant methionyl GH (Genentech, Inc.) at a dose of 0.1 mg/kg ideal body weight every 48 h to 10 obese adults for 11 weeks (24). These subjects were fed an 18 Kcal/kg ideal body weight reducing diet during therapy. Mean fasting blood glucose and serum insulin concentrations and 2-h postprandial glucose and insulin concentrations were not higher in the GH-treated than in control subjects. Likewise, no increment in 24-h urinary C-peptide was observed as a result of GH therapy. While these results are reassuring, they must be interpreted in light of the fact that dietary restriction might have attenuated any tendency toward carbohydrate intolerance.

We conclude from these data that it is rational to be concerned that GH treatment might cause patients to develop carbohydrate intolerance. It appears, however, that most GH recipients are able to compensate for the diabetogenic actions of GH by increasing insulin secretion. Perhaps these patients will not be at risk. On the other hand, patients who have pre-existing impairment of insulin secretory reserve may be at higher risk for carbohydrate intolerance and diabetes. More experience is needed to assess the accuracy of these conclusions, and to determine whether the increased insulin secretion in response to GH will have adverse effects.

RISK OF SALT AND WATER RETENTION AND OF HYPERTENSION

Plasma volumes are increased in patients with active acromegaly and return to normal when the disease is treated successfully (25-27). In addition, 20-30% of acromegalic patients develop hypertension (18). Injection of GH (10 mg) into normal adults reduces urinary sodium excretion and urine volume within 12 h (28), and 24-h urinary sodium excretion is decreased by 15-53 mEq/day (28) (Table 3). Likewise, GH given over several days causes persistent sodium and potassium retention and hypervolemia (28,29; Fig. 2). GH is believed to exert these effects by stimulating tubular reabsorption of sodium because it acts without increasing aldosterone (28) and in adrenalectomized patients (28). Furthermore, GH injections stimulate renal sodium-potassium-ATPase activation directly in hypophysectomized rats (30).

In our studies of the effect of GH injections on obese adult volunteers receiving restricted caloric intake, we have evidence for sodium retention (24). Unlike controls, subjects given recombinant GH (0.1 mg/kg/ideal body weight every other day) failed to lose weight during the first week of therapy. For the next 10 weeks of GH therapy, weight loss paralleled that of controls and when GH was stopped, a dramatic loss of weight occurred so that there was no difference between GH treated and control subjects in the mean total weight lost during dietary restriction. Several of these subjects developed mild peripheral edema during GH therapy.

The potential consequences of fluid retention due to GH therapy are obvious in some patients. While none of our obese volunteers suffered any significant ill effects, this might not be the case in older patients or in patients with preexisting cardiopulmonary disease. The link between sodium and water retention and hypertension in patients with acromegaly is not established, but it seems likely that the former contribute to

Table 3. Responses to one injection of
human growth hormone.*

Subject	hGH (mg)	Derivation from Control		
		Urinary N (gm/d)	Urinary Na (mEq/d)	Urinary K (mEq/d)
1	10	1.0	50	31
2	10	1.9	17	14
3	10	0.9	26	60
4	10	1.3	52	46.5
5	8.2	2.4	53	31
6	10	2.0	--	--
7	8.2	1.0	15	6
Mean		1.5	36	31

Na intake = 110–120 mEq/day
*From reference 28.

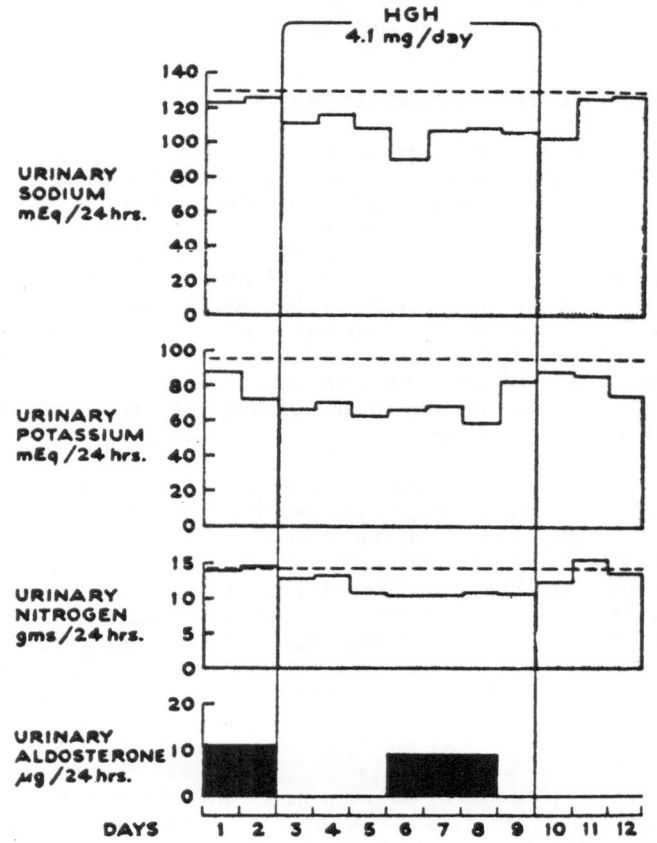

Fig. 2. Effects of prolonged injection of GH
in normal volunteers. From Reference 28.

hypertension and might be significant in GH-treated patients who have a predisposition to hypertension.

RISK OF ENHANCING TUMOR FORMATION OR TUMOR GROWTH

Several experimental studies suggest that GH might stimulate tumor formation. Although hypophysectomy produces changes in hormones other than GH, it has been shown that removal of the pituitary of rats causes regression of stem-cell erythroblastic leukemias that have been induced with 7, 8, 12-trimethylbenzanthracene (31). Also, hypophysectomy markedly decreases the tendency to form sarcomas in rats injected with methylcholanthrene (32). Furthermore, in hypophysectomized rats treated for 305-346 days with 0.4-2.5 mg of GH, there was almost complete absence of neoplasia (33), while intact rats treated in a similar fashion develop tumors of lymphoid tissue (34), adrenals (35), and other organs at a high rate (36).

The incidence of polyposis and carcinoma of the gastrointestinal tract is increased in humans with acromegaly. In 17 patients with acromegaly, Klein et al. (37) observed polyps in 9 (premalignant adenomatous polyps in 5). In 44 patients with acromegaly, 4 had colonic carcinoma, 2 had breast cancer, 3 had thyroid adenomas and single cases of renal cell, papillary thyroid, parathyroid, cervical, or uterine carcinomas were observed (37). Ituarte et al. (38) likewise observed that 3 of 12 acromegalic patients had colon carcinoma and 3 others had polyps. In another survey of 48 acromegalic patients, 7 were found to have had malignancies, producing ratios of observed/expected incidence for gastrointestinal malignancies of 4.55 (39).

While these observations on the relationship between GH and tumor formation are derived from special situations and do not make a compelling statement for increased likelihood of tumor formation in patients treated with GH, these data should be kept in mind as trials proceed.

RISK OF TREATMENT FAILURE

Studies on the use of GH in short children who are not GH deficient indicate that as many as 50% of the patients will have no significant improvement in growth rate (40,41). When considering treatment for such children, physicians and parents often forget that there is a substantial chance of treatment failure and that such failure may have adverse psychological effects on the child. Family members often have unrealistically high expectations of GH therapy (42), and even when linear growth velocity is increased, depression has been observed to occur in the patient (43), presumably because the growth achieved does not fulfill the family's expectations. Treatment often is begun in an atmosphere of great excitement and expectation, following a long period of observation, numerous lengthy discussions about the patient's growth problem, and batteries of tests of hormonal secretion. These activities tend to reinforce the child's belief that his shortness is undesirable and that he needs to be changed. During therapy, the family's interests, energy and financial resources are directed at obtaining GH, giving the injections and interacting with health care professionals. In this setting, it is not difficult to understand that failure of the child to grow faster will disappoint all parties greatly and will be interpreted by the child (and perhaps his parents) as another failure on his part. This may compound preexisting feelings of inadequacy. Because of the risk of failure, a trial of therapy with GH should never be considered a "nothing to lose" course of action. Rather, it is crucial that families be prepared for the possibility that treatment might not produce any beneficial effects and receive support and guidance in dealing with failure if it occurs.

OTHER POSSIBLE RISKS

In addition to the risks that have been discussed, a list of other possible risks of prolonged GH therapy can be derived from experience with patients with acromegaly. These include renal complications from GH-induced hypercalciuria, soft-tissue overgrowth leading to carpal/tarsal tunnel syndromes, chronic arthritis, atherosclerosis, skeletal muscle weakness and cardiac hypertrophy. As with some of the possible risks discussed earlier, it is difficult to assess the relevance of GH therapy to these complications of acromegaly, in which GH excess often is marked and prolonged. Because some of the undesirable effects of excess GH may be expressed within a few years of the onset of acromegaly (44), patients who participate in extended trials of GH therapy should be monitored carefully for these side effects.

SUMMARY

While GH has a good record as a safe, efficacious therapeutic agent, the ratio between benefits and risks may shift as its therapeutic use is expanded to conditions other than GH deficiency. It is important, therefore, that systemic studies of efficacy and safety be carried out for each potential therapeutic indication.

REFERENCES

1. Frasier SD. Human growth hormone (hGH) therapy in growth hormone deficiency. Endocr Rev 1983; 4:155-70.
2. Brown P, Gajdusek C, Gibbs CJ, Asher DM. Potential epidemic of Creutzfeldt-Jakob disease from human growth hormone therapy. N Engl J Med 1985; 313:728-31.
3. MacGillivray MH, Frohman LA, Doe J. Metabolic clearance and production rates of human growth hormone in subjects with normal and abnormal growth. J Clin Endocrinol Metab 1970; 30:632-8.
4. Alford EP, Baker HWG, Burger HG. The secretion rate of human growth hormone. I. Daily secretion rates, effects of posture and sleep. J Clin Endocrinol Metab 1973; 37:515-20.
5. Alford EP, Baker HWG, Burger HG, Cameron DP, Keogh EJ. The secretion rate of human growth hormone. II. Acromegaly, effect of chlorpromazine treatment. J Clin Endocrinol Metab 1974; 38:309-12.
6. Taylor AL, Finster JL, Mintz DH. Metabolic clearance and production rates of human growth. J Clin Invest 1969; 48:2349-58.
7. Thompson RG, Rodriquez A, Kowarski A, Blizzard RM. Growth hormone: metabolic clearance rates, integrated concentrations, and production. J Clin Invest 1972; 51:3193-9.
8. Jansson J-O, Albertsson-Wikland K, Eden S, Thorngren K-G, Isaksson O. Circumstantial evidence for a role of the secretory pattern of growth hormone in control of body growth. Acta Endocrinol (Copenh) 1982; 99:24-30.
9. Clemmons DR, Williams RW, Snyder DK, Underwood LE. Treatment with growth hormone conserves lean body mass during dietary restriction in obese volunteers. J Clin Endocrinol Metab 1987; 64:878-83.
10. Sakuma M, Knobil E. Inhibition of endogenous growth hormone secretion by exogenous growth hormone infusion in the rhesus monkey. Endocrinology 1970; 86:890-4.
11. Abrams RL, Grumbach MM, Kaplan SL. The effect of administration of

human growth hormone on the plasma growth hormone, cortisol, glucose, and free fatty acid response to insulin: evidence for growth hormone autoregulation in man. J Clin Invest 1971; 50:940–50.

12. Hagen TC, Lawrence AM, Kirsteins L. Autoregulation of growth hormone secretion in normal subjects. Metabolism 1972; 21:603–10.

13. Mendelson WB, Jacobs LS, Gillin JC. Negative feedback suppression of sleep-related growth hormone secretion. J Clin Endocrinol Metab 1983; 56:486–8.

14. Berelowitz M, Szabo M, Frohman LA, Firestone S, Chu L, Hintz RL. Somatomedin-C mediates growth hormone negative feedback by effects on both the hypothalamus and the pituitary. Science 1981; 212:1279.

15. Brazeau P, Guillemin R, Ling N, et al. Inhibition by somatomedin of growth hormone secretion stimulated by hypothalamic growth hormone releasing factor (somatocrinin, GRF), or the synthetic peptide hpGRF. C R Acad Sci [III] (Paris) 1982; 295:651–4.

16. Abe H, Molitch M, Van Wyk JJ, Underwood LE. Human growth hormone and somatomedin-C suppress the spontaneous release of growth hormone in unanesthetized rats. Endocrinology 1983; 11:1319–24.

17. Underwood LE, Voina SJ, Van Wyk JJ. Restoration of growth by human growth hormone (Roos) in hypopituitary dwarfs immunized by other growth hormone preparations: clinical and immunological studies. J Clin Endocrinol Metab 1974; 38:288–97.

18. Daughaday WH. The anterior pituitary. In: Wilson JD, Foster DF, eds. Williams textbook of endocrinology. 7th ed. Philadelphia: WB Saunders, 1985:600.

19. Beck JC, McGarry EE, Dyrenfurth IH, Venning EH. Metabolic effects of human and monkey growth hormone in man. Science 1957; 125:884–5.

20. Luft R, Ikkos D, Gemzell CA, Olivecrona H. Effect of human growth hormone in hypophysectomized diabetic subjects. Lancet 1958; 1:721–2.

21. Mason AS. Effects of human growth hormone on childhood diabetes mellitus. Acta Endocrinol (Copenh) 1962; 67(suppl):61.

22. Rosenfeld RG, Hintz RL, Johanson AJ, et al. Methionyl human growth hormone and oxandrolone in Turner Syndrome: preliminary results of a prospective randomized trial. J Pediatr 1986; 109:936–43.

23. Raiti S, Moore WV, Van Vliet G, Kaplan SL. Growth-stimulating effects of human growth hormone therapy in patients with Turner syndrome. J Pediatr 1986; 109:944–9.

24. Snyder DK, Clemmons DR, Underwood LE. The effect of growth hormone on nitrogen balance and body composition during caloric restriction (in preparation).

25. Stauch G, Lego A, Therain F, Bricaire H. Reversible plasma and red blood cell volume increases in acromegaly. Acta Endocrinol (Copenh) 1977; 85:465–78.

26. Falkheden T, Sjogren B. Intracellular fluid volume and renal function in pituitary insufficiency and acromegaly. Acta Endocrinol (Copenh) 1964; 46:80–8.

27. Deray G, Rieu M, Devynck MA, et al. Evidence of an endogenous digitalis-like factor in the plasma of patients with acromegaly. N Engl J Med 1987; 316:575–80.

28. Biglieri EG, Watlington CO, Forsham PH. Sodium retention with human growth hormone and its subfractions. J Clin Endocrinol Metab 1961; 21:361–70.

29. Venning EH, Dyrenfurth I, Giroud CJP, Beck JC. Effect of growth hormone on aldosterone excretion. Metabolism 1956; 5:697–702.

30. Shimomura K, Lee M, Oku J, Bray GA, Glick Z. Sodium/potassium dependent ATPase in hypophysectomized rats: response to growth hormone, triiodothyronine, and cortisone. Metabolism 1982; 31:213–6.

31. Huggins C, Oka H. Regression of stem-cell erythroblastic leukemia after hypophysectomy. Cancer Res 1972; 32:239–42.

32. Moon HD, Simpson ME, Evans HM. Inhibition of methylcholanthrene

carcinogenes by hypophysectomy. Science 1952; 116:331.

33. Moon HD, Simpson ME, Li CH, Evans HM. Neoplasms in rats treated with pituitary growth hormone. V. Absence of neoplasms in hypophysectomized rats. Cancer Res 1951; 11:535-8.

34. Moon HD, Simpson ME, Li CH, Evans HM. Neoplasms in rats treated with pituitary growth hormone. I. Pulmonary and lymphatic tissues. Cancer Res 1950; 10:297-308.

35. Moon HD, Simpson ME, Li CH, Evans HM. Neoplasms in rats treated with pituitary growth hormone. II. Adrenal glands. Cancer Res 1950; 10:364-70.

36. Moon HD, Li CH, Simpson ME. Effect of pituitary hormones on carcinogenesis with 9,10-Dimethyl-1,2-benzathracene in hypophysectomized rats. Cancer Res 1956; 16:111-6.

37. Klein I, Parveen G, Gavalu JS, Vanthiel DH. Colonic polyps in patients with acromegaly. Ann Intern Med 1982; 97:27-30.

38. Ituarte EA, Petrini J, Hershman JM. Acromegaly and colon cancer. Ann Intern Med 1984; 101:627-8.

39. Pines A, Rozen P, Ron E, Gilat T. Gastrointestinal tumors in acromegalic patients. Am J Gastroenterol 1985; 80:266-9.

40. Van Vliet G, Styne DM, Kaplan SL, et al. Growth hormone treatment of short stature. N Engl J Med 1983; 309:1016-22.

41. Gertner JM, Genel M, Gianfridi SP, et al. Prospective clinical trial of human growth hormone in short children without growth hormone deficiency. J Pediatr 1984; 104:172-6.

42. Grew RS, Stabler B, Williams RW, Underwood LE. Facilitating patient understanding in the treatment of growth delay. Clin Pediat (Phila) 1983; 22:685-90.

43. Rotnem D, Cohen D, Hintz RL, Genel M. When treatment fails: psychological sequele of relative "treatment failure" with human growth hormone replacement. J Am Acad Child Pyschiatry 1979; 19:505-20.

44. Csanady M, Gaspar L, Hogye M, Gruber N. The heart in acromegaly: an echocardiographic study. Int J Cardiol 1983; 2:349-57.

35

SUMMARY OF INTERNATIONAL GROWTH HORMONE SYMPOSIUM

Robert M. Blizzard, M.D.

Director, Children's Medical Center
University of Virginia School of Medicine
Charlottesville, Virginia

INTRODUCTION

The amount of material presented at this meeting is exceedingly large and complex. A summary can only collate and coordinate the major points covered. It is not the intent of this summary to give explicit details, and it is not even possible to present data from all of the investigators that have presented.

The participants have been most fortunate to learn much about the neuroendocrine regulation of growth hormone secretion. Dr. Tannenbaum has led the way in working out the interrelationship between growth hormone releasing hormone and somatostatin to produce growth hormone pulsatility. In addition, she demonstrated that antiserum against growth hormone releasing hormone elevates the basal levels of growth hormone; the trough levels are elevated. She and Dr. Martin demonstrated very convincingly that growth hormone releasing hormone is secreted in the posterior part of the hypothalamus (tubero-infundibular region). The ventromedial and arcuate nuclei are particularly involved. Somatostatin neurons are located primarily in the anterior hypothalamic region.

Galanin is a recently described neuropeptide of 29 amino acids and is additive in its action with that of growth hormone releasing hormone. Galanin also is produced in the ventromedial and arcuate nuclei. Somatostatin blocks the action of galanin as it blocks the action of growth hormone releasing hormone in humans.

Dr. Muller contributed also to our understanding and pointed out that if epinephrine release is blocked, galanin does not cause growth hormone release. Therefore, galanin action requires the presence of epinephrine. Dr. Muller emphasized the importance of the cholinergic system and demonstrated that atropine blocks the release of growth hormone to exercise, arginine, and clonidine. Dr. Muller presented data indicating the additive effect of GHRH and pyridostigmine, a cholinesterase inhibitor, in normal children, children with constitutional delayed growth and adolescence, familial short stature, and even growth hormone dependency. Muller and his group have applied their knowledge regarding clonidine, an alpha two adrenergic agent, to increase growth hormone production and increase growth velocity in at least some children with severe short stature over a 6-12 month period.

Other neurotransmitters such as L-dopa have been used in a limited number of patients by Lanes and co-workers, but further studies are indicated to determine if there is any significant therapeutic role for these agents. GHRH itself has been used as an effective therapeutic agent, as reported by Dr. Rogol for our group yesterday. Dr. Rogol stated, "A more potent analog is needed if GHRH is to be a valuable therapeutic agent." In the meantime, its use as a tool to study neuroendocrine interrelationships is very important, as demonstrated in the studies reported by both Dr. Rogol and Dr. Evans.

We were treated to scholarly presentations concerning the production of growth hormone by Doctors Phillips, Eberhardt, Baumann and Lewis. Dr. Phillips shared with us his knowledge of the growth hormone and chorionic-somatomammotropin genes on chromosome 17. Recently, there has been presented evidence that there is a placental growth hormone resulting from activity of the second growth hormone gene (the hGH-V gene). It has been suggested that this product which has the same number of amino acids as 22K pituitary growth hormone, but with 13 substitutions, might be a fetal growth factor. However, Dr. Frankenne and co-workers from Liege presented a poster reporting that the placental growth hormone is not found in amniotic fluid or in fetal serum, but is found in high quantities in maternal serum. The low pituitary growth hormone levels found in maternal serum may result from the high levels of placental growth hormone.

Dr. Phillips also shared with us how both 20K and 22K growth hormone can be produced in the pituitary by the same gene (hGH-N gene) at the transcription level. The 20K:22K growth hormone ratio is consistently 1:9. Dr. Phillips presented further information regarding the two hGH and three CSM genes on chromosome 17. The first CSM gene is inactive. Apparently none of these genes are necessary for survival, as neonates have been born without these genes. Dr. Rappaport has observed one patient who has only one of these five genes. The patient has only the inactive CSM-I gene.

Dr. Eberhardt presented his exciting studies regarding the regulation of the growth hormone genes by triiodothyronine and dexamethasone. Thyroid and dexamethasone positively affect the transcription of both the rGH and hGH genes. Dr. Eberhardt suggested that in humans, thyroid hormones exert a positive influence on growth hormone production at the level of secretion, but not at the level of transcription.

Dr. Baumann discussed with us the various forms of monomeric hormone in the pituitary. Dr. Lewis has spent over 20 years studying the various forms of growth hormone in the pituitary. Knowledge regarding the 20K growth hormone has come primarily from work in his laboratory. Interestingly, both immunologic and growth-promoting activity are minimal in this particular preparation, but there is diabetogenic activity present. Dr. Lewis concluded, "Although the number of growth hormone variants and modifications have reached eight, there are at least an equal number of unidentified forms in pituitary extracts."

Dr. Baumann discussed the multiple forms of growth hormone and serum including the 22K, the big growth hormone and the big big growth hormone. There were many others to which he alluded. He emphasized that we do not always know what we are measuring when we receive a report that 20 ng/ml of growth hormone is present in plasma. An exciting, relatively new presentation was given by Dr. Baumann who described two binding proteins in plasma for growth hormone. Growth hormone binding protein is specific for 22K and 20K growth hormones, although the binding capacity for 22K is limited (20 ng/ml) as compared to 20K growth hormone (450 ng/ml). The function, if any, of these binding proteins remains unknown, although several speculations are possible. One of these is that the binding protein(s) is tied in with the receptor protein. For example, a binding protein could be a degradation product of the hGH receptor, which has binding properties, or it could be an important part of a complex (GH+GHBP) that permits growth hormone to attach to its receptors. Dr. Bier told us of three patients with a growth hormone deficient-like phenotype who make growth hormone, but who have no binding protein. Those patients do not generate IGF-I, and do not grow when given growth hormone. We do not know what the tie-in is between the absent binding protein and the failure of growth hormone to act metabolically in these patients. Possibly the data presented by Spencer and co-workers at a poster session lend credence to this theory. These workers concluded from their data that the serum binding protein is part of the 130KB membrane receptor, which is released by proteolysis.

Dr. Imura gave an exciting report pertaining to the methodology used in measuring growth hormone. Dr. Imura described the eloquent sandwich enzyme immunoassay to measure growth hormone which he and his collaborators have developed. The lower sensitivity of this assay is 50 pg/ml, and growth hormone can be found using this assay in nearly all normal individuals. Dr. Imura uses this assay to assist in making the diagnosis of growth hormone deficiency and acromegaly,

This assay has been applied also for the measure of growth hormone in urine, as reported in the poster sessions by Dr. Hattori and co-workers of Tokyo. Dr. MacGillivray's group of Buffalo and Dr. Shizume's group of Tokyo also reported regarding the measurement of growth hormone in urine. This technique has enhanced our diagnostic capability and has revealed that the kidney plays an important role in the degradation of growth hormone. Growth hormone excretion is increased in patients with kidney disease. This should be kept in mind when measuring growth hormone in urine.

Not only were there exciting discussions regarding growth hormone in serum, but we had exciting discussions regarding the circulating insulin-like growth factors (IGF-I and IGF-II). Dr. Rechler reminded us that IGF-I and II are highly homologous, and that IGF-II in rats and MSA differ in only 3 of 63 sites. In the rat, IGF-II levels are very high in serum at birth and fall to adult levels by 25 days of age. Dr. Rechler and others are exploring the possibility, which seems to be becoming a probability, that IGF-II plays a role in fetal growth. The mRNA of IGF-II is demonstrated to be abundant in fetal tissues both before and at birth, and to fall rapidly. Heart, muscle, lung, intestine, and liver are particularly rich in this mRNA. Dr. Sussenbach and co-workers discussed the IGF-II gene which has 7 exons. During fetal development of the liver, IGF-II mRNA is expressed by exons 4-7, while exons 1-3 and 5-7 are expressed in adult liver. Dr. Czech discussed IGF-II receptors measured using Western blot techniques and told us that there is a marked fall in IGF-II receptors after birth, while there is no change in IGF-I receptors.

The action of growth hormone and insulin-like growth factors on bone and on metabolic pathways was discussed at great length by Doctors Isaksson, Froesch and Hizuka. Dr. Isaksson infused growth hormone locally on one of the epiphyseal plates of the right femur and demonstrated growth unilaterally in that femur. He, therefore, believes that growth hormone probably plays a role at the epiphyseal plate to initiate growth. He concluded that growth hormone stimulated colony formation of epiphyseal chondrocytes isolated from the area adjacent to the epiphysis, and IGF-I stimulates cells isolated both from the proximal and intermediate parts of the growth plate.

Dr. Hizuka and Dr. Froesch each reported the growth-promoting effect of IGF-I on the tibial plates of hypophysectomized rats. Dr. Hizuka demonstrated weight gain in hypophysectomized rats and in normal rats receiving IGF-I. An increase in body length also was noted in both hypophysectomized and normal rats. Dr. Hizuka and her co-workers demonstrated that the administration of IGF-I markedly increased the pituitary content of growth hormone, indicating a negative feedback on growth hormone release by the administration of IGF-I.

The metabolic action of growth hormone in relation to nutrition was explored by Dr. Clemmons. Dr. Clemmons reported that IGF-I levels in obese individuals do not fall with low-energy diets as they fall in individuals who are not obese. He and his co-workers also demonstrated that the administration of growth hormone over an extended period of time does not enhance weight loss in these individuals. The dosage of growth hormone used by Dr. Clemmons was 0.1 IU/kg/body weight and was given every other day.

Dr. Manson and co-workers examined the effect of 10 mg of growth hormone given each day to individuals who have undergone significant trauma and/or surgery. Increased nitrogen balance, potassium, sodium, and phosphate retention occurred. These studies need to be expanded by Dr. Manson and explored by other investigators.

This summary would be incomplete if we did not mention in some detail the presentations regarding growth hormone production and secretion in children and adults. Dr. Evans presented data regarding the characteristics of growth hormone secretion in young adults and older adults. Young adult females secrete more growth hormone than do individuals from the other three groups. The correlation of growth hormone secretion with various hormones was positive only in respect to estrogen concentrations in serum. Dr. Evans also presented preliminary data regarding the changes in growth hormone secretion during the menstrual cycle. The highest levels of secretion are during the midfollicular phase. These data also are suggestive that estrogen increases growth hormone concentrations in serum.

Dr. Albertsson-Wikland presented her studies suggesting that growth hormone concentrations are directly proportional to the height of children both in the pubertal and prepubertal stages. Further studies need to be done by other groups to, hopefully, confirm these data.

Dr. Bercu recapitulated for us his extensive studies in short children regarding growth hormone concentrations in serum over 24 h. Briefly, Dr. Bercu and his co-workers have described what has been termed an entity of growth hormone neurosecretory dysfunction (GHND). This topic deserves a few summarizing comments.

Nearly all investigators agree that this is an appropriate term for a definite entity such as the one which occurs in patients who have been exposed to cerebral irradiation and who acquire dysfunction in their growth hormone secretion. These patients have a pathological reason for a defect in growth hormone secretion. The problem many investigators have in the application of this term, growth hormone neurosecretory dysfunction, is to children who may be a variant of normal and not be abnormal; therefore, the application to children who may have a low normal growth hormone output, instead of an abnormality of growth hormone production. If we were sure these individuals had an abnormality of growth hormone production, we could accept the term "dysfunction," but many of these children, such as the patients with constitutional delayed adolescence with low growth hormone production, as tested by pulsatility studies, and discussed by Dr. Bierich, are probably variants of normal. We all admit that these children are perplexing. It is probably desirable that these children with low normal or low GH output and who have what could also be termed "partial and/or transient growth hormone deficiency" receive growth hormone therapy, although in my opinion only the most severe ones should receive growth hormone and only under specific protocol.

Growth hormone neurosecretory dysfunction certainly exists in a form that everyone can accept as a pathological entity and not a variation of normal and Dr. Rappaport discussed this. He and his group studied the effect of cranial irradiation on growth hormone secretion and growth. Dr. Rappaport reported that it usually takes 18 or more months following brain irradiation for slowing of growth to occur. Of course, it occurs sooner and more severely in those who have had cranial and spinal irradiation than in those who have had just cranial irradiation. These patients with GHND often have significant growth hormone release with pharmacological testing but have decreased pulsatility of growth hormone release over 12 or 24 h in the physiological setting. These patients, as described by Dr. Rappaport, do have growth hormone neurosecretory dysfunction. However, even in this group of patients the secretion of growth hormone may be reversible when sex steroids are given. We have recently observed a male who received both cranial and testicular irradiation 10 years ago for acute lymphocytic leukemia. This patient has gonadal failure, a low somatomedin-C, and a very slow growth rate. The determination of pulsatile growth hormone secretion indicated no significant growth hormone pulses. With testosterone administration because of the gonadal failure, growth hormone release had increased markedly when retested over a 24-h period. Testosterone then was discontinued and, after a period of one month, the pulsatility of growth hormone secretion was again determined. The pulsatility had returned to the pretestosterone levels. This is a fertile area for further investigation.

During this conference, questions were raised pertaining to patients who appear to be growth hormone deficient during childhood, but who make growth hormone after they have spontaneously gone into adolescence. The question has been raised whether these patients have transient growth hormone deficiency, partial growth hormone deficiency, or have recovered from growth hormone deficiency. We addressed this problem in identical twins studied in our clinic. One twin was growth hormone deficient and repeatedly had abnormal growth hormone secretion when stimulated pharmacologically. The pulsatility studies were compatible with those of a patient with growth hormone deficiency. Her normal sibling made normal amounts of growth hormone. The growth hormone deficient patient was treated over a number of years and eventually progressed into adolescence. Her ultimate height was several centimeters less than that of her non-growth hormone deficient sibling. Upon retesting after epiphyseal fusion occurred, the hypopituitary patient secreted growth hormone in the low but unequivocal normal range. Her sister secreted growth hormone in the high normal range. In both of the patients, sex steroids triggered an increase in growth hormone secretion, but in the hypopituitary patient not up to the high normal levels of her sister. Even in the presence of growth hormone dysfunction, androgens and estrogens may stimulate greater growth hormone production than was present prepubertally.

In this summary, nothing has been stated about growth hormone production at the time of puberty. Dr. Albertsson-Wikland demonstrated that there is increase in growth hormone secretion at puberty when longitudinal studies of growth hormone secretion were undertaken in prepubertal and pubertal children.

In terms of growth hormone treatment of growth hormone deficiency in non-growth hormone deficient patients, we have heard excellent presentations by Dr. Frasier regarding dosages vs. effectiveness, from Dr. Rosenfeld regarding the effect of growth hormone in the treatment of patients with Turner's syndrome, from Dr. Root regarding the use of growth hormone in various types of short stature, and from Dr. Kaplan regarding the use of growth hormone in the treatment of non-growth hormone deficient short stature. We would all agree that we need to be judicious in prescribing growth hormone, both in respect to patients who are selected and the dose that is used. From a personal vantage point, I would like to state the following: "Children who are not growth hormone deficient should be treated only under rigid protocol conditions." In my opinion, protocols should include at least those criteria used and carried out by Dr. Kaplan, as in the study which she reported.

The questions remaining to be answered are many. This is true in both the basic science and clinical areas. For example, in respect to questions pertaining to treatment, several participants have expressed concern that we know little about the psychological implications of our intervening in the lives of short children by giving them injections, and by alerting them to our concerns that they may not be normal. In this conference, only one poster, a poster from Buffalo, and one paper, that by Dr. Underwood, dealt with the psychological implications of treatment. In the future, this topic needs to be more fully addressed.

In closing, I would like to thank Dr. Barry Bercu, his committee, Dr. James Posillico, the University of South Florida, and the Serono organization for holding this stimulating and successful conference. All of us attending have improved our scientific acumen of the physiology and production of growth hormone and its related and controlling factors.

AUTHOR INDEX

SUBJECT INDEX

Iodoacetamide, 38
Iodotyrosine, 193
Irradiation, external
   cranial, 143–155
   spinal, total, 151

Jet lag syndrome, 175, 181

Kenny Caffey syndrome, 322
17–Ketosteroid, 289

Laron dwarfism, 61, 264, 265
Leucine oxidation, 190, 192
Leukemia, acute, lymphoblastic,
      143–144, 150–152
   and growth hormone secretion
         pulsatile, 122
Leupeptin, 193
Lipid synthesis
   inhibition by growth hormone,
      347–348
Lipolysis, 189, 190, 192
   and growth hormone, 347–355
Luteinizing hormone, 161
Lymphocyte radioreceptor assay, 264
Lysosome, 193, 195

Mannosidase II, 195
Median eminence, 77–79, 85
Medulloblastoma, 144–146, 148, 150,
      151
β–Mercaptoethanol, 37–38, 47
Methotrexate, intrathecal, 144
Methylhistidine, urinary, 266
Morquio disease, 320, 321
Mulibrey nanism, 320, 321

Narcolepsy, 181
Neuraminidase, 193, 196
Neuron, parvicellular
   immunoreactive, 73, 74
Neuropeptide
   and growth hormone, 83–88
   list of, 85
Neurotoxin fraction b4–2, 137
Neurotransmission, cholinergic, 88–
      90
   cotransmission, 83
Neurotransmitter
   and growth hormone secretion, 83–
      94
   and growth hormone-releasing hor-
         mone release, 85–86
   list of, 87
Nitrogen
   balance, 351
   conservation, 347–355
   loss in stress, 339
   urinary, normal, 266–268
Noonan syndrome, 322
Norepinephrine, 85–87, 89

Ornithine, 291
Osteochondrodystrophy, 319–321
Osteosarcoma, maxillary, 147
Oxandrolone, 160, 331–335

Pacemaker, circadian, 175–176
   and jet lag, 175
Panhypopituitary dwarfism, 61
Phenylephrine, 87
Pilocarpine, 89
Pirenzepin, 88
Pituitary gland, 33, 44, 61, 64,
      83, 84, see Growth hormone
Plaque assay, reverse, hemolytic,
      167, 168
Plasma membrane and enzymes, 196
Plasmin, 20, 38
Polyneuropathy, uremic, 135–140
Polypeptide hormone, see separate
      hormones
Potassium, urinary, 362
Prader–Willi syndrome, 320, 321
Preoptic area, 73–74, 77
Proinsulin, 13, 214
Prolactin, 43, 49, 76, 190
Propranolol, 85
Protein binding growth hormone, 19–
      20
Protein kinase, 197
Puberty
   precocious, 146
   retarded, see Delay of growth
Puromycin, 195
Pyridostigmine, 89–91

Rabbit
   chondrocyte, 200–202
   and growth hormone, 199–205
Radioimmunoassay, polyclonal, 263–
      266
Rat, 3–12, 166–168, 176–177, 189–
      199, 200, 201, 206–209,
      213–250, 341
Receptor of growth hormone
   structure, 189–199
Retinoblastoma, 149, 150
Rhesus monkey, 178
Ribonucleic acid, see RNA
Rickets, hypophosphatemic, 320
Rieger syndrome, 61, 64
Ring chromosome, 320, 321
mRNA, 15–16, 234, 238, 239
Russell–Silver syndrome, 311, 315–
      317
   and growth hormone therapy, 317,
      318
   and hyposomatotropism, 318

Sampling frequency in hormone
      studies, 161–164
Scatchard plot, 191